Aromatherapeutic
BLENDING

by the same author

Essential Oils
A Handbook for Aromatherapy Practice Second Edition
ISBN 978 1 84819 089 4
eISBN 978 0 85701 072 8

Listening to Scent
An Olfactory Journey with Aromatic Plants and Their Extracts
ISBN 978 1 84819 125 9
eISBN 978 0 85701 171 8

Fragrance and Wellbeing
Plant Aromatics and Their Influence on the Psyche
ISBN 978 1 84819 090 0
eISBN 978 0 85701 073 5

A Sensory Journey
Meditations on Scent for Wellbeing
Card Set
ISBN 978 1 84819 153 2
eISBN 978 0 85701 175 6

Aromatherapeutic
BLENDING

ESSENTIAL OILS IN SYNERGY

JENNIFER PEACE RHIND

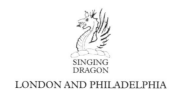

SINGING
DRAGON
LONDON AND PHILADELPHIA

First published in 2016
by Singing Dragon
an imprint of Jessica Kingsley Publishers
73 Collier Street
London N1 9BE, UK
and
400 Market Street, Suite 400
Philadelphia, PA 19106, USA

www.singingdragon.com

Library of Congress Cataloging in Publication Data
Rhind, Jennifer, author.
  Aromatherapeutic blending : essential oils in synergy / Jennifer Peace Rhind.
    p. ; cm.
  Includes bibliographical references and index.
  ISBN 978-1-84819-227-0 (alk. paper)
  I. Title.
  [DNLM: 1. Aromatherapy--methods. 2. Drug Synergism. 3. Oils, Volatile--therapeutic use. WB 925]
  RM666.A68
  615.3'219--dc23
                              2015008188

British Library Cataloguing in Publication Data
A CIP catalogue record for this book is available from the British Library

ISBN 978 1 84819 227 0
eISBN 978 0 85701 174 9

Printed and bound in Great Britain

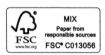

For Derek and Leeloo – always and forever in my heart

CONTENTS

PREFACE AND ACKNOWLEDGEMENTS

This book was originally conceived as a practical blending tool – a set of cards – that could be used to explore the relationships between essential oils when formulating aromatic prescriptions. I had an idea that these cards would contain colour-coded information, and that they could be laid out in patterns – rather like tarot spreads – to illustrate the different approaches to blending described in *Essential Oils: A Handbook for Aromatherapy Practice* (Rhind 2012); indeed, it was to be a companion to that text. As good an idea as that sounded, it quickly became clear that the intricacies of aromatherapeutic blending demanded a much fuller investigation, not only into what constitutes synergy from the perspective of holistic aromatherapy, but also of the recently published research into the biological and therapeutic actions of essential oils and their constituents.

When I began to explore the concept of synergy and aromatic plants, it was my 'inner biologist' that fuelled the search for evidence, and I accessed a considerable number of papers from a wide range of journals – keeping everything as current and up to date as possible. As the first chapter progressed, I was becoming more and more aware that this robust but reductionist approach was revealing only a small, albeit important, facet of synergy; and that to give us a meaningful exploration of how we formulate aromatherapeutic blends, this approach was too narrow. This made me reflect upon what makes aromatherapy vibrant and special for us – it is not only about chemistry and biology, but also about our relationships with aroma, the natural world and indeed one another. Aromatherapy is a unique therapy – we are promoting health and wellbeing with aromatic plants, the very same species and scents that were used by our ancestors for healing. We have thousands of years of collective wisdom to help inform our practice, and we can explore some of the ancient traditional aromatic formulae too, giving us a deeper insight into what, exactly, constitutes synergy.

It was with this holistic perspective that I proceeded with my work. I broadened my vision to integrate concepts of synergy as experienced via the senses, in the natural world, within therapeutic relationships, within perfumery, within our relationships with odours; I explored 'aromatic signatures', and how aromatherapy draws upon traditional philosophies to give models for synergistic blending, and how we can gain esoteric insights via meditation on the aromas of essential oils. At this point, I was beginning to feel that I was no longer deconstructing the therapy that has formed such a very big part of my life; the magic was still very present.

However, it had also become clear that this book was not just about aromatherapeutic blending! A literature search, focusing on the evidence for essential oil actions, was long overdue. This involved many hours of searching and extracting information relevant to the quest – and inevitably the inner biologist surfaced again! This all culminated in Part II, where a selection of the 'evidence for actions' is presented. It was very important to me that this should be accessible and useful, as it forms the basis of the information that we need in order to select appropriate essential oils, even before considering their potential synergistic interactions. This is why the actions are presented in loose groupings, and either related to physiology (e.g. pain) or directed to specific systems (e.g. respiratory), or to the psyche. Although this is, essentially, a biomedical/reductionist approach, I do feel that if we aspire to be holistic, we must be able to understand the detail, and respect the microcosm, because this can help us formulate effective aromatic prescriptions with the confidence that we are basing our practice on evidence from a variety of life and social science disciplines.

Part III is presented as a series of full and abbreviated essential oil profiles, and is an attempt at synthesising the philosophical theories presented in Part I with the evidence in Part II, revealing the opportunities for essential oil synergy. These profiles are based on the evidence for biological actions revealed in the literature search, but the blending suggestions are also informed by wider holistic and energetic perspectives, as well as my nose.

Throughout the book, I have attempted to present the 'hard' science in an accessible way. Aromatherapy is such a very broad subject, with its foundations in several disciplines, and very few of us are experts in all aspects. I do not claim or pretend to be an expert in anything, but I do love to explore, think, debate, communicate and write. The more you do this, the more you understand just how much you still have to learn, and I relish this journey! Where I have needed to improve upon my own education, I have shared this with you in the form of footnotes, and a glossary, which, for me, was a very useful reminder when I was on less familiar territory. I hope that you too will find this helpful. I stopped myself preparing a reference section on the known actions of specific constituents. This might have been very helpful, but it would have been the very antithesis of what this book is all about – an exploration of ideas, and a synthesis of these, to give each and every aromatherapist, regardless of their favoured or default *modus operandi*, an unprecedented opportunity to join me on this journey, and to dissect, analyse, reflect, and then emerge a more knowledgeable and insightful practitioner.

No book is a solo endeavour – even though the process of writing can feel somewhat lonely at times. There are several special individuals that I would like to thank: Tamara Agnew for contributing a reflective case study that probably illustrates synergistic blending better than anything else, for creating a model for blending, and for being my 'critical friend'; Jonathan Hinde and Malte Hozzel of Oshadhi, who shared their unique philosophy and supplied many of the more unusual essential oils for sensory appreciation and description; Megan McGeever for sharing her pilot study exploring the role of the client in essential oil selection; Christine Donnelly for ensuring that the areas where my knowledge of physiology was murky became clarified; Kareen Hogg, a shining example of a practitioner who combines her understanding of essential oils with deep tissue massage and myofascial release; Anita James for her interest in and support of my work; and Lora Cantele for giving me the opportunity to contribute regularly to *The International Journal of Professional Holistic Aromatherapy*. My husband Derek is always my rock, and for an architect he can really hold his own in a conversation about the philosophical aspects of aromatherapy. Our 13-year-old Tibetan terrier Leeloo has had a difficult year, but her vitality, sparkling presence and unconditional love continue to pervade our lives; indeed many of our conversations about how this book was progressing were undertaken during her daily walks! Also, I extend my thanks to all at Singing Dragon, especially Jessica Kingsley, Jane Evans, Victoria Peters, Linda De Angelis and Anne Oppenheimer: you have given me, yet again, the chance to write about what I care about; thanks also for publishing books that 'make a difference'. All of you have made this a better and more comprehensive book, but you have also been wonderful companions; I value your professionalism and friendship.

I hope that you will embark on this book with excitement and an open mind. You will find that evidence of my inner biologist is scattered throughout – but it happily co-exists with my love of the esoteric, symbolism, the natural world and its inhabitants, plants and all things scented – and I sincerely hope that I have managed to strike a balance between science and traditional wisdom. This is a book to be read first, and then used as a reference and companion – and as your practice evolves, you might return to it on occasions for reflection and review. It has been written for every aromatherapy student and practitioner, and it is my honour to accompany you on your professional journey. Make an aromatic difference to our world!

With love,

Jennifer
14 February 2015

Introduction

The synergistic blending of essential oils is at the very heart of aromatherapy practice. Here, the aim is to examine the concept and the underpinning hypotheses, and from this provide informed and accessible guidance on how to formulate aromatherapeutic blends, with an evidence-based and philosophically sound approach. To this end, the information is presented concisely, and from the theoretical perspective. This book has been written primarily for the professional practitioner and student; however, it is hoped that it may also be of value to those who want to use essential oils for personal purposes, outside the realm of professional practice.

In Part I, prevalent philosophical approaches are explored, and in Part II, supportive research and traditional practices are presented. In Part III, full and abbreviated essential oil profiles are offered, in order to inform and facilitate the formulation of individual essential oil prescriptions. Explanatory footnotes are supplied throughout Parts I and II.

Throughout, student and professional aromatherapists are guided and encouraged to reflect upon various aspects of their practice. This book will help practitioners explore their beliefs and approaches, and appraise the goals and intended outcomes of their blends and treatment plans.

Finally, and perhaps most important, the book will help and inspire all those who work with, or simply enjoy essential oils to be responsible, mindful and creative in their use.

Part I

PRINCIPLES AND PRACTICE

Chapter 1

Essential Oil Synergy

We will begin by asking a seemingly simple question – in aromatherapy, why do we usually blend essential oils rather than use them singly? To answer this, we need to look at how the practice originated, and its theoretical basis and evidence.

Perhaps the earliest example of aromatics used in combination can be found in the pharmacopoeia of ancient Egypt, circa 1500 BCE – the gum resins frankincense and myrrh. In traditional Chinese medicine they are always simultaneously prescribed for the treatment of blood stagnation and inflammation, swelling and pain (Shen and Lou 2008). It is difficult to mention one without the other; they have become inextricably linked in the collective psyche. Recent research has confirmed what the ancient Egyptian and Chinese healers must have observed – that this combination of aromatics had greater therapeutic effects than each could exert on its own – and this phenomenon is often referred to as 'synergy'.

De Rapper *et al.* (2012) investigated the *in vitro* antimicrobial effects of three species of Ethiopian frankincense (*Boswellia rivae*, *B. neglecta* and *B. papyrifera*) and two of myrrh (*Commiphora guidottii* and *C. myrrha*) essential oils. Their study demonstrated enhanced efficacy against a range of pathogens; indeed, most combinations displayed synergistic effects, and strong synergism was noted between *B. papyrifera* and *C. myrrha*. However, Chen *et al.* (2013) explored the activities of frankincense and myrrh, and, in contrast, did not find any evidence of synergistic interactions. From this we could postulate that synergistic activity is context dependent.

Across the globe, folk medicines and herbal healing traditions feature 'synergistic formulae' – for example, the traditional Indian Ayurvedic herbal combination *Chitrakadivati*, where *Ferula asafoetida* resin (asafoetida), *Zingiber officinale* rhizome (ginger) and *Glycyrrhiza glabra* root (liquorice) are combined to treat flatulence, gut microflora imbalances and indigestion. Ch and Smitha (2011) were able to demonstrate that this combination exhibited synergistic antimicrobial activity against both bacteria and fungi. However, they also suggested that the elements present in the mixture consisted of not only active substances, but also co-effectors and matrix formers – and that their presence and interaction actually protects the active ingredients; this is perhaps why ginger and long pepper (*Piper longum*) feature in so many traditional formulae. Indeed, the Ayurvedic compound medicine *Trikatu*[1] contains both ginger and long pepper – and it has been suggested that they increase the bioavailability of active ingredients by promoting absorption in the gut, and/or by protecting the active principles from being metabolised during the first pass in the liver (Chauhan *et al.* 2011).

In ancient Rome, medicine was influenced by both Egyptian and Greek practices. Here too we can see how aromatic plant ingredients were used in specific combinations – again illustrating an awareness of synergy. The word '*medicamentum*' had various meanings – cosmetic, perfume, magic potion, drug, and remedy – and many perfumes, made with aromatic plant extracts, were used not only for pleasure and personal care, but also as medicines. Indeed, aromatics were present in almost every drug formula, and the aromas themselves were understood to have a therapeutic effect. From this, it is easy to make comparisons with what we now call 'aromatherapy', where essential oils are combined for their therapeutic impact on the mind, body and spirit.

In the early 1970s, Paolo Rovesti was possibly the first to demonstrate the clinical efficacy of aromatic essences in the treatment of anxiety and depression (Tisserand 1988). However, Rovesti had also noted that individuals appeared to respond better to essential oil combinations rather than single oils. There could be several reasons for this. Perhaps it was because the odours of some undiluted essential oils can be very strong, and sometimes perceived as unpleasant. If these oils are diluted, and/or used in combination with others, the aroma of the mixture could well be perceived as being more pleasant and thus acceptable. Nobody responds positively to an odour that they dislike! It could be argued that Rovesti's observation has further underpinned the aromatherapy practice of prescribing blends of essential oils, rather than single aromatics. Marguerite Maury, a pioneer of holistic aromatherapy, was one of the first to explore and promote the blending of essential oils. She developed her concept of the 'Individual Prescription', taught it to the first generation of holistic aromatherapists, and wrote about it[2] – and so the practice of blending essential oils became central to contemporary holistic, clinical aromatherapy.

Synergism, additivity and antagonism: the evidence

At the core of the practice of blending is the concept of *synergy*. Put very simply, synergy is the term used to describe the phenomenon where the effect of the whole is greater than the sum of its component parts. Williamson (2001) explained that

---

1   *Trikatu* contains black pepper, ginger and long pepper – the 'Three Pungents' – and is used for increasing digestive fire, treating cold and fevers, and relieving respiratory congestion. Piperine is a pungent alkaloid, and is an important constituent in both black and long peppers; it is thought to be implicated in many of their medicinal and health-promoting benefits (Meghwal and Goswami 2013). It is not found in the essential oil.

2   Maury published *Le Capital Jeunesse* in 1961; the English version, *The Secret of Life and Youth*, was published in 1964. Two of her students, Micheline Arcier and Danièle Ryman, brought her holistic perspective on the subject to the UK in the 1960s (Ryman 1989).

synergistic interactions are considered to be of 'vital importance' in phytomedicine; indeed, synergy is the foundation of herbal medicine's philosophical approach, where whole or partially purified plant extracts are considered to be more effective than single isolated constituents. In her 2001 review, Williamson explored both positive (synergistic) and negative (antagonistic) interactions, and identified some of the methods used to identify and measure synergy and antagonism. It is unsurprising to read that there are difficulties in measurement and methodology; however, she suggested that the preferred method is the 'isobole method', where the effects of doses of individual constituents and their combinations are measured and the results plotted on a graph. Synergy is identified by a concave isobole (curve), and antagonism by a convex isobole. The resulting picture can be complex, because it is possible to find synergy at one dose combination, and antagonism at another. This results in an isobole with a wave-like or elliptical appearance.

Synergy is also fundamental to aromatherapy philosophy, where it is thought that the whole, complete essential oil is more effective than its individual components. This could be described as 'intrinsic' synergy. There is some supporting evidence for this belief. For example, in an animal study exploring the anxiolytic effects of inhalation of a range of lavender essential oils, Takahashi *et al.* (2011) determined the efficacy of various constituents, and concluded that linalyl acetate works synergistically with *l*-linalool – and that the presence of both is essential for the anxiolytic effect of inhaled lavender oil. However, when we begin to look at applying this concept in the context of essential oil blends, a greater degree of complexity is encountered; this is because each essential oil is itself a mixture of several (sometimes many) different chemical constituents, and in a blend the number of potentially active components and co-effectors may be increased considerably. As always, abstract concepts are best explored by looking at examples which illustrate them.

Delaquis *et al.* (2002) stated that combinations of individual essential oils can lead to additive, synergistic or antagonistic effects, and when discussing mixtures of essential oils and the interactions of compounds therein, Tisserand and Young (2014) discuss the concepts of additivity, synergism and antagonism.

Beginning with *additivity*: if two or more substances are administered at the same time, additivity describes the situation where the actions and potency of a mixture can be predicted by the properties of its constituents.

Synergy describes the outcome where the components potentiate[3] one another – and the outcome is significantly greater than what might be predicted by additivity. Tisserand and Young (2014) cite research conducted by Itani *et al.* (2008), where three compounds found in the essential oil of Lebanese sage (*Salvia libanotica*) were tested singly, in pairs and all together to assess their activity against two human colon cancer cell lines.

The results were suggestive of synergism, as shown in Table 1.1.

---

3   Potentiate, in this context, means increase the effects of each other.

Table 1.1 Lebanese sage: synergistic constituents

Constituent	Antiproliferative activity
Linalyl acetate	Minimal activity
Terpineol	No activity
Camphor	No activity
Linalyl acetate + terpineol	A moderate effect (33% and 45% reduction in cell proliferation in the two cell lines)
Linalyl acetate + terpineol + camphor	A significant effect (50% and 64% reduction in cell proliferation in the two cell lines)

Antagonism is the very opposite of synergism. Although the concept could be viewed as negative, in aromatherapy practice, antagonism can have beneficial effects! To illustrate this, Tisserand and Young (2014) cite several essential oil studies which highlight how the effects of toxic or sensitising constituents are mitigated by the presence of other constituents within the same oil. For example, the toxicity of carvacrol, a phenol found in some chemotypes of *Salvia officinalis* and *Thymus* species, is significantly lessened by the presence of its isomer, thymol (Karpouhtsis *et al.* 1998), and the sensitizing effect of cinnamaldehyde is ameliorated by *d*-limonene and also eugenol, which itself is a sensitizer (Guin *et al.* 1984). When antagonism is observed in relation to skin sensitisation, the phenomenon is sometimes called 'quenching'. Tisserand and Young (2014) suggest that a specific property found in many essential oils may be at the root of these anti-toxic effects – and that is their anti-oxidant activity. This is implicated in other beneficial and protective effects of essential oils, and will be explored later.

Returning to the concept of intrinsic synergy, there are numerous studies which demonstrate that 'complete' or 'whole' essential oils can have more pronounced actions than their main constituents have singly. Astani, Reichling and Schnitzler (2010) found that mixtures of some monoterpenes[4] which are present in tea tree oil (*Melaleuca alternifolia*) have significantly greater antiviral action[5] and lower toxicity than individual isolated monoterpenes. Another study, investigating the anti-cancer activity of the essential oil of *Anemopsis californica*[6] roots/rhizomes, found that although its main components inhibited the growth of two human cancer cell lines,[7] the complete essential oil showed a specific bioactivity against both lines – perhaps the result of 'a synergistic relationship' between the combined major and minor components (Medina-Holguin *et al.* 2008). This supports the argument than in aromatherapy, as in phytotherapy, whole, complete extracts should be

---

4   The monoterpenes were α-terpinene, γ-terpinene, α-pinene and *para*-cymene, and their oxygenated derivatives terpinen-4-ol, α-terpineol, thymol, citral and 1,8-cineole – also found in *Eucalyptus* species and *Thymus* species.

5   *In vitro*, against HSV-1.

6   A member of the Saururaceae family; a medicinal plant that is traditionally and culturally used to treat uterine cancer.

7   AN3CA (uterine) and HeLa (cervical) cancer cell lines; also investigated in relation to A549 (lung), MCF-7 (breast), PC3 (prostate) and HCT116 (colon) cell lines.

used rather than fractions or isolated constituents. This is because, apart from the positive synergistic relationship between the active constituents, it is possible that some constituents protect others (for example, by acting as anti-oxidants), that some of the active constituents have not actually been identified, and equally that some constituents have, as yet, unidentified activities.

Many essential oils have antibacterial and antifungal (antimycotic) activity, and this is yet another area where research reveals additivity, synergism and antagonism. For example, Cassella, Cassella and Smith (2002) demonstrated that tea tree (*Melaleuca alternifolia*) and lavender (*Lavandula angustifolia*) formed a synergistic combination with enhanced activity against two dermatophytes – *Trichophyton rubrum* and *T. mentagrophytes* var. *interdigitale*.[8] Later, in 2004, Edwards-Jones *et al.* explored the antimicrobial activity[9] of lavender in combination with tea tree, patchouli (*Pogostemon cablin*) and geranium[10] (*Pelargonium × asperum*), finding that lavender, geranium and tea tree had an increased inhibitory effect on the growth of methicillin-resistant *Staphylococcus aureus* (MRSA), but that lavender and tea tree was less active against MRSA, suggestive of antagonism. So, it is clear that what might be a synergistic combination in some circumstances might actually be antagonistic in others – it all depends on the context.

Fu *et al.* (2007) demonstrated that the essential oils of rosemary (*Rosmarinus officinalis*) and clove (*Syzygium aromaticum*) both had, individually, a wide spectrum of antimicrobial activity against bacteria, yeasts and fungi. However, they found that if the oils were used in combination against the same test organisms, the combination exerted additive effects on the test bacteria (*Staphylococcus epidermidis*, *S. aureus*, *Bacillus subtilis*, *Escherichia coli*, *Proteus vulgaris* and *Pseudomonas aeruginosa*), a synergistic effect in the case of *Candida albicans*, and antagonism with *Aspergillus niger*.

Evidence for synergism in an essential oil blend was provided by an *in vitro* study to support the development of a hand sanitizer for use in infection control. Here, Caplin, Allan and Hanlon (2009) investigated the comparative activities of a blend of *Thymus zygis* cultivar essential oils[11] and a single linalool chemotype of thyme against two strains of methicillin-sensitive *Staphylococcus aureus* (MSSA). They noted that it was already believed that thymol and carvacrol were synergistic, and that most of the antimicrobial activity in thyme oils is associated with the

---

8   *Trichophyton rubrum* is the fungus responsible for *Tinea pedis* ('athlete's foot'), *Tinea cruris* ('jock itch') and dermatophytosis ('ringworm'); fungal nail infections are caused by *T. mentagrophytes* var. *interdigitale*.

9   Tested against methicillin-resistant *Staphylococcus aureus* (MRSA), using the inhibition zone method, with both direct and vapour contact (administered on dressings for burns).

10   According to Tisserand and Young (2014), most of the commercial geranium essential oil is obtained from *Pelargonium × asperum*, a hybrid of *P. capitatum* and *P. radens*, not the frequently cited *P. graveolens* (which is the source of an *iso*-menthone-rich essential oil).

11   The blend comprised four UK-grown cultivars of *Thymus zygis*; it was designed to contain a high concentration of thymol (31.1%) and linalool (23.6%), and a relatively high concentration of α-terpinene (13.2%) and terpinen-4-ol (11.7%) – the latter two are usually found as very minor components of some thyme oils. The blend also contained 1.1% carvacrol.

thymol and carvacrol chemotypes (Rota *et al.* 2008). It had also been shown that linalool, too, has strong activity against some bacteria and fungi, but especially so in the presence of other constituents such as α-terpinene, γ-terpinene, limonene, terpinen-4-ol and α-terpineol (Pattnaik *et al.* 1997). However, Rota *et al.* had demonstrated that an essential oil of *T. zygis* which contained 39% linalool had no activity against strains of *Escherichia coli* – except when thymol or carvacrol were also present. Building on these observations, Caplin, Allan and Hanlon (2009) demonstrated that a specially formulated *T. zygis* blend, based on these suspected synergies between constituents, showed 'substantial' anti-staphylococcal activity compared with the linalool chemotype. They hypothesised that this was due, in part, to the strong antimicrobial activity of the terpinen-4-ol in synergy with, for example, thymol and linalool.

At this point, it is worth noting that results from studies such as these, which include the use of the agar disc diffusion assay, will also be affected by the solubility of essential oils in hydrophilic growth media. This assay will tend to favour the more water-soluble essential oil constituents over the lipophilic (fat-soluble) ones.

Recent evidence for additivity, synergism and antagonism in essential oil blends can be found in research conducted by de Rapper *et al.* (2013). They report the results of a comprehensive study which set out to explore the interactive *in vitro* antimicrobial[12] properties of 45 essential oils when combined in various ratios with lavender (*Lavandula angustifolia*). In this study, the 'microdilution minimum inhibitory concentration' (MIC) method was used rather than disc diffusion assay; this was deemed to be more suitable for the purpose. They reported a 26.7% incidence of synergism, and 48.9% incidence of additive effects. There was only one instance of antagonism – a combination of lemongrass (*Cymbopogon citratus*) and lavender (*L. angustifolia*).[13] Some combinations were singled out as worthy of comment. These included lavender with cypress (*Cupressus sempervirens*), lavender with may chang (*Litsea cubeba*) against *Candida albicans*, and lavender in 1:1 combinations with carrot seed (*Daucus carota*), Virginian cedar (*Juniperus virginiana*), cinnamon (*Cinnamomum zeylanicum*) or sweet orange (*Citrus sinensis*) against both *C. albicans* and *Staphylococcus aureus*. In some instances, ratios were also significant. For example, if carrot seed dominated in a combination with lavender, synergistic activity against *C. albicans* was observed, but simply additive effects against *S. aureus* were noted. A lavender and cinnamon combination with a dominance of lavender showed synergistic activity against *C. albicans*; but if tested against *S. aureus*, additive effects were observed with all ratios, except when cinnamon was dominant (3:7) and synergy was observed. They suggested that this supported the use of this particular combination for the treatment of topical

---

12   Once a broad spectrum profile of lavender had been established, pathogenic strains of *Staphylococcus aureus* (a Gram-positive bacterium), *Pseudomonas aeruginosa* (a Gram-negative bacterium) and *Candida albicans* (a yeast) were selected as the test organisms. The Gram stain is a test that differentiates bacteria into two large groups based on the properties of their cell walls.

13   Based on equal ratios, 75.6% of the combinations showed either synergistic or additive activity, notably against *Candida albicans*.

infections. They also commented on sweet orange – which by itself had relatively poor antimicrobial activity, but if combined with lavender, synergism was observed with all ratios; this supports the use of a sweet orange and lavender combination in the treatment of respiratory infections. Other notable synergistic combinations were lavender with Virginian cedar as a possible treatment for bacterial respiratory infections and candida infections such as thrush.

It has been demonstrated that some essential oils and their components form synergistic combinations with antibiotics – this could perhaps become an alternative strategy to deal with infections caused by drug-resistant bacteria. Langeveld, Veldhuizen and Burt (2014) reviewed the evidence for interactions between antibiotics and essential oils containing carvacrol, cinnamaldehyde, cinnamic acid, eugenol and thymol, amongst others. They suggested that the observed synergistic effect might be due to several factors, such as by affecting multiple targets, by physicochemical interactions and by inhibiting antibacterial resistance mechanisms.

Liapi *et al.* (2008) investigated the anti-nociceptive actions of 1,8-cineole and β-pinene (noted as two monoterpenes from *Eucalyptus camadulensis* essential oil), and again evidence of synergism and antagonism was found, this time with morphine and naloxone.[14] In this animal study, 1,8-cineole had an anti-nociceptive[15] action similar to morphine, but naloxone did not antagonise it. It was suggested that there was a 'significant synergism' between 1,8-cineole and morphine. The findings with β-pinene were somewhat surprising. It was thought that β-pinene also had anti-nociceptive activity – as a partial agonist of some opioid receptors – but this activity was very weak. It did have supraspinal[16] activity in rats but not mice, but it reversed the anti-nociceptive effects of morphine and naloxone (Liapi *et al.* 2008, cited by Adorjan and Buchbauer 2010).

So, it is accepted that additivity, synergism and antagonism occur not only within essential oils, but also in their combinations, and with analgesic drugs and antibiotics – but can this theory be applied in aromatherapy? If two or more essential oils are combined, will the same phenomena be witnessed in the blend?

Synergism in aromatherapy: a broader interpretation of the theory

Blending with the aim of producing positive synergistic effects has become an accepted aromatherapy practice.[17]

---

14 Naloxone is an analgesic narcotic antagonist, used to counteract morphine overdose – especially the effect of respiratory depression.

15 The anti-nociceptive effect is a reduction in pain sensitivity made within neurones when a substance, such as an opiate or endorphin, combines with a receptor.

16 'Supraspinal' refers to the area of the medulla and midbrain.

17 This is not unique to aromatherapy; this is a type of 'polypharmacy' which is also practised in herbal medicine.

The synergistic rationale for using combination products looks to producing a dynamic product that has multiple modes of action, respecting the principle that the action of the combined product is greater than the sum total of known and unknown chemical components. (Harris 2002, p.179)

However logical and lucid this rationale is, the practice is less well defined. It is certainly easier to apply when we are dealing with essential oils which have significant levels of constituents with known actions, and more difficult when we are using oils that have no predominant constituents, and perhaps with unknown, or suspected, or yet to be established properties. We also need to consider ratios, and be aware that what is synergistic in one context may be antagonistic in different circumstances! As the Chen *et al.* (2013) study on the anti-cancer activities of frankincense and myrrh illustrated, synergy may be context dependent. It also raises another question – can we only discuss synergism in relation to chemistry?

Harris (2002) was the first to publish guidelines regarding the formulation of potentially synergistic blends of essential oils specifically for holistic aromatherapy practice – an area that, despite its importance, was somewhat murky and populated by numerous anecdotal accounts. She suggested that the selected oils should complement one another in terms of chemistry, activity and direction; that the number of oils in the formula should be restricted to between three and seven, so that the active components in the blend would dominate; and that the therapeutic purpose should be clear, and not attempt to encompass too many goals. Harris noted that the base or carriers would have an impact on the synergistic potential. However, she also suggested that synergism and antagonism might exist on other levels, such as the interaction between the therapist and client, and even between the client and their blend – perhaps witnessed in their cognitive and emotional responses to the odour of the prescription. Therefore, we could say that synergism and antagonism also exist in interpersonal relationships, and that the synergistic potential of a blend could be affected by our individual reactions to its aroma. Holistic aromatherapy often involves massage and various bodywork modalities. So here is yet another factor that can have a significant impact on the intervention – as the psychological, physiological and physical effects of bodywork will undoubtedly impact on the treatment outcome! Consequently, we also need to consider the case for synergy between essential oils and the nature of their application.

Plant aromatics and bodywork: is there evidence for synergism?

There is some evidence that acupressure and massage can potentiate the effects of essential oils and plant extracts. Taking their cue from the 'combined acupuncture and herbs therapy' of traditional Chinese medicine, Zhou *et al.* (2008) investigated whether auricular acupressure[18] could increase the absorption of the flavones[19] in a bitter orange (*Citrus aurantium*) peel aqueous extract. The extract was administered orally. They found that specific acupoints[20] could significantly improve the absorption of the flavones naringenin and hesperitin in the human body.

The case for massage and essential oil synergy is supported by a preliminary study conducted by Kuriyama *et al.* (2005). They demonstrated that although massage with and without essential oils could both decrease short-term anxiety, only aromatherapy massage[21] showed beneficial effects on serum cortisol levels and on the immune system. In this study, aromatherapy massage elicited a significant increase in peripheral blood lymphocytes and CD8+ and CD16+ lymphocytes – suggesting pharmacological benefits (such as improving resistance to infection) of using essential oils with massage. In 2008 Takeda *et al.* explored the differences between the physiological and psychological effects of aromatherapy massage[22] in comparison with non-aromatic massage after a stress-inducing task. The result suggested that massage, with or without essential oils, was more advantageous than rest alone in terms of psychological and subjective evaluations, but not in terms of physiology. In both cases, salivary cortisol was unchanged and secretory immunoglobulin A (sIgA)[23] increased significantly. However, it was noted that aromatherapy massage elicited stronger and more continuous relief from fatigue – especially mental fatigue.

However, perhaps the most striking example of essential oil/bodywork synergy was revealed in a study which investigated the effects of Shirodhara[24] with and without lavender essential oil (Xu *et al.* 2008). The study demonstrated that Shirodhara with plain sesame oil has an anxiolytic effect, but that Shirodhara with lavender and sesame oil had a greater effect. It was hypothesised that the psycho-physiological effects were due to the relaxing effect of lavender via olfaction, the pharmacological action of the substances absorbed through the skin, and

---

18 Auricular acupressure was developed by Paul Nogier, a French practitioner; the use of auricular acupoints was described originally in *Huangdi Neijing* – the 'Yellow Emperor's Classic of Internal Medicine'.

19 Flavones form a group of phytochemicals, including flavonoids such as luteolin (an anti-inflammatory agent), which are found in cereals and herbs, notably parsley, celery and also citrus peel. They are thought to have health benefits and may be of use in cases of atherosclerosis, osteoporosis, diabetes mellitus and some cancers.

20 The acupoints were Sympathetic (AH6A), *Shenmen* (TF4), Adrenal gland (TG2p), Subcortex (AT4), Endocrine (CO18), Kidney (CO10), Heart (CO15) and Liver (CO12).

21 The aromatherapy massage was conducted with 10–15ml of lavender (0.15ml), sweet marjoram (0.1ml) and cypress (0.05ml) essential oils in sweet almond; the control was conducted with sweet almond oil.

22 In this study, the aromatherapy massage was conducted with a blend of sweet orange, true lavender and sweet marjoram (2:1:1 at 1%).

23 Secretory IgA works with lysozomes to combat infection.

24 Shirodhara is an Ayurvedic treatment where herb-infused sesame oil is dripped onto the forehead over the region related to the 'third eye' or *ajna chakra*. This is reputed to produce profound relaxation, or an altered state of consciousness.

the physiological effects elicited by the dripping action on the thermosensors and pressure sensors via the trigeminal nerve. Xu *et al.* call this a 'complicated pharmaco-physio-psychological action' (p.956), but it might also be seen as a manifestation of essential oil/bodywork synergism.

Aromatherapeutic blending: is there any evidence of synergy?

The importance of the therapeutic relationship and bodywork skills in holistic clinical aromatherapy must never be underestimated, and should always be included when reflecting on practice. However, here our focus is on essential oils and the ways in which we can approach blending for the maximum benefit to our clients. It would be fair to say that the synergism hypothesis is of relevance to aromatherapeutic blending, but there is little *direct* scientific evidence to support its practice.

Most published investigations on the impact of essential oils on human wellbeing, or in the broader aromatherapy context, focus on single essential oils or absolutes. Only a few studies[25] have investigated blends, and in such cases the same blend is used on all participants. This is because blending different oils for individual participants who take part in such studies introduces an experimental variable that would undermine the results and make it impossible to draw valid conclusions. This is a problem which is inherent in aromatherapy research design. One of the few studies to explore the aromatherapeutic potential of blending was conducted by Hongratanaworakit (2011). It was hypothesised that a blend of essential oils could be used to treat depression or anxiety. A combination of lavender and bergamot was used in abdominal massage, and a range of autonomic parameters and emotional responses were analysed. Compared with the placebo group, the lavender and bergamot blend caused significant decreases in pulse rate and systolic and diastolic blood pressure, indicating a decrease in autonomic arousal. The aroma group also reported that they felt 'more calm' and 'more relaxed' than the control group of participants, suggesting a decrease in subjective behavioural arousal. However, although we can see why lavender and bergamot might be a synergistic combination from the chemistry perspective (both contain linalool and linalyl acetate), and both oils are strongly associated with relaxation, this study did not include an investigation of each oil used singly, so we do not know if the combination had synergistic effects.

There is the temptation to put all of these positive aromatic combinations under the umbrella of synergy…but we also need to consider that we might be

---

25 Komori *et al.* (2006) conducted the first clinical trial to evaluate the use of fragrance in the discontinuation of the long-term use of the hypnotic drugs of the benzodiazepine type. A fragrance was constructed, using aromatic plant extracts/fragrances that had shown the best results during a preliminary animal study. The fragrance was adjusted to suit most preferences, and consisted of sandalwood (35%), juniperberry (12%), rose (8%) and orris (6%). This study demonstrated that fragrance is a feasible, non-pharmacological treatment for primary and secondary insomnia.

witnessing simply additivity! Is it possible to create a synergistic blend of essential oils for application in holistic practice? Certainly, this is possible, but if we were asked for evidence of synergy, we would probably not be able to provide it. We have no robust studies to support the synergism theory when applied in aromatherapy, thus we have no published scientific evidence, so it must, for the time being, remain a hypothesis. However, it is a hypothesis that provides our very foundation for practice, and so demands careful examination and consideration by the aromatherapy profession – however unsettling this may be. We must be able to stand up to scrutiny from all angles!

So far, the argument for synergism has been grounded in science. What would happen if we were to consider synergy as an abstract concept, from the perspective of the senses?

An experiential perspective on synergy

To a large extent, our lives are experienced through our senses – sight, hearing, touch, taste, smell. Perhaps we should digress and consider how we might experience manifestations of synergy in our world. There is little doubt that sight is our dominant sense, so it is easy for most of us to 'see' synergy, for example, in the natural world. We can look at a sunflower, its centre composed of numerous seeds, which in themselves are visually unremarkable – but when arranged in the sunflower head they form a beautiful natural 'mandala' surrounded by an uplifting yellow halo. The arrangement of the seeds corresponds to the Fibonacci sequence,[26] which manifests throughout the natural world. How does observing a sunflower make us feel – is this not greater than the sum of a collection of seeds, petals and other plant tissues?

Turning to sounds, it is equally easy to find examples of synergy – for example, in music. Whether we choose to listen to a single instrument playing a series of notes within a composition, or a myriad of instruments playing a symphony, or a collection of individuals manifesting a unique musical signature in a rock band, we can be aware of synergism. It can change how we are feeling, perhaps moving us to tears or engendering feelings of exaltation and exhilaration. It is the same with the human voice. Perhaps the novel jazz harmonies sung by the American wartime trio, the Andrews Sisters, who sang the parts that were written for the saxophones to create something different, or the close harmonies popularised by the Everly Brothers, allow us to experience synergy through popular music. Indeed, on the death of Phil Everly, the singer Linda Ronstadt mentioned that the best close harmonies are sung by those with shared genes, a contemporary example being the Secret Sisters. However, this phenomenon might also be evident in performers

---

26 The numerical sequence: 1, 2, 3, 5, 8, 13…was proposed by Fibonacci in 1202 CE, where each number in the sequence is the sum of the two preceding numbers. It was considered an important numerical sequence for many years; recently it has been shown to play a fundamental role in the growth of plants. For more information, see www.popmath.org.uk/rpamaths/rpampages/sunflower.html.

who have close emotional and artistic links, such as Emmylou Harris and Gram Parsons. We all have different 'tastes' in music, but whatever your preferred genre, you can easily find synergy.

Staying with the idea of taste, the world of food also offers numerous examples of synergism. Eating involves sight, touch, texture, taste, smell and sound. If we have the choice, we will elect to cook and eat what brings us most enjoyment, and again, there are huge variations in what brings such pleasure to individuals. However, it is clear that it is the *combinations* of seasonings, herbs and spices, the aromatic elements and the other ingredients that contribute tastes and textures, which form the identity and characteristics of the foods that we like to eat. Entire cultures can be identified with their cuisines! Many dishes can be enjoyable, but those that are memorable are possibly the ones with synergy – the optimum combinations of ingredients, spices and herbs, the cooking techniques, and the creativity, vision and palate of the chef are all parts of the greater whole!

This naturally leads us to the world of scent – where numerous cross-modal associations link olfaction with our other senses. We do not experience smells in isolation, at least not under normal circumstances. To begin with a simple example: Burr (2007) wrote about an interview with the perfumer Jean-Claude Ellena, who is renowned for his skill in creating an olfactory impression with comparatively few ingredients. During this interview, Ellena demonstrated that if ethyl vanillin (a 'gourmand' vanilla-scented aromachemical) is mixed with cinnamon, orange and lime essences, a realistic impression of 'coca cola' is created. Mixtures of even a few perfume materials can give rise to completely new olfactory impressions. Some of the great perfumes have been described as works of art, defined by skilful combinations of aromachemicals and aromatic plant extracts, although, as Lawless (2009) commented, 'I concur fully with Roudnitska's[27] statement that quality in perfume (or any other endeavour) is entirely dependent upon an educated consumer' (p.13). So, yes, olfactory synergy exists too – but maybe it is a little more elusive, and its appreciation can be enhanced by cultivating the olfactory palate.

The sense of smell itself is integral to aromatherapy – indeed, aromatherapy is the only healing modality that harnesses (or exploits) the multiple effects of olfaction. Perhaps we might speculate that its profound effects on the body and psyche are a consequence of quasi-pharmacological, hedonic valence, semantic and placebo mechanisms[28] acting in a synergistic manner.

When we examine the concept of synergy from this alternative and indeed wider perspective, we realise that one of the ways in which we are aware of its presence is through beauty – the beauty of our world and its inhabitants, and our

---

27 Edmond Roudnitska (1905–1996) was a well-known, highly respected, influential perfumer and theorist; he composed many 'classic' fragrances including Dior's *Diorissimo*, *Eau Sauvage* and *Diorella*.

28 The perfumer Stephan Jellinek (1997) suggested that there are four ways in which smells can exert their effects on our states of mind. He named these the *quasi-pharmacological*, *semantic*, *hedonic valence* and *placebo* mechanisms.

creations – as witnessed through our senses and feelings. This surely is no less valid than the scientific perspective on synergy.

POINTS FOR REFLECTION

✳ How much importance do I currently attach to synergy when creating aromatherapeutic blends?

✳ Do I take any special measures to ensure that my blends are synergistic, or do I tend to rely on instinct and intuition?

✳ Do I consider additivity?

✳ Do I tend to focus on chemistry, or the broader interpretations of synergism in aromatherapy practice? And, perhaps, do I need to reach a balance in my approach?

✳ Where are my strengths and weaknesses? Do I need to become more cognisant of the science, imperfect as it is, or do I need to adopt a more holistic mindset?

✳ Looking to the natural world and art forms, what other examples of synergy can I find?

Chapter 2

The Individual Prescription

Leaving synergy aside, just for the moment, if we look at other forms of evidence to inform the therapeutic use of essential oils, we find a rich diversity of supportive data. There is little doubt that both single aromatics and essential oil blends applied in the aromatherapy context have beneficial physiological, cognitive and emotional effects, and so we now need to look at another concept central to holistic and clinical aromatherapy practice – the 'Individual Prescription'.

It could be said that the most enduring part of Marguerite Maury's legacy is the preparation of a blend of essential oils specific to an individual. She called this the 'Individual Prescription' (often abbreviated to I.P.), and this was based on 'the physiological and psychic[1] identity of the individual'. The I.P. would reflect weaknesses, compensate for deficiencies and reduce excesses, and normalise rhythms and functions (Maury 1989); in other words, it should restore equilibrium, and it was not curative *per se*. However, it was not just the choice of oils that was important; it was their balance, their relative proportions in the formula. Maury also conveyed that the I.P. should be dynamic, and could be altered as the individual progressed over a course of treatments; this is sound therapeutic practice, but a researcher's nightmare! We shall use the abbreviation I.P. to denote an individualised aromatherapeutic blend.

An I.P. can only be formulated after a thorough case history has been taken, and realistic short-term aims as well as appropriate and achievable longer-term goals have been established. It is also important to identify appropriate assessment tools – without which there is no way to monitor reactions, outcomes and progress, and consequently no way of knowing whether the therapy is effective, or whether changes are appropriate. The therapeutic relationship and the therapeutic conversation, integrated with clinical awareness, allow for the development of an aromatherapy treatment plan that includes the formulation of personalised aromatic prescriptions. These are all crucial elements in aromatherapy practice, and core aspects of professional education programmes.

We can generalise, up to a point, about the likely effects of specific essential oils, and indeed some research is very supportive of the concept that specific aromas could be prescribed to elicit specific and reproducible effects. However, as aromatherapists, we must remain cognisant of the philosophy that essential

---

1   Here, the word 'psychic' is used to denote the cognitive, emotional and non-physical aspects of the individual.

oil blends can have synergistic or additive potential, and that if they are prepared specifically for an individual, this therapeutic potential may be further enhanced.

It is clear that the starting point for formulating an aromatherapeutic blend is the identification of some of the essential oils that could benefit the individual. This process can be somewhat overwhelming, because of the multiple properties of many essential oils, the uniqueness of each individual and the complexity of each pathophysiological process! It is important to be able to see the overall picture as well as the detail; the 'macro' perspective will often determine many of the appropriate oils, while the 'micro' view can be significant when 'fine-tuning' the prescription.

If we take a step back at this stage, and consider how aromatherapy has developed in recent years, it becomes apparent that aromatherapists have 'imported' or adopted and adapted philosophies from related and allied medical and therapeutic modalities, on which to base their own practices. By doing this, we can begin to see how the essential oil selection process can be achieved.

Adopted, adapted and novel aromatherapy paradigms

Aromatherapy – or *aromathérapie* – has its origins in France in the early 1920s. Tisserand (1993) credits the chemist and perfumer René Maurice Gattefossé with the development of this new therapeutic discipline. Gattefossé's aromatherapy was influenced by the prevalent medical approach – and he was responsible for introducing the idea of synergy in aromatherapy, for the importance of the percutaneous absorption of essential oils and the dermal route of their application, and he also acknowledged the psychotherapeutic benefits of fragrance. These concepts continue to underpin contemporary, holistic aromatherapy practices (Tisserand 1993; Schnaubelt 1999).

Gattefossé presented his work in a medical and scientific way, focusing on the pharmacological activities of essential oils and relating these to their active constituents; because of this, aromatherapy initially developed in the medical domain. This trend continued in France; in the 1960s practitioners such as Jean Valnet fostered the idea of relating functional groups[2] with therapeutic potential, and Maurice Girault developed the aromatogram[3] which paved the way for further investigation into the antimicrobial potential of essential oils and their application in the clinical arena. Paul Belaiche further developed the use of essential oils in the clinical domain, specifically in the treatment of infection, later collaborating

---

2   A 'functional group' is an atom or small group of atoms on a molecule that is important in its identity and classification (e.g. alcohol, aldehyde, ketone) and is implicated in its odour, properties and biological activities. In essential oil chemistry, functional groups are attached to carbon frameworks (terpenoid and phenylpropanoid) and they usually contain one or more oxygen atoms.

3   This is a laboratory technique that can elucidate the antimicrobial activities of specific essential oils in relation to specific microbial pathogens. The aromatogram, because of the watery nature of agar, the matrix of the growth medium, does favour the more water-soluble essential oil constituents, and can be seen as biased against the more fat-soluble ones.

with others to develop treatments for a range of infectious diseases. Like Valnet, Belaiche advocated that essential oils could be classified according their dominant functional groups. So developments in France from the 1920s to the early 1980s have given us our foundations – dermal application and absorption, clinical and psychotherapeutic aspects, synergy and the functional group hypothesis.

In France in the 1940s, Marguerite Maury, who was not medically qualified, focused on the external applications of essential oils, as the internal prescription and medical use of essential oils was, and is, legally restricted or prohibited in most Western countries (Schnaubelt 1999; Bensouilah 2005). It was Maury's style of aromatherapy that flourished in English-speaking countries. It is also of significance that her holistic approach encompassed the clinical potential, but was infused by her interest in Tibetan and Chinese medicine, so here we witness the trends that were to influence the evolution of our contemporary aromatherapy practices.

The medical practitioner and naturopath Daniel Pénoël, in collaboration with the chemist Pierre Franchomme, developed what they termed 'scientific aromatherapy', practised within a holistic context. Pénoël introduced the concept of the terrain[4] to aromatherapy and developed Franchomme's functional group hypothesis[5] into what he called the 'molecular approach' – a model for constructing synergistic blends of essential oils. Mainly through Franchomme and Pénoël, the use of chemotypes[6] was introduced in aromatherapy, although the practice was not universally accepted; for example, Jean Claude Lapraz disputed their significance, proposing the 'Law of All or Nothing', where the entire essential oil is of importance, not its individual constituents. Lapraz, in conjunction with Christian Duraffourd, also developed the 'endobiogenic concept', which emphasised the importance of the root causes of pathology, and the terrain of the patient, in the determination of the optimum phytotherapeutic/aromatic treatment.

Meanwhile, therapists who were practising aromatherapy as a complementary therapy were becoming exposed to relevant research in the life and social sciences, mainly due to the influential *International Journal of Aromatherapy*, founded and edited[7] by Robert Tisserand. This journal also featured articles written by practitioners such as Peter Holmes and Gabriel Mojay, who were exploring and developing alternative approaches to aromatherapy based on traditional, vitalistic

---

4   Claude Bernard (1813–1878) was a physiologist who suggested that it was the condition of the body and its internal environment that determined the individual's healing capacity; for example, an infection could only develop if the conditions are favourable. Pénoël called this the *terrain*.

5   The functional group hypothesis attempted to explain and predict the physiological and biological activities of essential oils based on their dominant functional groups. The hypothesis was based on an electrochemical experiment, where chemical constituents of essential oils were sprayed between 'electromagnetic plates'; later Schnaubelt (1995) presented 'structure effect' diagrams which applied this theory to practice.

6   *Chemotypes* are essential oils from plants bred or selected for their ability to produce significant amounts of key active constituents.

7   Bob Harris continued as editor in its later years, founding the excellent but short-lived *Journal of Essential Oil Therapeutics* after the demise of the *International Journal of Aromatherapy*.

medicine. As a result, the evidence base and philosophical basis of aromatherapy became broader, and new avenues for practice were introduced, such as Holmes' 'Fragrance Energetics' and Mojay's 'Five Elements Aromatherapy'.

By now it will be very clear that aromatherapy encompasses diverse practices, based on a plethora of hypotheses – synergism, functional groups, the terrain, endobiogenics and also philosophies such as holism and vitalism. The impact of global healing practices – ethnomedicine, phytotherapy, Western biomedicine and Eastern medicine, including Unani Tibb, Ayurveda and Chinese medicine – can be seen too. All of this has given rise to diverse styles of practice within the discipline as it has grown…and has influenced approaches to blending and the creation of the I.P.

We will next consider the science-based molecular approach and reveal its relevance and potential, and then explore some vitalistic approaches to aromatherapy. Before progressing, here are some questions we can ask ourselves, or perhaps discuss with our peers and mentors.

POINTS FOR REFLECTION

* Aromatherapy has borrowed theories, philosophies and even evidence for practice from multiple disciplines. How do I feel about this?

* Should we be focusing on developing a stronger, more unified identity, or continue to embrace the relevant parts of other practices? After all, aromatherapy is already a sort of hybrid therapy, fusing bodywork with aromatic prescriptions, which are inherently related to both phytotherapy and perfumery!

* Do we look to other disciplines to support our perceived 'weak' scientific evidence base; do we have an option?

* Should we look to other disciplines to diversify our scope of practice? What might be the positive and negative implications of this?

Chapter 3

A Spectrum of Approaches

Science-based, Psychosensory and Vitalistic Paradigms

In this chapter we will review some of the prevalent approaches to aromatherapeutic blending. These range from the reductionist, science-based, 'molecular approach', and the psycho-aromatherapeutic perspective, to holistic psychosensory and vitalistic approaches that have been inspired by traditional practices. Throughout, we can reflect on how these philosophical approaches are relevant to, and could be applied in, clinically and holistically focused aromatherapy practice.

The science-based molecular approach: synergy in the clinical realm

At first glance, the molecular approach could be seen to epitomise reductionism and be more allied to biomedicine than complementary and alternative medicine (CAM). However, if we are to embrace holistic principles, we do need to explore the microcosm as well as the macrocosm, and the molecular approach allows us to do just this!

Pénoël (1998/1999) maintained that his speciality – medical aromatherapy – may have curative purpose and preventative action, or may simply assist someone who feels well, but wants to feel better and improve their potential in general or specific areas. He also considers that 'aromatic care' can be emergency, intensive, or regular for chronic states. In holistic/clinical aromatherapy, we are not able to offer cures, but we can contribute to the maintenance and enhancement of wellbeing; we can also apply essential oils intensively for short periods or in lower concentrations over a longer time frame to address specific concerns.

The molecular approach to creating a synergistic prescription relies on knowledge of the likely properties of functional groups, and combining essential oils to create blends that have high concentrations of the desired active constituents. Pénoël (1998/1999) suggested that essential oil blends can be created for either 'horizontal' or 'vertical' synergistic actions. *Horizontal synergy* may be found in a blend of several essential oils containing similar functional groups, for a single specific purpose. For example, a blend rich in monoterpene alcohols such as linalool, terpinen-4-ol and α-terpineol should have enhanced antimicrobial action. *Vertical synergy* may be found in a blend of essential oils containing different functional groups, intended for more than one purpose. Vertical synergy might be more appropriate for holistic aromatherapy practice, where usually clients present with more than one need, and the terrain requires consideration. Even a single disease normally entails several different pathophysiological processes, such as inflammation and pain. As each essential oil in the blend will contain more than one type of functional group, there is scope for further overlap of properties. However, unlike the case of horizontal synergy, where, for example, antimicrobial activity can be measured, vertical synergy does not lend itself so easily to research and investigation.

Since its emergence in the early 1990s, the functional group theory has had its detractors, mainly because of the prevalent tendency to over-generalise about the properties attributed to functional groups, and also because of the opposing 'all or nothing' viewpoint. The most sensible way forward is to use the molecular approach in the appropriate circumstances, where each constituent has a known action, and essential oils (and possibly their chemotypes) are combined to create a demonstrable synergy – as in the blend of *Thymus zygis* cultivars investigated by Caplin, Allan and Hanlon (2009), or in the findings reported by de Rapper *et al.* (2013). We can also look at the known activities of specific molecules (which may or may not be due solely to the influence of their functional groups) within oils, be cognisant of the potential for intrinsic essential oil synergy,[1] and create the dynamic, multi-functional blends as described by Harris (2002).

However, it might seem that if we adopt the molecular approach, we could lose sight of the potential impact of the aroma of essential oils on the senses and psyche, and indeed the energetic perspective. Psychosensory approaches to blending offer an alternative, so that we are not only contemplating synergy from the chemistry/pharmacology perspective, but also from the individual/aroma perspective – although the latter might also be a manifestation of the former!

Synergy in a holistic context

Having reflected upon the molecular approach, where the hypothesis of aromatherapeutic synergy is perhaps closest to its scientific origins, we now need to look at how it sits within the holistic context, as this is how most contemporary aromatherapy is practised. In reality, we are now applying the synergy hypothesis in a diffuse realm, seemingly without boundaries. This is a very interesting philosophical exercise, where we must, at times, explore concepts such as the psyche and vitalism – which is very much at odds with science and orthodox medicine.

We can start by exploring the effects of aromatics on the psyche, where we find some interesting research that can support 'psycho-aromatherapy', and some

---

1 Intrinsic essential oil synergism was named the 'Kaleidoscope Principle' by Schnaubelt (1999). He gives the example of the monoterpene/terpene alcohol/1,8-cineole synergy in the essential oils of ravintsara (*Cinnamomum camphora* leaf, 1,8-cineole chemotype), niaouli (*Melaleuca quinquenervia*) and *Eucalyptus radiata* – calling this the 'cold' and 'flu' synergy – recognisable by its medicinal aroma and association with antiseptic and expectorant properties.

theories that might explain how odour can have such a remarkable impact on cognition and emotions.

The psycho-aromatherapeutic perspective

Via the sense of smell, odours can act directly on the psyche, and different odours can enhance, modify or stabilise cognitive and emotional states. Aromatherapy is the only contemporary therapeutic modality that has developed around this particular observation, and in practice the different odour characteristics of plant essential oils and absolutes are used to impart positive mood benefits. This aspect of aromatherapy is sometimes termed 'psycho-aromatherapy', to differentiate it from the wider health-enhancing effects of essential oils, but in reality it is an integral part of holistic aromatherapy practice.

In 1923 Giovanni Gatti and Renato Cajola published a comprehensive review of the effects of essential oils on the nervous system, and their influences on moods and emotions (Tisserand 1988). They had investigated the states of anxiety and depression, and identified specific oils as sedatives, which would counteract anxiety, and stimulants, which counteract depression. They also documented, for the first time, the phenomenon that an aroma which was stimulating on initial light exposure sometimes brought about a state of sedation if exposure was prolonged or repeated. Later, in 1973, Professor Paolo Rovesti of the University of Milan identified that specific essential oils could be used to alleviate depression and anxiety (Tisserand 1988).

There have since been numerous studies which have investigated the effects of essential oils on human and animal behaviour, mood and cognition, most of which support the belief that essential oils can be used as olfactory therapeutic agents. Some of these studies have been concerned with the effects of the odours, while a few explore the ways in which these odours might be producing their effects. Most of this research is very supportive of the aromatherapy concept that specific aromas could be prescribed to elicit specific and reproducible effects. For example, Moss, Hewitt and Moss (2008), in a study on the effects of aroma on cognition,[2] supported a quasi-pharmacological mechanism of action, suggesting the concept of substance-specificity, where each odour would deliver a unique pattern of influence. In 2012 Moss and Oliver reported the results of a study which elucidated the relationship between absorbed 1,8-cineole rosemary essential oil, cognitive performance and mood. It was found that the plasma concentration of 1,8-cineole was significantly related to cognitive performance – the higher the concentration, the better the performance in terms of both speed and accuracy. The effects of 1,8-cineole plasma concentration levels on mood were less clear, although it was observed that there was a significant negative correlation between

---

2   This particular study focused on the effects of ylang ylang and peppermint, two oils that are commonly used in aromatherapy, and supported the use of ylang ylang as a relaxing scent, and peppermint as a scent that does not slow down reaction times and can perhaps increase task motivation.

change in subjective feelings of 'contentment' and 1,8-cineole levels. Moss and Oliver suggested that compounds absorbed from the diffused rosemary affect both cognition and mood, but that this happens independently via different neurochemical pathways. However, there are other factors at work, apart from the quasi-pharmacological mechanism – our responses are also influenced by semantics, hedonics and placebo/expectation.[3]

The body of research has highlighted the many ways in which odour affects us at physiological and psychological levels, and that the mechanisms are intricate and interrelated, and indeed inextricable. Generally, essential oil aromas fall into three categories – activating, deactivating and 'harmonising'. It is clear, then, that the activating or stimulating oils would be more suited to depressive states, while the deactivating or sedating oils might be useful for anxiety. However, it has been found that many oils are 'harmonising' – meaning that they can be relaxing on the physical level, while uplifting the spirits or arousing the emotions – so their effects are not always clearly defined, and are certainly not 'polarised'.

However, the studies have also shown the many ways in which hedonically pleasing odours can contribute to wellbeing – an aspect that should not be overlooked in holistic aromatherapy practice. In stark and simple terms: a recipient should like, very much, the aroma of their I.P. The exception might be a prescription for home use, which might smell 'medicinal' – but even then, if the blend includes an element that is attractive when applied, improved compliance of use might be encouraged; or we might witness the placebo/expectation phenomenon, where there might be the belief that if something has a medicinal smell, it will have a medicinal or therapeutic effect.

The principal aim of psycho-aromatherapy is to restore balance to the mind and emotions, and perhaps to redress symptoms of anxiety, depression and stress. At the outset, it must be emphasised that both anxiety and depression are complex conditions which have an impact on our physical, physiological, cognitive, emotional and spiritual wellbeing, and so, although the scents of many aromatic oils have been shown to have a positive impact, they should not be considered as a 'stand-alone' treatment, especially if specific and serious mental health problems have been identified. However, this caution is in no way meant to detract from the considerable benefits of odours on cognition and emotions, and thus upon our physical health and spirits. The psychotherapeutic properties of essential oils and absolutes can certainly be used to enhance feelings of wellbeing, and can be particularly beneficial when anxiety and depression are experienced.

---

3   *Hedonics*: where the effects of an odour depend on the subject's state of pleasure or displeasure with that odour. *Semantics*: we usually experience smells in the context of life situations, and smells, memory and associations quickly and irreversibly become linked. Each odour thus carries an emotional memory, the impact of which can lead to physiological changes such as an increase in heart rate or blood adrenalin. *Placebo/expectation*: if an individual is told that a certain odour will have a specific effect, and this becomes a belief, then the chances are that the odour will indeed elicit the expected effect.

The selection of potentially synergistic essential oils and absolutes is based upon the evidence that supports their psychotherapeutic benefits, but perhaps it should also involve the recipient in this choice, in order to create a blend that is hedonically pleasing. For the aromatherapist, a good familiarity with the odours of plant aromatics is essential – we need to know how they will interact with each other, not just initially, but as the blend evolves over time. The aroma part of the therapy is so important! When working in this way, we also need to ensure that we have a thorough understanding of the mechanisms that underpin our responses to odours, because this will help us understand individual reactions and responses.

If these reactions are positive, we can use aroma alone, perhaps delivered by an 'aroma stick', between aromatherapy treatments, harnessing the power of positive olfactory conditioning – a therapeutic intervention derived from the classical concept of conditioning first observed in Pavlov's dogs. In essence, classical conditioning relates to the pairing of a neutral object with an emotional and/or physiological reaction. In 1983 King demonstrated that with unconscious conditioning, odour could be paired with a positive emotional state, and so future exposure to the odour produced the same emotion. Kirk-Smith, Van Toller and Dodd (1983) showed that it was also possible to pair an odour with a negative emotional state, and that the emotion could be evoked at a later stage in response to the odour. In 1988 King observed that odours quickly become linked with emotional meanings, which can be very personal – and unique to the individual. A decade later, Alaoui-Ismaïli *et al.* (1997) demonstrated that there was a strong link between hedonics and autonomic nervous system responses, and thus emotion. The individual's expectations can also influence reactions to specific odours (Knasko, Gilbert and Sabini 1990, cited by Ilmberger *et al.* 2001; Robbins and Broughan 2007). Therefore, using odour as an evocative agent has enormous therapeutic potential, and aromatherapists are in a very strong position to harness this.

An intuitive element

We could take the view that research and observations over a long period of time give credible support to psycho-aromatherapy. However, we have yet to explore the intuitive element that pervades the practice of not only psycho-aromatherapy, but aromatherapy generally, and we can begin by taking a very brief look at the work of Philippe Mailhebiau. He developed a concept which he named the '*characterologie*' of essential oils, linking their olfactory characteristics and 'personalities' with the olfactory affinities and temperament of the individual and describing this as 'aromatic typology'. It would seem, therefore, that this is closely allied to psycho-aromatherapy, but Mailhebiau combines aromatic typology with the practice of science-based aromatic medicine, to refine and personalise his aromatherapy treatments so that they not only address clinical symptoms, but also aim to restore balance and equilibrium. His approach is, however, intuitive rather than based on research and evidence, and as such has been compared to the work of Hahnemann, the founder of homeopathy (Clerc 1995). Mailhebiau's comment that 'this approach opens the door to personalised treatments which go beyond the scope of symptomatic aromatherapy by combining efficient physiochemical action with a decisive psycho-sensory effect' (Mailhebiau 1995, p.xi) echoes what we have already noted about the I.P. It is sometimes the detail, the 'micro' perspective, that is important in 'fine-tuning' an I.P., and Mailhebiau also states that 'nuances are imperative in assigning a patient a specific characterology' (cited by Clerc 1995, p.16). This approach is broadly aligned with the holistic underpinnings of aromatherapy, so we can adapt *characterologie* to prepare I.P.s that address not only clinical concerns but also the psyche – but we need a genuine 'rapport' with our essential oils and their aromas, as well as an understanding of their therapeutic actions. This connection can only be achieved by actively working with the sense of smell; with reference to Mailhebiau's work, Farrer-Halls (2014) explores how we can use meditation and mindfulness to expand intuitive aromatherapy practice.

The energetic dimension: vitalistic approaches

Michel Lavabre (1990) suggested that psychosensory philosophy should be central to aromatherapy practice, and that we should develop an appreciation of aromatic plants – their morphology, physiology and growth habits – because this gives an insight into their nature and fragrances. Mojay maintains that it is the fragrance of essential oils that has the most immediate and generalised effect on the body and mind. If we are to use the psychosensory model, it is therefore vital to engage directly with the essential oils in terms of their scents, experiencing the diverse fragrances of essential oils from rhizomes and roots, stems and leaves, grasses, needles and cones, woods, resins, flowers, fruits and seeds. This requires the active use of the sense of smell, from which we gain tangible insights into aromatic influences.

There are several distinct styles of aromatherapy that have emerged from the blend of science, traditional healing practices, observation and intuition – and these include Five Elements aromatherapy, Ayurvedic-inspired aromatherapy and Fragrance Energetics. They do have one thing in common, however, and that is that they all consider the individual's interactions with essential oils. They are holistic approaches, and also have a vitalistic element. For example, Chinese Five Elements and Ayurvedic approaches are derived directly from traditional and complete healing systems.[4] The Fragrance Energetics model is closely aligned with holistic aromatherapy and includes elements of several classical traditional medicine practices. These philosophies certainly offer alternative and viable approaches to aromatherapy practice, including the construction of individualised essential oil prescriptions.

---

4   It is advised that if such alternative approaches are to be used in aromatherapy practice, further specialist studies are undertaken.

Chinese Five Elements

The theory of the Five Elements is central to traditional Chinese medicine. The Five Elements are symbolic of phases or movements of *yin* and *yang* energy, and manifest in the natural world, including the seasons, the climate and human emotions. The Five Elements are named Earth, Metal, Water, Wood and Fire; they are interrelated, and these relationships are described symbolically by the *sheng* cycle and the *ke* cycle.

Gabriel Mojay, who pioneered the use of the Chinese Five Elements framework in aromatherapy, also emphasises the importance of the impact of aroma on the psyche. Mojay (1996) explains that this approach encompasses the botanical, traditional and energetic aspects of essential oils and oriental medicine to define their unique healing potential. He uses the framework of the Chinese Five Elements to explore the fragrance energies of essential oils, proposing that Five Elements theory allows the aromatherapist to align the actions of essential oils with holistic therapeutic intentions that encompass the body, emotions and spirit.

The *shen*, or spirit, equates to the psyche – the emotional, mental and spiritual aspects of a human being. The spirit is expressed through many emotions, such as feeling love and compassion, joy when witnessing beautiful natural phenomena, or being moved by music. If the health of the spirit is adversely affected by stress, there is a knock-on effect that can result in mental and physical illness. So the health of the spirit is of vital importance (Hicks, Hicks and Mole 2011; Mojay 1996). The Five Elements approach can engender a deeper understanding of the human condition and our relationship with the natural world. It can allow insight into the root causes of disharmony and dysfunction, and it certainly offers an alternative way of looking at essential oils and their interrelationships. However, Chinese Five Elements assessment is based on detailed observations and an understanding of the underlying theory, and it is only with an understanding of this perspective that a practitioner can construct a philosophically sound individual prescription and treatment plan.

Ayurveda

Ayurvedic medicine of the Indian subcontinent originates from the ancient Sanskrit sacred texts known as the Vedas (Caldecott 2006). The four books that compose the Vedas date from around 3000 BCE and give detailed instructions on how a human being should live a spiritual life – a path with heart, which will ultimately lead to enlightenment. Ayurveda, meaning 'the knowledge of life', forms just one strand of the Vedas, and details how humans can live healthily in body, mind and spirit through an understanding of their own nature and interactions with the world. This is a system of medicine that is completely individualised; and although it gives great therapeutic detail on the treatment of illness through herbs, oils, massage, diet, and so on, it is more about prevention of disease through correct living. There is a rich history of the use of aromatic oils in the prevention and treatment of disease in Ayurveda – we could say that this too is part of aromatherapy's ancestry, significantly preceding Gattefossé! Some aromatherapists elect to study Ayurveda in order to incorporate their aromatherapy practice within this system of healing, while others will use some of the philosophical principles to gain an understanding of their clients and inform essential oil prescription. Like Chinese Five Elements, and Greek Four Elements, this is another example where parts of a philosophical system are integrated within another discipline, thus introducing new or alternative perspectives on theory and practice. It is often the Ayurvedic concept of the doshas that are related to essential prescribing.

In the Ayurvedic texts, the elements are combined into pairs, giving three doshas – *Vata* (Ether and Air), *Pitta* (Fire and Water) and *Kapha* (Water and Earth) (Frawley and Lad 1986). Each and every human being, as part of nature, has their own particular mix of the three doshas which gives rise to that individual's unique constitution or *pakriti* (Svoboda 1984). We all need the principle of motion that is Air, the principle of illumination that is Fire and the principle of cohesion that is Water and Earth (Pole 2006). However, our constitution or pakriti will be dominant in either one or two of the doshas; rarely there is an individual with balance of all three doshas, a *tridoshic* individual. The doshas have behavioural, emotional, cognitive and physical/physiological correspondences; a good practitioner of Ayurvedic medicine will recognise that each of the doshic predominances will generally display differing emotional responses. From this, we can see how we could begin to explore how essential oils might be prescribed to restore balance and promote health and wellbeing.

Fragrance Energetics

Peter Holmes suggests that we can base aromatherapy practice on an energetic system of essential oil fragrance pharmacology (Holmes 1998/1999). Considering the philosophical foundations of Chinese, Greek and Ayurvedic medicine,[5] he points out that they all embrace the concept that healing relies on a vital energy – *chi* (*qi*), *pneuma* and *prana* respectively. He describes vitalism as 'the principle or dynamo that runs life and so connects all life-forms in a living web of interconnections' (Holmes 2001, p.18).

Fragrance Energetics (Holmes 1997) is a model which aligns the scents of essential oils with their impact on the psyche. Holmes suggests that it is the energetic dimensions of a fragrance that elicit responses within an individual and will manifest on cognitive, emotional and spiritual levels. He proposes that if the root of a disease is in the psyche, the fragrance of essential oils will work via the

---

5   He includes the Four Element, Four Fluid (Humors) and Four Constitutional models (from traditional Greek medicine), the Five Elements and Eight Principles models (from traditional Chinese medicine), and the Five Elements, Three Dosha and Six Prakriti models (from Ayurvedic medicine), and also Specific Symptomatology (from homeopathy).

psychoneuroendocrine pathway, thus healing the physical dimension. Conversely, if the origin of the disease is in the body, the essential oils work via the body's physiology up to the mental and emotional levels, healing the whole person (Holmes 2001).

With his fusion of traditional practices and insight into fragrance pharmacology, Holmes has given us a comprehensive and viable model for holistic clinical aromatherapy practice; perhaps he has identified and encapsulated our own unique, hybrid philosophy. He maintains that we should 'let science be science and holism, holism' (Holmes 2001, p.14), and suggests that we do not rely solely on our knowledge of essential oil chemistry to rationalise our choice of essential oils. The solution is to practice a whole systems approach, because if we confuse essential oil pharmacology with therapeutics, aromatherapy is 'reduced to a science based therapy' (p.15).

Molecular Energetics

Dr Malte Hozzel is a teacher and lecturer in essential oils, and founder of the Oshadhi brand. He has been instrumental in developing and popularising an understanding of the actions of essential oils based on a synthesis of their energetics and their chemistry.

For example, he explains that we can view ketones as having a kind of 'anti-matter' energy. Speaking in terms of vibrations or field-energies, they lift us up from a mere physical existence, opening us to 'spirit' and spiritual experiences. It is no wonder that in ancient times many highly ketonic plants were used in sacred rituals; for example, the members of the *Artemisia* genus, sagebrush, thuya and hyssop. However, ketonic plants such as santolina and sage were also simply used to free the physiology from intestinal wastes, such as parasites, thus allowing humans (and animals) to purify the system in a very rapid way.

Metaphorically, we can consider ketones to be the 'dis-incarnators' of Mother Nature, a principle which is confirmed when we think of ketones increasing naturally in humans with age, for example; or, in the same direction, when we are fasting. In this sense, it is utterly comprehensible why children, who are humans in their incarnative phase, should not use ketonic oils. This principle is equally valid for pregnant and nursing mothers. Ketonic oils are appropriate in situations where, in some sense, we want to reduce 'physicality'. This explains also their value for reducing mucosal secretions and cellulite, dissolving phlegm, and so on.

From the energetic perspective, ketonic oils are highly valued for meditation and spiritual pursuits; that is, where the attention is drawn away from the physical towards the spiritual level. It is noteworthy that when Christ was on the cross he was given hyssop, a sacred plant of the Hebrews, which allows us to detach from the body, lifting the spirit up to the Divine in man. Meditation on the essential oil of hyssop afforded further insight into the energetic nature of ketones:

I poured the hyssop in my hands and much more poured out than I expected. I breathed in very deeply several times from my cupped palms. In about ten minutes I felt my body being rocked from inside – as if I were knocking against the container of the body – and visually, the room jolted a bit. I sat down and relaxed for a while. About 20 minutes later, we drove back to our hotel, and within an hour of breathing in the hyssop we were in bed.

When I lay down with my head on my partner's shoulder, at once the roof of the room had gone, and I was floating with the stars. I was out in the night sky surrounded by the stars of the night. I could have explored this place, and chose to just be with the incredible peace and soothing feeling that I experienced while floating amongst the stars.

I opened my eyes and was immediately back in the room with the ceiling over my head and walls around us. Closing my eyes again, I was in the open starry sky surrounded by night sky's stars, all around me. The feeling was comforting, and I was aware that I had no sense of hot or cold; it felt physically comfortable, mentally soothing and very peaceful. (Hinde and Hozzel 2015)

Here, through our sense of smell, with meditation and mindfulness, the molecular and the energetic dimensions become fused, allowing us deeper insights into the actions of essential oils on ourselves – our senses are the interface between the physical and non-physical realms.

POINTS FOR REFLECTION

In Chapter 3 we have reviewed just some of the prevalent philosophies from the West and the East that underpin the creation of aromatic prescriptions. It would seem that although they are diverse and come from seemingly disparate realms, there is a remarkable degree of connectivity – especially when viewed from the perspectives offered by Holmes, and Hinde and Hozzel. This is a very good point at which to pause, and reflect upon our philosophical roots and our current ways of practising. We could ask ourselves:

* How do I feel about the reductionist element that is inherent in the molecular approach? Is it at odds with my personal philosophy of healing, or does it bolster my need for scientific credibility?

* Am I adequately conversant with essential oil chemistry in order to use it to build additivity or synergism in my blends?

* Could the molecular approach enhance my clinical practice?

* How much importance do I attach to psycho-aromatherapy?

* How much attention do I pay to the scent of essential oils? Do I, or should I, involve my clients in the choice? How could I go about this?

﹡ How do I feel about vitalism, and could I, or would I, defend its incursion into aromatherapy practice?

﹡ What is my personal view on intuition? Does it influence my work consciously or unconsciously? Do I need a model on which to base intuitive practice? Is intuition influenced by prior knowledge?

﹡ In this section it was stated, several times, that it is vital to actively use our sense of smell to gain a deeper understanding of essential oils. Do I agree, and indeed is our intuitive capacity enhanced by developing our olfactory capabilities?

﹡ Do any of the energetic approaches strongly appeal to me? Can I see how they might enhance my practice?

﹡ How do I feel about picking and choosing small parts of traditional systems of healing to suit my purposes? How would I feel if practitioners of other disciplines started to use essential oils in their work, especially without formal study?

﹡ Peter Holmes (2001) asks 'Where does science end and aromatherapeutics begin?' (p.15). How would you reply to him?

Chapter 4

Aromatherapeutic Blending

Having explored the paradox of the significance of synergy in aromatherapy (where the importance attached to it is somewhat undermined by the paucity of evidence when the hypothesis is applied specifically within the context of holistic practice), and then considered a few of the philosophical principles which underlie the various therapeutic paradigms, we now need to focus on the principles that underpin the practice of aromatherapeutic blending. These principles revolve around both practical and theoretical considerations, so we do have a 'chicken and egg' scenario to negotiate here. We will begin with the theoretical underpinnings; the practicalities follow.

Assessment: core information for the I.P.

An essential oil prescription is based on the aromatherapist's assessment of their client. Systems of client assessment vary, but there would appear to be three broad approaches. First, the 'biomedical' approach has a focus on dysfunction and disease, and the identification and characterisation of presenting symptoms. Second, the 'biopsychosocial' approach allows consideration of physical and physiological, and cognitive, emotional and behavioural concerns – with perhaps a humanistic element, a focus on the client's lived experiences, geared to helping the client reach their full potential. Third, the 'energetic' or 'vitalistic' approaches to assessment can offer therapists the opportunity make their assessments and treatment plans from an alternative perspective – perhaps based on Eastern traditional medicine or vitalistic philosophies.

In holistic clinical aromatherapy, a client may often have two or more aromatic prescriptions – for professional application (usually with massage or allied bodywork), and also for home use between treatments, such as a prescription for pain relief, immune support, or a psychotherapeutic inhalation (for example, to alleviate insomnia, anxiety or low mood). It should be emphasised that an appropriate method for measuring treatment outcomes must always be established, and the choice of an assessment tool that involves the input of both parties is recommended. This ensures that the aromatherapeutic treatment is dynamic, and can evolve as the client progresses.

Sometimes it can be difficult to establish our clients' priorities. Sometimes a great deal of detailed information is divulged, and sometimes the reverse. This depends on the client – some clients 'open up' easily, others are very reserved, some have a high level of self-awareness, and others do not. Are there any tensions or coherences with your own observations and impressions? It is preferable to agree the short- and medium-term aims of the treatment, focus on one or two issues at any one time, and, if possible, try to find the root of any problems and address these as well as the symptoms. For example, if pain is an issue, inflammation may well be a contributing factor – so what is causing or contributing to the inflammation? How and where is this manifesting? How is it impacting on the client? In other words, we should try to explore the terrain.

Here, we will discuss the formulation of an I.P., models for practice, and the potential olfactory, biological and energetic responses that could refine our approach.

Formulation of an Individual Prescription

If we look back at Harris's guidelines, offering two or more prescriptions is sometimes advantageous – this helps us avoid trying to force too many objectives into one formula. However, in many cases, especially if maintenance or enhancement of general wellbeing is the overall aim, one I.P. might be all that is required. In addition to clarifying the aim/s of the prescription, the overall 'direction' should be clear. This can mean that the prescription is directed to a body system by including essential oils (or constituents) that are known to have effects on a specific system, or directed towards overall stimulation or sedation, activation or deactivation, for example.

An exploration of essential oils in terms of their chemical constituents, or their expected therapeutic actions, or their energetic activities, can begin to suggest the synergistic, additive or antagonistic potential of a prescription. Sometimes you might find that one or two oils encapsulate several of the therapeutic properties that you are looking for, and your blend can be constructed around these; so if you can identify even just one essential oil or a small range of oils that are strongly indicated for inclusion in the I.P., you can then identify any opportunities for synergism; and this can be refined further with the addition of a few more aromatics to produce an individualised and holistically focused blend.

Three models for aromatherapeutic blend creation

There are many ways of explaining how we might go about creating an I.P. The three models presented below are simple and practical, and can be applied to the biomedical/clinical, biopsychosocial and vitalistic approaches to practice.

THERAPEUTIC POSITIONS

Mojay (1996) created a clear and imaginative method of constructing a synergistic, clinical prescription, using the idea of essential oils occupying 'therapeutic positions' in a blend. Using terminology inspired by Chinese medicine (the 'Officials'[1]), he suggested that each prescription should contain an Emperor, which brings all-round benefits to the condition; a Minister, which reinforces one or more properties of the Emperor; Assistant/s, to enhance one or more benefits of the Emperor–Minister combination, and a Messenger, which gives the blend direction.

SYNERGISTIC ACCORDS

We could also consider the idea of building a blend using a series of integrated synergistic accords. If we establish one essential oil which has actions that address most of our aims, and then select another one or two oils that share its dominant constituents and characteristics, we can combine these to form our principal accord – the 'heart' of the blend. Then we can prepare another two accords (with a maximum of two oils in each) that reflect the different facets of the principal accord, and take the blend in the preferred direction. We should ensure that there are 'bridges' – olfactory and therapeutic connections between the accords – before combining them in appropriate ratios.

THE FIBONACCI SEQUENCE

The Fibonacci sequence, 1, 2, 3, 5, 8…, found throughout the natural world, can be used to inspire an aromatherapeutic blend.

- **1:** Beginning with the number one, there is absolutely nothing wrong with using a single aromatic rather than a blend. Indeed, sometimes this might even be preferable – for example, when we would like to harness the exquisite and unadulterated scent of a floral absolute in our therapy; or when we are working with an aromatic that is 'complete' in itself, such as osmanthus; or when we select a single essential oil which encompasses all of the desired properties, has the optimum balance of active constituents and an olfactory signature that resonates with the client.

- **2:** A combination of just two oils, carefully selected to work in harmony, but each retaining their own unique influence, such as sandalwood and

---

1   With similarities to a Daoist concept, the 12 organs of Chinese medicine can be described as 'Officials' in a court, each with a particular role or area of responsibility. According to Hicks, Hicks and Mole (2011), the Officials are: *Lord and sovereign, or the supreme controller* (Fire, held by the heart, and responsible for the radiance of the life spirit); *civil servants* (Fire, held by the pericardium, responsible for elation and joy; the triple burner responsible for harmony and balance and the small intestine responsible for receiving and making things thrive); *minister, chancellor* (Metal and held by the lung, regulation of the vital network); *general of the armed forces* (Wood and held by the liver, responsible for assessment and conception of plans), *official of justice* (Wood and held by the gallbladder, responsible for determination and decision); *the controller of storehouses and granaries* (Earth, held by the stomach and spleen, responsible for transforming and transporting, rotting and ripening, and the five tastes); *official of transport* (Metal, held by the large intestine, responsible for the residue of transformation); *controller of water/creation of power* (Water, held by kidney, responsible for skill and ability) and *office of regions and cities* (Water, held by the bladder, responsible for the power derived from transformation of *qi* or energy).

rose, might also be appropriate – and this combination can be seen in the beautiful attars which form part of Unani Tibb medicine.

- **3:** As already mentioned, when three oils are combined we are still aware of their individual presences within the blend, but a new accord or 'collective identity' will be created, with additive or synergistic therapeutic potential.

- **5:** We can use this trio as the 'heart' of our blend, and then add a further two essential oils, ensuring that these enhance the heart in terms of actions, direction and scent – giving us a blend based on the number five.

- **8:** If a further three oils are added to this, giving a total of eight essential oils, we might find that we have created a unique, personalised blend for a client, but from the molecular perspective, there will be the risk that desired active components will be diluted.

However, this is much more than a cerebral, paper exercise. We should also use our senses, and our sense of smell can be of enormous assistance when selecting and blending essential oils. We have already alluded to the significance of engaging with the aromas of essential oils and absolutes in order to gain understanding of their effects on the psyche, and of the role of olfaction in intuitive practice; now we shall explore how this can enhance the process of creating an aromatherapeutic blend.

Olfactory expertise

In 1998 the late and influential perfumer Guy Robert (1998) wrote that the nose was 'a perfumer's tool'. As aromatherapists, we too need to use our noses. There are two different aspects to consider when harnessing the sense of smell in our learning process. Both are experiential, and thus perfect tools for 'deep' rather than superficial learning. The first aspect is the acquisition of olfactory expertise, and the second is meditation on essential oil scents.

Dalton (1996) suggested that olfactory expertise was characterised by differences in the ways in which odour memory is stored and organised, and in the ways in which this information is evaluated and applied. Perfumers need to train their cognitive processes, which produce the associations between the sensory impact of an odour and the ability to recognise it, label it and then compose with it. This ability is described by Barkat *et al.* (2012) as requiring both a perceptual and a semantic[2] knowledge of odours. If aromatherapists adopt a similar approach, the sensory impact of essential oils can become associated with their chemistry and therapeutic actions. As a consequence, the process of composing synergistic,

---

2   Semantic is derived from the Greek word *semantikos* – the study of meaning, usually applied to language. It focuses on the relationship between things, such as signs and symbols, what they stand for, what they represent. In olfaction, the semantic mechanism is where an odour acquires a meaning and a label, and it thus enters the semantic odour memory.

aromatherapeutic blends is greatly assisted. There are no shortcuts to developing the olfactory palate – it takes a lot of practice, smelling essential oils and absolutes on blotters, and learning the language of scent.

We also need to smell our oils with awareness and enquiry. The essential oil trader and artisan perfumer Alec Lawless compared the experience of smelling with 'awareness and enquiry' with the 'just sitting' method of meditation. In order to still the mind, awareness is deliberately shifted to the body which is always 'present', unlike our thoughts; and with practice, mind and body become harmonised (Lawless 2010). When we fully engage with a scent, and it becomes our focus, we can detach from busy, distracting thoughts, or what Bloom (2011) calls our 'monkey mind', and experience a state of mindfulness and reflective awareness.

If olfactory awareness is integrated with essential oil studies, the entire learning experience can be enhanced. Students who have experienced scent meditations in conjunction with theoretical material have often reported that they feel more engaged with their studies and more connected with the oils. Smelling[3] essential oils and absolutes with awareness enables us to recognise and give verbal labels to olfactory sensations, and also brings the opportunity to identify some of the individual constituents by odour. This gives us considerable advantage in understanding the chemistry and biological actions of essential oils.

Take, for example, the aldehyde citronellal, present in essential oils such as citronella (*Cymbopogon nardus*), lemon-scented eucalyptus (*Eucalyptus citriodora*) and petitgrain combava (*Citrus hystrix* leaves). Citronellal has a distinctive odour, which we can experience while associating it with its therapeutic properties – namely a marked depressant action on the central nervous system, sedative and sleep-inducing properties, anti-nociceptive actions, anti-inflammatory effects and anti-oxidant activity (Melo *et al.* 2010a; Quintans-Júnior *et al.* 2010; Quintans-Júnior *et al.* 2011a). Thus, citronellal enters the semantic memory, and when citronellal-rich essential oils are encountered it is much easier to recall their properties because of these olfactory associations. Taking this one step further, we can consider another aldehyde – citral. Just by smelling citral-rich oils such as lemongrass (*Cymbopogon citratus, C. flexuosus*), may chang (*Litsea cubeba*) and lemon balm (*Melissa officinalis*) we can easily understand that citral has structural similarities to citronellal because of the 'aldehydic lemon' odour. Again, by olfactory association, it is unsurprising that citral too has anti-nociceptive actions, and is effective against inflammatory pain (Quintans-Júnior *et al.* 2011b). We might also begin to recognise specific hazards via olfaction – both citronellal and citral are associated with skin sensitisation – and so essential oils which contain significant

---

3   Active smelling should focus on sniffing the essential oil after it has been applied to a blotter, working quickly before olfactory fatigue sets in.

amounts of these constituents should be used with caution on hypersensitive, diseased or damaged skin (Tisserand and Young 2014).[4]

Meditating on the scents of essential oils can allow first-hand experience of their potential effects on the psyche. Here the aroma is the focus of the meditation, and, inevitably, the vapours will be inhaled as well as sniffed. If inhalation is prolonged, effects on the psyche may be more pronounced; for example, drowsiness or heightened sensibilities. For most of us, this experience is much more meaningful than simply reading that, for example, rosemary (*Rosmarinus officinalis*) is activating, lavender (*Lavandula angustifolia*) has calming effects and ylang ylang (*Cananga odorata* var. *genuina*) has uplifting, euphoric effects.

In order to practise, we really do need to engage with our aromatic *Materia Medica*. We must take an experiential approach; we need to form olfactory relationships with our essential oils. This could be compared to the process in which we learn how to prepare, cook and flavour foods. It is unsurprising that many respected perfumers are also said to be good and enthusiastic cooks. We can learn a lot from how herbs and spices are combined – and often find that many of these tried and tested culinary combinations can also be applied in aromatherapy with their essential oil counterparts!

The I.P.: olfactory attributes

When blending oils to restore emotional and mental balance, Mojay (1996) suggested that no more than three oils constitute the blend, because the 'unique and subtle influence of each oil will only emerge if the blend is kept relatively simple' (p.133). However, if the intent is also clinical, up to seven or eight essential oils might be included. In a simple binary mixture, it will be relatively easy to identify the two oils that give rise to the olfactory impression, and with three, the olfactory impression and influence of each will still be apparent. With four or more oils, we are more likely to produce new odour impressions, and as the number of oils increases, it will become more and more difficult to identify their individual presences.

A brief look at some perfumery principles can help us understand the olfactory perspective on aromatherapeutic blend construction. Perfumes contain top, middle and base notes, and are constructed of aromatics with varying volatility, diffusivity and intensity. Perfumes also will contain fixatives, or fragrance retarders, which are slow to evaporate and can hold the other components together, so that the top notes contain some of the body notes and the base contains some of the middle notes. Some of these principles of perfumery can be applied to aromatherapeutic formulation.

Alec Lawless (2009) wrote that 'in Ottoman cooking, the cultivation of taste is preferred to following recipes' (p.42), and he applied this premise to olfaction

---

4   Tisserand and Young (2014) suggest using no more than 0.5% in cases of dermatitis, and perhaps a maximum of 1% for sensitive individuals (p.335).

and artisan perfumery. It is equally applicable in aromatherapeutic blending. Yes, we do need to understand the therapeutic properties of our aromatic ingredients, but without cultivating our sense of smell, we are lost. With olfactory experience, however, instinct can guide us in blend construction, and lead us to the optimum olfactory ratios in our blends. It will afford us another way of appreciating the beauty of fragrance. Olfactory expertise is indeed necessary when we are creating a hedonically pleasing I.P. However, we also need to explore how individuals might respond to their I.P. on both conscious and unconscious levels, how the imposed odour of their prescription might affect their behaviour and physiology, or even their biological and energetic signatures.

Olfactory, biological and energetic responses to an aromatic prescription

As we have already established, the overall scent of an aromatic prescription is important – it should resonate with the recipient. For this reason, odour preferences and dislikes can be addressed during the consultation, simply by offering the recipient a selection of potential essential oils and absolutes, and asking for a simple yes or no, while also observing non-verbal signals.

Despite the many studies that have asked subjects to report their emotional reactions to odours using tools such as the established and reliable Geneva Emotion and Odour Scale (Chrea *et al.* 2009), the verbal measurement of odour-evoked feelings had not, until fairly recently, been explored. Porcherot *et al.* (2010) used the following words in their revised, quick and efficient questionnaire:[5]

Pleasant feeling – happiness, wellbeing, pleasantly surprised

Sensuality – romantic, desire, in love

Unpleasant feeling – disgusted, irritated, unpleasantly surprised

Relaxation – relaxed, serene, reassured

Sensory pleasure – nostalgic, amusement, mouth-watering

Refreshment – energetic, invigorated, clean.

It is a reasonable suggestion that this type of vocabulary could be utilised within the therapeutic conversation when exploring essential oil aroma preferences beyond the initial 'like/dislike' response, although even the yes/no practice is considerably better than denying clients the opportunity to express their opinions at all. It could be argued that in professional practice there really should be more discussion about the client's involvement in their I.P. It is obvious that the aromatherapist's knowledge of essential oils should direct the process, but – and this is a big 'but' – there is evidence which suggests that individuals respond very much better

---

5   The questionnaire was developed to establish consumer preferences for fragranced products.

to *chosen* fragrances rather than to *imposed* ones. Are we, as aromatherapists, sometimes 'guilty' of imposing scents on our clients?

The application of a fragrance can affect self-perception and also the way in which an individual is perceived by others. On a superficial level, fragrance choice is perhaps not thought to have a major impact on social activities, but at a deeper level, an imposed rather than a chosen fragrance can reduce the quality of social interactions (Freyberg and Ahren 2011). The anthropologist Jan Havlíček suggested that there is a strong interaction between perfume and individual body odour, and that individuals select fragrances which complement their own odour. He found that when people apply self-selected fragrances, the effect is rated as more pleasant than when they apply a scent chosen by another (Gray 2011; Lenochová *et al.* 2012). The view that self-selected perfumes can work with body odours to enhance their biological signal was shared by Milinski and Wedekind (2001). In addition, Lenochová *et al.* (2012) suggested that there was interaction between body odour and perfume rather than a simple masking effect. It was suggested that this interaction creates an individually specific odour mixture. These findings support the hypothesis that we choose scents that interact positively with our own body odour, and can explain why our perfume preferences are so highly individual; perhaps, rather than 'replacing' our biological olfactory signature with a chosen scent, we are actually reinforcing, amplifying and complementing it. Could this be seen as physiology/fragrance synergism? If so, we might conclude that it is important to allow our clients a degree of choice – and to do this, we must ourselves develop olfactory expertise in order to be able to guide our clients.

McGeever (2014) conducted a pilot study exploring whether (or not) there was a role for the client in the selection of essential oils during the consultative process. The study incorporated both quantitative and qualitative questions; thematic and comparative statistical methods were used to analyse the data. Despite the small sample size, it was clear that the aroma of their blend was important to most clients – but the way in which this manifested varied between individuals. All of the participants had been involved, to some degree, in their selection, but opinions were mixed in terms of their views on this experience. The quantitative analysis revealed that clients do want to engage in the selection process; however, the qualitative data suggested that clients view the therapist as integral to the choice, and indeed a positive therapeutic outcome. Although the research questions were not aimed at the therapeutic relationship, this became a recurrent theme throughout. McGeever concluded that although the aroma of the I.P makes a significant contribution to the treatment outcome, the therapeutic relationship could be considered as an 'inseparable element' in aromatherapy treatment. She recommends that, based on this small study, aromatherapists should offer clients the opportunity to participate in essential oil selection.

This leads us to another phenomenon regarding the interface between our biology and scent. Most of us will have noticed that a fragrance does not smell the same on the skin of different individuals; for example, a simple combination of essential oils of rose, sandalwood and citrus might smell very sweet on one person and more vibrant or woody on another. The aroma of an I.P. will change as time elapses and the different notes emerge, but the change can also sometimes happen very quickly and unexpectedly. It is more difficult to explain this in terms of its construction or 'skin chemistry', simply because of the speed with which this happens. In aromatherapy practice, the phenomenon of sudden and often incongruous changes in odour characteristics has been observed (Rhind 2014). Perhaps this is due to genetics, or perhaps these transient olfactory impressions are expressions of our body odour interacting with the imposed odour of the I.P.? Or is the I.P. facilitating and amplifying the expression of our own odour, as it is shifting and changing under the influence of the touch and massage elements of the therapeutic intervention, or indeed the client–therapist interaction? Is this a further, highly complex, dynamic, sensory manifestation of synergism and antagonism? Again, if this is the case, it would seem sensible to allow the client a degree of choice regarding the aroma of their I.P. – because it might have more far-reaching effects than we realise!

The anosmic client

Occasionally we might find anosmic or hyposmic clients presenting at our practice. Given the emphasis that has been placed on the importance of olfaction in aromatherapy, what does this mean for these clients? To answer this, we need to think about the quasi-pharmacological model, and the fact that very many animal studies support the therapeutic use of essential oils. For example, there is little doubt that inhalation of lavender essential oil has anxiety-relieving effects in humans and animals. This is thought to be due to two mechanisms. First, if aromatic molecules such as linalool are inhaled, they can be absorbed by the lungs and nasal mucosa and then transported in the bloodstream to the central nervous system (CNS), where they act on neurotransmission. Second, they can be transmitted via the nose and olfactory system, bypassing the blood–brain barrier, and thus reach the CNS; by activating olfactory neurons which are intricately connected with regions in the brain associated with cognition and emotion. Chioca *et al.* (2013) demonstrated that in mice with induced anosmia, lavender inhalation produced an anxiolytic effect, suggesting that olfactory stimulation was not necessary. They commented that a previous study with anosmic mice (Kagawa *et al.* 2003) had indicated that cedrol, found in cedarwood oils, did not require olfaction to exert effects, but the sedative effect of a lavender and Roman chamomile mixture was impaired by anosmia. Essentially, it would appear that anosmics can experience mood benefits from aromatherapy, even when olfaction is removed from the equation. It is just that their experience will be different. Some anosmics might experience olfactory-type sensations via the trigeminal nerve too, but usually only with penetrating aromas, such as peppermint and camphor.

REFLECTION

The philosophical and theoretical aspects of aromatherapeutic blending have been explored, and many points for reflection have been raised. We owe it to our profession to explore, evaluate and question established practices. We might feel concerned, for example, at the lack of hard evidence for synergism, specifically in aromatherapeutic practice, but that is not to say that it does not exist, and it is a sound hypothesis on which to base our aromatic prescriptions.

Another concern might be the number of essential oils in our blends. It is clear that if more than three oils are selected, we can create some interesting and beautiful aromas. However, Bowles (2003) argues that this practice 'borrows more from perfumery than science' and that by including many oils, we are 'dealing with polypharmacy at a scale unimagined in mainstream pharmacy' (p.131). She supports her argument with a sobering figure. If we blend several oils, each of which might have as many as 300 constituents (some with unknown actions), we are faced with the scenario where many of these components will be present in tiny quantities – perhaps as small as a nanogram (0.000000001g). So how do we know if there is the potential for additivity or synergy? Therefore it could be argued that if you elect to use the molecular approach, or select your oils based on the known qualities of their constituents, the number of oils in your blend should be sensibly restricted. If, however, you prefer to use a psychosensory approach, when the olfactory impact on wellbeing is important, a larger number of oils would be perfectly acceptable.

However, a recent study counters Bowles' concerns, offering us an alternative perspective, and indeed support for our penchant for polypharmacy. Komeh-Nkrumah *et al.* (2012) investigated the anti-arthritic activity of an essential oil ointment on rats in a placebo-controlled study. The essential oils were selected for their analgesic and anti-inflammatory actions, and incorporated in an ointment with corn oil and beeswax. The results were positive – local application of the ointment reduced the severity of adjuvant arthritis[6] in the rats; the clinical and histological features of arthritis were suppressed, and these observations were supported by a significant reduction in both the immunological and biochemical mediators of inflammation. The results were considered significant, and it was concluded that essential oil therapy showed potential for the treatment of inflammatory arthritis in humans. However, the aromatic preparations used in this research did not reflect the commonly presented guidelines for aromatherapeutic blending, at least not in relation to the number of essential oils and concentration for a topical preparation. The ointment contained 16 essential oils, which constituted 20–40% of the preparations under investigation. The essential oil component contained basil, bitter orange, black pepper, clary sage, ginger, nutmeg and clove bud, each at

---

6   Adjuvant arthritis is an induced, sub-chronic form of the disease.

8.9%; eucalyptus, foraha,[7] sweet fennel, immortelle, lavender, pine, rosemary and sage at 4.4%; and Virginian cedarwood at 2.2%. The 20% concentration ointment proved most effective, and was applied to the rats' paws twice daily. From this we learn that, despite all of our theorising, we can observe clinical efficacy with a high concentration of a blend of many essential oils selected purely on their anti-inflammatory and analgesic actions, with no special consideration given to synergy *per se*!

---

7   *Calophyllum inophyllum.*

Chapter 5

Applications, Carrier Media,
Dosage and Ratios

In order to build on the theoretical principles of aromatherapeutic blending, we now need to address methods of administration, carrier media, dosages and ratios. Essential oil prescriptions are applied topically, often with massage or simply local applications, and via inhalation.

Massage and carriers

For massage, vegetable 'fixed' oils are the most suitable carriers; 'skin feel' and slippage are important, as is rate of absorption. The choice will be determined by the individual's skin condition, and the style and duration of the massage. For example, localised frictions, finger/thumb kneading or compression will require a base that will be rapidly absorbed but with limited slippage, while a slow-stroke, effleurage-based massage will be more effective with a slowly absorbed carrier that provides good lubrication.

It is important to select the fixed oils that are best suited to meet the therapeutic aims. See the appendix for a summary of commonly available carrier oils and acerated herbal oils; very often, a blend of these will be appropriate.

Local applications and inhalation

For local applications, either as prescriptions for home use or for more intensive bodywork, fixed and macerated herbal oils are also suitable carriers, perhaps packaged in a container fitted with a 'roller ball' applicator. However, creams, gels, waxes and patches might be appropriate. Therefore, we also need to consider suitable packaging for home treatments. For example, aroma sticks are a convenient and safe way to deliver essential oils for inhalation.

If, however, natural therapeutic perfume prescriptions are to be used, attractive bottles/packaging can encourage better compliance (James 2014); cultural expectations should be taken into account. Studies in the field of phytocosmetology support this observation. For example, Lodén, Buraczewska and Halvarsson (2007) recommend that the placebo and the test product should both be presented in the same packaging, and that the packaging should be attractive in appearance, easy to use, and suggestive of a high-end cosmeceutical – because product presentation can positively influence compliance, but affects self-evaluation to a much lesser extent.

Dosage

There is a huge variation in the percutaneous absorption rates of different essential oil components, and it is difficult to estimate the amount of essential oil that will enter the body after dermal application – there are many intrinsic and extrinsic factors that affect not only absorption, but also their distribution and metabolism.

Bowles (2003) gives some useful figures in relation to dosage; in a typical aromatherapy massage,[1] the potential dose range is anywhere between 1.2 and 16.0mg/kg. Inhalation for 5–15 minutes could result in 0.7–1.1mg/kg, baths could be 1.1–3.7mg/kg; and neat application of 1.0–2.0ml to small areas gives the greatest potential dose of 12.8–25.7mg/kg (p.132). Tisserand and Young (2014) suggest that we could assume 10% absorption. This means that a relatively low 'dose' of essential oil is absorbed when essential oils are diluted in a carrier and applied to the skin – normally no more than 0.1ml – and this is considerably less than the figure given by Bowles (2003).

When aromatherapy literature is examined, it emerges that different writers and practitioners hold differing views on dosage and application. Tisserand and Young (2014) suggest that for massage purposes, when large areas of skin are covered, it is generally recommended that a concentration of 2.5–3.0% is used, and that 5.0% should be the maximum. For the young and elderly, 1.0–2.0% is recommended, and for relaxation purposes or more regular use, 2.0–2.5% is sufficient. We do not know whether this falls below what might be described as a 'therapeutic' dose; and it is also possible that very small doses, in some cases, are as effective as larger doses. For example, an early study conducted by Boyd and Pearson (1946), which investigated the expectorant action of lemon oil, established that the optimum dose was 50mg/kg, but that even 0.01mg/kg was effective. Doses within that range were less effective. Another view is presented by Balacs (1995), who made a comparison of blood plasma concentrations of lavender essential oil constituents with the effective levels for a range of psychoactive drugs. He concluded 'the oft-quoted opinion that during treatment, essential oils reach the blood in amounts too small to have pharmacological effects, is not supported by the evidence'. In other words, aromatherapy massage can deliver sufficient active constituents to exert biological effects.

We have already mentioned Komeh-Nkrumah *et al.* (2012), whose animal study demonstrated the efficacy of an anti-inflammatory essential oil prescription, and established that the optimum dose was given by a 20% concentration. Therefore, it could well be that the 'optimum' or therapeutic dose is dependent on the desired outcome – low for psychotherapeutic effects and for some clinical

---

1 This is defined as 1–5% concentration essential oils, 10–25ml carrier, duration 5–90 minutes, involving skin (major) and lungs (minor) routes of absorption.

effects such as expectorant action, and perhaps for prescriptions delivered (mainly) via inhalation; and much higher for other clinical effects, such as anti-inflammatory action. Indeed, Schnaubelt (2011), who fuses scientific, clinical and vitalistic perspectives in his work, sometimes suggests much higher doses in specific circumstances, including the application of undiluted essential oils.[2] Aromatic 'frictions',[3] as described by French aromatherapist Nelly Grosjean (1992), also involve the application of up to 30 drops of essential oils directly to the skin – often over the solar plexus or the adrenals – with the intent of increasing 'protection, harmony, vitality and regeneration' (p.78), or for specific reasons such as pain relief or improving circulation.

Given the lack of hard evidence and consensus amongst practitioners regarding the question of dosage, it would seem logical that several aspects need to be considered, including the desired therapeutic outcomes, how and where the prescription is to be applied, and the limiting factors. Clearly, when we are deciding on the concentration of essential oil, and assuming our client does not fall into a vulnerable category,[4] the limiting factors are safety, toxicity and the potential of any oil in the blend to cause skin irritation and sensitization. Both scientific and professional literature suggest that:

- low concentration/doses – that is, a concentration in the region of 1.0–2.5% for topical application, or brief/intermittent exposure to the vapour of undiluted aromatics – are suitable for psychotherapeutic effects via inhalation/absorption by the olfactory system

- smaller doses, including evaporation of undiluted essential oils, are appropriate for inhalation and actions on the respiratory tract

- mid-range concentrations, in the region of 2.5–5.0%, are suitable for aromatherapy massage where systemic absorption occurs via the skin, inhalation and olfaction

- higher concentrations, in the region of 20%, are appropriate for local applications for some clinical effects such as analgesia and anti-inflammatory actions

- high doses of 1.0–2.0ml of specific undiluted essential oils can be applied to small areas of skin; for example, to relieve pain.

For massage, it does seem that the 2.5–3.0% range has become accepted in aromatherapy practice. For practical purposes, essential oils are usually dispensed in drops. This is convenient, quick, hygienic and sufficiently accurate for most purposes. It is well known that these drops vary in volume depending on the

---

2   These oils are clearly identified, and self-administered (e.g. in the shower), as part of a lifestyle choice.

3   Here, the term is from the French, meaning 'rubbing'.

4   For example, age (children under 15 and the elderly), skin integrity, skin health, compromising health problems (e.g. liver and kidney disease).

viscosity and specific gravity of the essential oil or absolute and the dimensions of the dropper insert (Svoboda *et al.* 2001). The volume of a drop of essential oil is very approximately 0.05ml. For accuracy, it would be far better to prepare blends by weight, using a laboratory balance, or by volume with pipettes and calibrated glassware, and this is certainly how blends for research purposes should be prepared. However, in the therapeutic environment, and for the preparation of an I.P., drops are appropriate and fit for purpose. The concentration used and the method of application should be the educated choice of the individual practitioner, bearing in mind their realm and scope of practice and experience.

Ratios

We can look to the world of perfumery to gain understanding of the concept of ratios. Jean Carles, an influential perfumer and theorist, developed a systematic way of creating fragrances based on blending accords (Lawless 2009). An accord is, quite simply, the combination of two or more perfume materials, but the odour of the accord will vary depending on the relative proportions of each material in the mixture, that is, their ratios. Carles would experiment extensively with ratios to create his base, heart and top note accords and then, when the final choices, based on olfactory evaluation, were made, he would repeat the process with the accords, again to establish the best ratios for the final composition.

Ratios are expressed in 'parts', and a part can be a drop, or measured in millilitres or grams, or litres and kilograms – it doesn't matter, just so long as each part is measured by the same standard. If we were to blend three oils in equal proportions, say one drop of each, the ratio would be expressed as 1:1:1. However, if we were to mix mild-scented sandalwood (*Santalum album*) with geranium (*Pelargonium × asperum*), which is distinctive and more diffusive, and Roman chamomile (*Anthemis nobilis*) which has a very strong and highly diffusive odour, we might elect to go with a 4:2:1 ratio. It is easy to see how we can vary the ratios of essential oils in blends, but we are usually doing this from olfactory and perhaps safety[5] perspectives. However, when we consider the findings of de Rapper *et al.* (2013), we realise that ratios also affect the potential for synergism, and very occasionally can contribute to antagonism, at least in terms of antimicrobial activity. This is an area that has not been researched in relation to aromatherapy, although this particular study did support the practice of blending.

Falling into the broad domain of ratios is the 'phenol rule' which gives some guidance on the use of 'phenolic' essential oils such as thyme (*Thymus vulgaris*, *T. zygis* and *T. serpyllum*), clove bud (*Syzigium aromaticum*), oregano (*Origanum* species and *Thymus capitatus*) and savory (*Satureia hortensis* and *S. montana*). As well as having antimicrobial activity, some phenolic oils are noted for their analgesic and anti-inflammatory potential, but they are also irritating to the skin

---

5   For example, we might keep the proportion of irritant or sensitising oils such as clove bud in a blend low, and use non-irritant oils such as lavender in higher proportions (e.g. 1:9).

and mucous membranes. In order to harness their therapeutic potential while reducing these risks, Guba (2000) proposed the 'phenol rule'. This applies up to a 10% concentration, and relates to dermal use only. The ratio of phenolic oils to non-irritant oils should not exceed 1:9, and the total concentration of phenolic oils should not exceed 1% of the blend. However, there is an exception to this: if cinnamon bark (*Cinnamomum zeylanicum*) or cassia (*C. cassia* or *C. aromaticum*), both rich in cinnamaldehyde, are to be used, the concentration should not exceed 5%, and they can be used in conjunction with oils such as clove bud that have a high eugenol content, or oils with a high *d*-limonene content – because eugenol and *d*-limonene can quench the sensitising potential of cinnamaldehyde (Guin *et al.* 1984).

The concept of ratios is also useful when calculating the percentage of active constituents in a blend. This is arguably more important if the molecular model is being used to inform blend construction, but nonetheless can also be used to identify potential synergy or additivity in blends created using other paradigms. The calculation is straightforward, best illustrated by an example – see Table 5.1.

Table 5.1 Calculating the composition of a blend of clary sage, lavender and bergamot (ratio 1:2:2)

Essential oil ratios	Constituent 1 % and volume (in 100ml)	Constituent 2 % and volume (in 100ml)	Constituent 3 % and volume (in 100ml)
Clary sage (*Salvia sclarea*) 1 part	Linalyl acetate 65% (65ml)	*l*-Linalool 10% (10ml)	Germacrene D[1] 9% (9ml)
Lavender (*Lavandula angustifolia*) 2 parts	Linalyl acetate 42% (42ml) (42×2=84)	*l*-Linalool 45% (45ml) (45×2=90)	Lavandulyl acetate 3% (3ml) (3×2=6ml)
Bergamot (*Citrus aurantium* subsp. *bergamia*) 2 parts	Linalyl acetate 30% (30ml) (30×2=60)	*l*-Linalool 15% (15ml) (15×2=30ml)	*d*-Limonene 35% (35ml) (35×2=70ml)
Total 5 parts	Linalyl acetate 65+84+60=209ml in 500ml (209/500)×100= 41.8%	*l*-Linalool 10+90+30=130ml in 500ml (130/500)×100= 26%	Germacrene D (9/500)×100=1.8% Lavandulyl acetate (6/500)×100=1.2% *d*-Limonenel (70/500)×100=14%

Composition of blend	Linalyl acetate	41.8%	Other constituents
	l-Linalool	26.0%	
	d-Limonene	14.0%	
	Germacrene D	1.8%	
	Lavandulyl acetate	1.2%	
	Total	*84.8%*	*15.2%*

1. Germacrene D is a sesquiterpene; it is chemically related to cadinene isomers; it is fairly widespread; no information was found regarding its therapeutic actions.

Chapter 6

Acne Vulgaris

A Case Study

Tamara Agnew

Part I concludes with a case study which reflects upon the process of creating an aromatherapeutic blend. Here Tamara Agnew discusses the challenges encountered during its formulation, analyses the outcomes, and proposes a model for synergistic blending.

Introduction

Health is a complex phenomenon. There are often multiple dimensions of one condition; physical signs, or what we 'see', which includes aetiology and pathophysiology; and then there are the invisible or comorbid symptoms which are often an equally significant burden, including social, emotional and spiritual effects. Essential oils may be nature's perfect medicine; an intricate and perfect synergy of hundreds of chemicals in a single bottle, the essential oil has multiple therapeutic consequences. In this single bottle, there is the *potential* to heal multiple aspects of one condition, regardless of the blending approach you use to address it.

In clinical aromatherapy practice, we work hard to increase the healing potential of the blend without causing harm – but how do we judge success or failure? Is it a reduction of the presenting symptoms, or improvements in quality of life? Of course, there is no right or wrong answer; just as a person experiences symptoms in a very personal way, 'healing' is also very unique. There is some good, strong supporting evidence of synergism emerging in aromatherapy. However, it is a difficult theoretical concept to evaluate, and this was at the forefront of my planning when I embarked on my PhD in 2011.

In aromatherapy practice, we aim to create positive synergism to strengthen the overall therapeutic effect of the blend, quench irritant compounds and avoid antagonism. I like to think of synergy being more than what happens in the bottle, and so the definition 'the interaction of *elements* that when combined produce a total effect that is greater than the sum of the individual elements' (Dictionary. com n.d.) is an inclusive one; it includes the *person* as part of the synergy.

One criticism of aromatherapy research is that often it is not transparent; researchers fail to present parts of the methodology or the data, or are selective when presenting the findings (Cooke and Ernst 2000; Posadzki, Alotaibi and Ernst 2012). Transparency is critical in research (Rennie 2001) and in aromatherapy practice. Amongst other things, we needed to be able to justify the inclusion of some essential oils, and the exclusion of others to safeguard against injury or harm; informed consent is based on clear and precise information about the treatment; and finally, there is a legal obligation to maintain treatment records for a defined length of time (depending on which country/state you are working in).

The CLEANsE trial

The CLEANsE trial was a randomised controlled trial (RCT) with three parallel arms. Participants were randomly assigned to one of three groups:

- the essential oil (E/O) group: participants received a preconceived essential oil product, based on the physical symptoms of acne

- the aromatherapy group (Aromatherapy): people in this group attended a private health consultation appointment and the bespoke product was based on their individual needs

- the usual care (UC) group: continued their usual treatment (but received product at the end of the observation period).

The aim of the study was to assess outcomes in the two intervention groups, compared to usual care. This pragmatic, community-based RCT evaluated the effectiveness of the two interventions in a 'real world' setting, to reflect, as much as possible, the real experience of the aromatherapy consumer.

Data was collected over a three-month period and outcome measures included the AACNE (Adelaide Acne CliNical Evaluation Scale) Scale for measuring the physical symptoms of acne (severity), and the Acne-Specific Quality of Life (ASQoL) instrument, a disease-specific tool for assessing quality of life.

The oils were generously donated by the Sydney Essential Oil Company (www.seoc.com.au).

Acne

Acne vulgaris (acne) is a multifaceted condition, which has no 'cure'. Symptoms will spontaneously resolve, usually at the end of adolescence. However, more and more adults are experiencing a continuation of acne symptoms, and some an onset during their early 20s; this is especially prevalent for women (Agnew, Leach and Segal 2013; Dréno *et al.* 2012; Khondker *et al.* 2012; Perkins *et al.* 2012). Normal presentation is a combination of inflammation, seborrhoea, comedones, papules, pustules, nodules and often, scarring (Fabbrocini *et al.* 2012). There are four contributing factors: seborrhoea (over-production of sebum), hypercornification (over-production of keratin), colonisation of the follicular duct by *Propionibacterium acnes* (*P. acnes*), and inflammation (Thiboutot *et al.* 2009; Williams, Delavalle and Garner 2012).

It is a non-life-threatening, chronic condition, with acute outbreaks that are often severe. The psychosocial impact can be devastating, with reduced quality of life (Hanstock and O'Mahony 2002; Mallon *et al.* 1999), reduced self-esteem, self-consciousness, stress, frustration and anger (Hassan *et al.* 2009; Magin *et al.* 2006; Mulder *et al.* 2001; Papadopoulos *et al.* 2000), body dysmorphic disorder (Bowe *et al.* 2007; Dalgard *et al.* 2008; Uzun *et al.* 2003), social withdrawal (including relationships, sport, employment), alienation, bullying (Joseph and Sterling 2009; Magin *et al.* 2008; Timms 2013), suicidal ideation and actions (Halvorsen *et al.* 2011; Purvis *et al.* 2006).

There are literally hundreds of acne products available to the consumer, ranging from over-the-counter (OTC) washes, creams or lotions (Bowe and Shalita 2008) to prescription medications for internal or external use (Thiboutot *et al.* 2009). Combination treatment is often prescribed, to target multiple factors. The risk of side-effects is high, ranging from local skin irritations, reddening and peeling, to irreversible skin pigmentation, possible harm to an unborn child, depression and suicidal tendencies (Joint Formulary Committee 2010).

Synergy and CLEANsE

The following synergistic blending flowchart and checklist illustrate the process I took to develop essential oil blends for the CLEANsE trial.

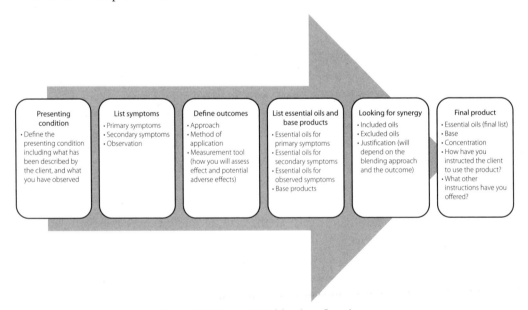

Figure 6.1: Synergistic blending flowchart

Checklist items

1. **Presenting condition:** Identifying the presenting condition is the starting point for developing the blend. This may be clear and obvious, or it may require a little more exploration in the consultation process to determine what is most important to the client/patient. Considering the potential for antagonism, a good general instruction is a 'per goal' standard; that is, one blend to achieve one therapeutic goal.

2. **Symptoms:** Following consultation, and in conjunction with the client, you can isolate the primary and secondary symptoms associated with the presenting condition. This may include physical and emotional symptoms. You may also wish to include any observations that you make which may not have been verbalised by the client. At this point, you may want to include more than two primary symptoms, or you may wish to exclude the observed symptoms.[1]

3. **Outcome:** This is the purpose of the blend; what does the client/patient expect from the appointment/product? Again, this may require a little investigation; in doing so, you are helping to inform the blend of essential oils, and you are helping the client to identify the various aspects, and address the most urgent part. At this stage, you will also think about the approach to treatment, the method of application, and the tool you will use to measure benefit.

4. **Essential oils and base:** This is the point at which you start to consider the oils for achieving the therapeutic purpose of the blend. It is helpful when developing a synergistic blend to think about the oils you might use for the individual symptoms. It is also important to consider the base product/s; thinking about synergy, remember that the properties of the base product may influence the therapeutic effect of the essential oil blend (Harris 2002). This list can be as long or as short as you like.

5. **Looking for synergy:** At this stage, you will start to determine which oils you will include and exclude from the blend, and keeping a written record of your justification may be beneficial. It is very easy to blend the first seven oils on your list, but if you are looking for positive synergy, you will need to consider the approach you are taking, and then look at how the oils may positively or negatively affect the outcome. Synergy is a difficult concept to calculate; however, if you keep to the Harris rule of between three and seven

---

1 When thinking about the presenting condition and the symptoms, always ruminate on how one may be influencing the other; consider this hypothetical situation– the client is experiencing pain related to stress, and is feeling lethargic in the afternoons. How might one be the antecedent of the other? If you try to address both of these (in one blend or two) you may cause discord. Think about the client *and* their symptoms as part of your synergy.

oils (Harris 2002) and keep focused on the therapeutic objective, you will develop a purposeful blend.

6. **Final product:** Now you will develop and record your final product, including the concentration of the essential oil blend in the base, and the instructions for the use of the product. This record is an important part of your clinical note-taking for future appointments with this individual, and also for your professional records for legal purposes.

Case study: Female, age 20

Presenting condition: *Acne vulgaris* (acne)

Symptoms: Primary – visible facial lesions, and comedones; secondary – often feels fairly 'down'; observed – oily skin around the T-zone; redness.

Outcome: Reduced acne symptoms. I adopted a biopsychosocial approach which incorporated the molecular approach for the physical symptoms, and the psychosensory approach described by Michel Lavabre (Rhind 2012) for mood. The product was applied directly to the affected area; measurement tools included AACNE Scale and ASQoL.

Essential oils and base: The chemical components indicated for the treatment of the specific aspects of acne (Table 6.1) determined which essential oils would be best to treat the physical symptoms (Table 6.2).

Table 6.1 Chemical components and therapeutic value

Functional group	Therapeutic value	Chemical
Terpenes		
Monoterpenes	General tonic, analgesic, quenching and hormone effects (Price and Price 2007); skin penetration enhancing (Bensouilah and Buck 2006)	Limonene; myrcene; α-pinene; Δ-3-carene; limonene + α-phellandrene; sabinene; β-pinene; camphene; terpinene
Sesquiterpenes	Anti-inflammatory, calming, analgesic (Price and Price 2007); antiseptic and antibactericidal, antihistaminic/anti-allergic (Bensouilah and Buck 2006)	E-β-farnesene; γ-himachalene; α-himachalene; germacrene-D; (E,E)-α-farnesene; α-bulnesene; α-guaiene
Esters	Calming and tonic; anti-inflammatory	Linalyl acetate; α-terpinyl acetate; geranyl acetate; menthyl acetate; benzyl salicylate; benzyl benzoate
Ketones	Wound healing (Bensouilah and Buck 2006)	Camphor

Alcohols		
Monoterpenols	Antibacterial; vasoconstrictive; analgesic; tonic and stimulant; sedative	Linalool; himacholol; citronellol; geraniol; α-terpineol; menthol; terpinen-4-ol
Sesquiterpenols	General tonic; phlebotonic; cardiotonic; neurotonic; oestrogenic; anti-inflammatory; antiviral; antimalarial	Patchoulol; t,t-farnesol; α-bisabolol; α-santalol
Oxides	Expectorant; antispasmodic	1,8-Cineole; α-bisabololoxide
Aldehydes	Calming to CNS; anti-inflammatory; antimicrobial; antifungal	Santalal; neral; citronellal
Cyclic Ethers	Not researched for therapeutic effects (Bowles 2003)	Menthofuran

Table 6.2 Essential oils for treating acne

Common and botanical name	*Key chemical components*	Anti-inflammatory	Antibacterial	Reduce redness	Cicatrisant	Astringent	Wound healing	Calming	Uplifting
Bergamot (*Citrus bergamia*)	Limonene 38% Linalyl acetate 28% Linalool 8% (Bowles 2003; Russo *et al.* 2012)		●		●			●	
Cardamom (*Elattaria cardamomum*)	1,8-Cineole 48.4% α-Terpinyl acetate 24% Limonene 6% (Bowles 2003)	●							
Cedarwood (*Cedrus atlantica*)	Himacholol 42.20–46.32% γ-Himachalene 13.95–15.80% α-Himachalene 6.10–8% (Saab, Harb and Koenig 2005)				●				
Clary sage (*Salvia sclarea* L.)	Linalyl acetate 29.5–51.6% Linalool 17–28.8% Geranyl acetate 1.7–2.8% (Cai *et al.* 2006)	●	●						

Common and botanical name	Key chemical components	Anti-inflammatory	Antibacterial	Reduce redness	Cicatrisant	Astringent	Wound healing	Calming	Uplifting
Cypress (*Cupressus semipervirens*)	α-Pinene: 21.4–46.0%; δ-3-Carene 16.0–27.0% Germacrene-D 2.1–13.0% (Emami *et al.* 2006)		•			•			
Frankincense (*Boswellia carteri*)	α-Pinene 37.3% Limonene + α-Phellandrene 14.4% Myrcene 7.3% (Woolley *et al.* 2012)	•	•		•				
Geranium (*Pelargonium graveolens*)	Citronellol 33.9–42.1% Geraniol 7.2–14.9% Linalool 0.8–2% (Nejad and Ismaili 2013)	•	•		•	•			
German chamomile (*Matricaria chamomilla*)	E-β-Farnesene 42.6% α-Bisabolol oxide A 21.2% (E,E)-α-Farnesene 8.32% (Heuskin *et al.* 2009)	•			•				
Juniperberry (*Juniperus communis*)	α-Pinene 51.4% Myrcene 8.3% Limonene 5.1% (Höferl *et al.* 2014)					•		•	
Lavender (*Lavandula angustifolia*)	Linalool 33.35–52.59% Linalyl acetate 9.27–25.73% Camphor 6.81–8.79% (Danh *et al.* 2013)	•	•		•		•	•	
Niaouli (*Melaleuca quinquenervia*)	1,8-Cineole 53.8% Sabinene 14.9% α-Terpineol 8.1% (Sfeir *et al.* 2013)	•	•						
Patchouli (*Pogostemon cablin*)	Patchoulol 36.6% α-Bulnesene 13.95% α-Guaiene 11.96% (Albuquerque *et al.* 2013)	•	•		•				

Peppermint (*Mentha piperita* L.)	Menthol 53.28% Menthyl acetate 15.10% Menthofuran 11.18% (Saharkhiz *et al.* 2012)	•	•	•				•	
Petitgrain (*Citrus aurantium* var. *amara*)	Linalool 34.4–36.8% Linalyl acetate 11.3–22.1% α-Terpineol 6.6–11.7% (Boussaada and Chemli 2006)	•	•					•	
Rosemary (*Rosmarinus officinalis*)	α-Pinene 43.9–46.1% 1,8-Cineole 11.1% Camphene 8.6–9.6% (Jamshidi, Afzali and Afzali 2009)	•	•		•				
Rosewood (*Aniba rosaeodora*)	Linalool 82.15% α-Terpineol 3.6% Geraniol 1.33% (Fidelis *et al.* 2012)				•	•		•	
Sandalwood (*Sandalwood spicatum*)	t,t-Farnesol 31.6% α-Bisabolol 10.7% α-Santalol 9.1% (Brophy, Fookes and Lassak 1991)	•	•		•			•	
Sweet orange (*Citrus sinensis*)	Limonene 90.66% Linalyl acetate 2.8% β-myrcene 1.71% (Singh *et al.* 2010)		•						•
Tea tree (*Melaleuca alternifolia*)	Terpinen-4-ol 40.1% γ-terpinene 23.0% α-terpinene 10.4% (Carson, Hammer and Riley 2006)	•	•						
Ylang ylang (*Cananga odorata*)	Benzyl benzoate 33.61% Linalool 24.5% Benzyl salicylate 12.89% (Sacchetti *et al.* 2005)	•	•					•	

Looking for synergy: The aim of the blend (Table 6.3) was to treat the physical symptoms of acne: redness, bacteria and inflammation. Although the participant described eczema and dermatitis, peppermint was included. Its known cooling effects would help reduce redness; and despite it being a slight skin irritant (Bowles 2003), the antihistaminic/anti-allergic properties of the sesquiterpene content of lavender should act as a quencher against the irritant menthol of peppermint (Harris 2002). Although tea tree has strong evidence for reducing acne symptoms, the participant did not enjoy the medicinal aroma. Juniper is depurative, and so may be suitable in the treatment of acne (Rhind 2012). Potential synergy includes strong antibacterial and anti-inflammatory value and significant calming effect. Considering Lavabre's philosophy, the blend should also have an effect on mood; primarily from the flower, fruit and leaves families of oils, together they should relieve stress and anxiety – especially recovering self-image and confidence, and helping to stimulate and revitalise (Rhind 2012).

Table 6.3 The therapeutic blend

Blend	Anti-inflammatory	Antibacterial	Reduce redness	Cicatrisant	Astringent	Calming
Bergamot × 12		●		●		●
Clary × 16	●	●				
Cypress × 12		●			●	
Juniper × 12						●
Lavender × 12	●	●		●		●
Peppermint × 16	●	●	●			●

Base: The base product for the CLEANsE trial was pre-blended for all participants, regardless of their allocation. The formulation included jojoba wax (*Simmondsia sinesis*), sunflower oil (*Helianthus annuus* L.), evening primrose oil (*Oenothera biennis*) and grapeseed oil (*Vitis vinifera*).

The final product: 5% concentration; 100ml of product. Participant was instructed to apply twice daily, to skin after cleansing.

Measures

Table 6.4 AACNE and ASQoL scores

	Appointment 1	Appointment 2	Appointment 3
AACNE	4/7	4/7	3/7
ASQoL	38.5	123	132

Please refer to Table 6.4. At the second appointment, the participant described an almost immediate reduction in redness, and reduced symptoms by about week three. She noticed that the healing rate of individual lesions was improved, and her skin did not get any worse at the time of her menses. She was happy with the product, it made her feel good, and her skin felt fresh and soft. She did not want to make any changes.

At the final appointment, she said that her skin was continuing to improve and it 'felt great'. She enjoyed the ease of the product, which was applied directly to the face after washing, and she felt that this worked with her lifestyle.

The participant experienced a one-point reduction in symptoms; this is neither statistically nor clinically significant; however, her QoL scores increased dramatically (where a larger score indicates improved quality of life).

Conclusion

Acne is a severe, chronic skin condition which is more than skin deep; psychosocial sequelae are considerable, and the significance of this is often missed by primary health-care providers. The side-effect profile for commonly available acne products is substantial and despite claims of positive effect, acne is still highly prevalent in the population.

Aromatherapy is described as a holistic approach to healing. Side effects from topical applications are usually allergy based, and this can be teased out in the consultation; if a mild adverse event does occur, this can be managed by the professional aromatherapist, who can tweak a preparation for the individual. Serious adverse events are rare and are usually associated with misuse of oils, so the risk of any further damage caused by the aromatherapy professional is very small.

Synergy is difficult to measure; without the necessary gas chromatographic instrument, we can only estimate the total effect of blending. It is also difficult to determine antagonism – after all, how much is too much?

For the practising aromatherapist, assessing whether we have created synergy will be evident from the effect of the product for our client. It is necessary to remember that creating synergy in the bottle is not necessarily synergistic for the client. Therefore, it may be easier to measure synergy by considering adherence. The academic literature tells us that a person will adhere to the treatment if they are satisfied with the practitioner and the product; that is, they require an empathetic ear, they do not want to experience any negative adverse events, and they need the symptoms to improve (Baldwin 2006; McEvoy, Nydegger and Williams 2003; Renzi *et al.* 2002). If these needs are not met, the person is less likely to be compliant and the product will fail. So, considering this, an equation for synergy may be:

Synergy = (client + practitioner + product + therapeutic outcome)

All parts are equally important, and so the focus should be a holistic one.

For the individual described in my case study, there was no clinical worsening of symptoms, and there were no adverse reactions; I think that I created a good rapport with the client, who was able to talk openly with me about some very personal issues in her life; she found the product easy to use, and she enjoyed using it. This case study describes a positive outcome for this participant who, despite only a small change in skin condition, experienced significantly improved quality of life.

Perhaps it is the nature of acne that makes it a difficult case study? Regardless, this lady left the trial feeling much better about herself, her life, and her skin. So did *we* create positive synergism? I think so…

ESSENTIAL OILS AND ABSOLUTES

Actions and Evidence

In Part II the confirmed and suspected therapeutic effects of essential oils are presented, based not only on their traditional uses and observations from aromatherapy practice, but also on research from a variety of disciplines. You will find that in some cases, research in social and life sciences is highly relevant and supportive, but also that evidence presented from some studies relates to *in vitro* research, or is derived from animal studies, and might, or might not, be directly applicable to holistic aromatherapy practice. This is neither a definitive nor an exhaustive review, but it is representative of the therapeutic possibilities offered by a wide range of accessible and commercially available essential oils and absolutes.

Here the specific actions of a selection of essential oils and absolutes – including the commonly used ones, as well as those which are lesser known but have aromatherapeutic potential – are identified. Where possible, evidence that supports the aromatherapeutic use of these oils is provided; this is drawn from research and established traditions of use. This facilitates the identification of essential oils that share important characteristics, and which may be used together with synergistic or additive potential. For more detail of selected oils, blending suggestions, and to identify other oils that might enhance your blends, from both therapeutic and olfactory perspectives, refer to Part III.

In Part II the actions and evidence are presented in a series of short chapters and reference tables, with the essential oils listed in alphabetical order, and by common name.

To facilitate a deeper awareness of mechanisms of action, and the actions of specific constituents, each table is preceded by some explanatory notes. Broadly speaking, it is thought that when essential oils are inhaled, or applied to the skin, their lipophilic components act on the lipid parts of the cell membranes, and thus modify calcium and potassium ion channels, effectively changing the permeability of the cell membranes and the substances that can pass in and out. However, the nature of these interactions depends upon the properties of the individual essential oil constituents, and the effects on various functions can be witnessed – for example, on transport systems, enzymes, ion channels and receptors (Saad, Muller and Lobstein 2013). These notes will be particularly relevant if the molecular approach is being adopted, and might also facilitate an evidenced-based approach to clinical practice. However, please bear in mind that although an essential oil's constituents will probably give a good idea of its actions, very often the essential oil will have greater therapeutic potential!

Chapter 7

Pain and Inflammation

In this chapter we will look at how essential oils and their constituents act as pain-relieving and anti-inflammatory agents. These actions can have a therapeutic impact across body 'systems' but are perhaps of particular interest in problems with muscles and joints. We shall look more specifically at visceral pain in Chapter 8, inflammation in the respiratory system in Chapter 11, and the skin and soft tissues in Chapter 12.

Pain

Conventional analgesics are opioids (such as morphine and codeine), which bind to opioid receptors in the central nervous system (CNS), and non-opioids (such as aspirin and non-steroidal anti-inflammatory drugs, or NSAIDs), which inhibit prostaglandin production and inhibit cyclooxygenase (COX) enzymes in the peripheral nervous system. Side effects are commonplace, especially with opioids,[1] and so there has been a longstanding search for novel analgesic agents, including studies of the monoterpenes and their derivatives found in essential oils.

In general terms, analgesics can work in either of two ways. The first is the 'gate control' mechanism, where pain impulses are interrupted at the spinal or supraspinal (medulla and midbrain) level. The second is via peripheral mechanisms that inhibit the influx of nociceptive[2] impulses. This is known as the anti-nociceptive effect – a reduction in pain sensitivity made within neurones when a substance such as an opiate or endorphin combines with a receptor. Several studies have indicated that essential oils and their constituents have anti-nociceptive effects, and a few of these studies have explored the molecular mechanisms for this activity. This effect is often found in combination with analgesic and anti-inflammatory activity.

Some essential oil components appear to have multiple modes of action, which means that they might be very useful for the treatment of different kinds of pain. Guimarães, Quintans and Quintans-Júnior (2013) conducted a systematic review of papers published between 1990 and 2012, and summarised the current knowledge based on *in vitro* studies and *in vivo* animal studies. The conclusion was, from an aromatherapist's perspective, very welcome, in that out of the

---

1   These include nausea, vomiting, pruritus, constipation, miosis (constriction of the pupils of the eyes), drowsiness, respiratory depression and an increasing tolerance to the drug.

2   A nociceptor is a pain receptor that responds to stimuli by sending nerve signals to the spinal cord and brain.

27 monoterpenes[3] in the review, only one did not have analgesic activity, and that was *d*-menthol. The authors reported that 'the great diversity of mechanisms that may be associated with the analgesic effect of these monoterpenes is amazing' (p.11). A very brief summary of just some of the evidence for the analgesic effects of monoterpenes and their oxygenated derivatives follows.

l-**Linalool** is possibly the most-studied acyclic monoterpenoid and has multiple and diverse sites of action – it can modulate ten systems[4] (Guimarães *et al.* 2013). It has been demonstrated that *l*-linalool (and also *l*-carvone) can produce marked anti-nociception against glutamate-induced pain in mice, via a non-opioid central mechanism (Batista *et al.* 2008). The effects of *l*-linalool on pain caused by inflammation and oedema are thought to be due to the reduction of nitric oxide synthesis or release, thus preventing its accumulation in tissues. Nitric oxide (NO) contributes to oedema, nociception and pain by stimulating the release of cytokines and free radicals, which are pro-inflammatory mediators (Rivot, Montagne-Clavel and Besson 2002, cited by Guimarães *et al.* 2013). Studies (Behrendt *et al.* 2004; Batista *et al.* 2011) have also revealed some of the molecular mechanisms[5] behind its nociceptive effects.

Linalyl acetate is a derivative of linalool that has been shown to possess anti-nociceptive activity; however, its anti-inflammatory activity was not as strong as either *l*-linalool or a racemic mix of *d*- and *l*-linalool (Peana *et al.* 2002, cited by Guimarães *et al.* 2013).

Geranyl acetate is a derivative of geraniol;[6] it displayed a 'discrete' analgesic profile,[7] with anti-nociceptive action and some anti-oxidant activity; it does not impair motor activity (Guimarães *et al.* 2013).

d-**Camphene** is a bicyclic monoterpene that has a significant anti-nociceptive effect; it displayed good anti-oxidant and scavenging potential *in vitro*; this and anti-inflammatory activity is related to inhibition of prostaglandin synthesis; it does not impair motor activity (Guimarães *et al.* 2013).

---

3   These were the acyclic monoterpenes and monoterpenoids citral, citronellal, citronellol, *d*- and *l*-linalool, linalyl acetate, myrcene; the monocyclic monoterpenes and monoterpenoids carvacrol, *d*- and *l*-carvone, *p*-cymene, hydroxydihydrocarvone, *d*-limonene, *d*- and *l*-menthol, α-phellandrene, *d*-pulegone, α-terpineol, thymol, thymol acetate, thymoquinone; the bicyclic monoterpenes and monoterpenoids carvone epoxide, 1,8-cineole, *l*-fenchone, limonene oxide, α- and β-pinene, pulegone oxide, rotundiflone.

4   Including muscarinic, opioid, dopaminergic, adenosinergic and glutamatergic receptor systems, ATP-sensitive K^+ ion channels, and nicotinic receptor-ion channels at the neuromuscular junction (similar to some anaesthetic drugs).

5   l-Linalool inhibits TRPA1 (transient receptor potential A1) and N-methyl-D-aspartate (NMDA) channels, thus reducing induced nociception (Batista *et al.* 2011). Behrendt *et al.* (2004) and Proudfoot, Garry and Cottrell (2006) suggested that chronic nerve pain might be controlled via its activation of TRPM8 (transient receptor potential cation channel 8).

6   Geraniol is an isomer of linalool and nerol.

7   *In vitro*, and at higher doses than *d*-camphene, one of the other compounds in this study.

β-**Myrcene** is an acyclic monoterpene with anti-nociceptive properties. It acts at central and peripheral sites, perhaps by mediating endogenous opioids[8] and α$_2$-adrenoreceptors[9] (Rao, Menezes and Viana 1990, cited by Guimarães *et al.* 2013). It has been shown to have a strong analgesic effect on some types of induced pain, but this is dependent on the route of administration. It has been postulated that myrcene causes an increase in cGMP,[10] which in turn modulates ion channels (Guimarães *et al.* 2013). β-Myrcene also has anti-inflammatory action, perhaps via the inhibition of lipopolysaccharide-induced inflammation, cell migration and synthesis/release of NO, c-interferon and interleukin-4[11] (Souza *et al.* 2003, cited by Guimarães *et al.* 2013).

Citronellal has a marked depressant action on the central nervous system, coupled with sedative and sleep-inducing properties, and it has anti-nociceptive actions (Melo *et al.* 2010a; Quintans-Júnior *et al.* 2010). Further studies revealed that it is also an anti-inflammatory and anti-oxidant agent[12] (Quintans-Júnior 2011a). It was suggested that the anti-oxidant actions may rely on the anti-nociceptive and anti-inflammatory mechanisms.

Citronellol has analgesic properties; Brito *et al.* (2012) suggested that this was probably mediated by inhibition in peripheral and central systems.

Citral is a mixture of two chiral isomers, the aldehydes neral (cis-citral) and geranial (trans-citral). Stotz *et al.* (2008) noted that citral was a partial agonist of some members of the TRP (transient receptor potential) channel family with prolonged inhibition in some types. This prompted the suggestion that because of this broad spectrum and prolonged sensory inhibition, citral might prove very useful in the management of pain that involves superficial sensory nerves and the skin, such as allodynia[13] or itching. Quintans-Júnior *et al.* (2011b) demonstrated that it has anti-nociceptive activity, and can also reduce induced oedema and inflammation. Therefore, citral might be very useful in the treatment of pain with accompanying oedema and inflammation.

Carvacrol is a phenol derived from the terpene pathway, noted for its pronounced anti-oxidant actions (Mastelic *et al.* 2008). In their review, Guimarães *et al.* (2013)

---

8   Endogenous opioids are psychoactive and pharmacologically active opiate-like chemicals produced by the body, such as endorphins.

9   These are found in the central nervous system and on blood vessels.

10   Cyclic guanosine monophosphate (cGMP) is a regulator of ion channel conductance at the cell surface.

11   Interleukin-4 and c-interferon are pro-inflammatory cytokines – signalling chemicals involved in the immune response and inflammation.

12   Bhardwaj *et al.* (2009) speculated that if oxidative stress is implicated in pain pathophysiology, the use of anti-oxidants might relieve pain, via similar anti-nociceptive and anti-inflammatory mechanisms.

13   Allodynia is pain that results from a stimulus (such as temperature, or a physical stimulus such as brushing) which does not normally cause pain. It can manifest as a 'burning' sensation, and can be a feature of, for example, fibromyalgia, migraine and postherpetic neuralgia.

noted that it has anti-nociceptive actions, and this, along with the anti-oxidant activity, can contribute 'significantly' towards analgesia, possibly via the inhibition of prostaglandin synthesis, inhibition of pro-inflammatory cytokines and inhibition of NO release, all of which are also indicative of its anti-inflammatory effects. It is possibly a strong agonist of an ion channel (TRPV3, found in dorsal root ganglia, the brain and spinal cord) which is implicated in hyperalgesia, inflammation and skin sensitisation (Xu *et al.* 2006).

Thymol is an isomer of carvacrol, and also displays anti-nociceptive activity. Guimarães *et al.* (2013) cite studies which suggest that this is possibly via modulating ion channels, receptors and prostaglandin synthesis.

***para*-Cymene** is a cyclic monoterpene with analgesic action, and 'excellent' anti-nociceptive potential in cases of neurogenic and inflammatory pain. It appears to work via the opioid system (Santana *et al.* 2011, cited by Guimarães *et al.* 2013). Santana *et al.* (2011) also noted that *para*-cymene does not affect motor activities or performance, eliminating the suggestion that it has a non-specific muscle relaxing effect. Quintans-Júnior *et al.* (2013) demonstrated that *para*-cymene had strong anti-nociceptive activity, but had relatively poor anti-oxidant potential[14] and was not active against NO; however, it did display mild activity against superoxide, which could attenuate damage due to NO.

Carvone is a cyclic monoterpene ketone that exists as two chiral forms. Both have analgesic action; *l*-carvone has anti-nociceptive activity that does not involve the opioid system and *d*-carvone can also reduce nociception. Both are believed to modulate Na⁺ ion channels. De Sousa *et al.* (2007) found that *l*-carvone was slightly more active than *d*-carvone.

***d*-Pulegone**, another cyclic monoterpene ketone, appears to have similar actions to carvone. It has also been demonstrated that it is a COX inhibitor, and possibly inhibits the production of pro-inflammatory mediators.

***d*- and *l*-Menthol** are cyclic monoterpene alcohols. Menthol is well known as a topical analgesic, and some human studies have indicated that it has analgesic activity in headaches (Gobel, Schmidt and Soyka 1994) and in postherpetic neuralgia (Davies, Harding and Baranowski 2002). The *d*- form was the only compound in the systematic review that did not display analgesic action. The *l*-form appears to suppress pro-inflammatory mediators and cytokines. However, menthol is probably best known for its ability to produce a cooling and numbing sensation on the skin – at least when low concentrations are applied – because ion channels are activated. However, at higher concentrations, menthol induces warmth, or burning and even painful sensations; this is because the higher concentration leads to a reversible ion channel block (Guimarães *et al.* 2013).

---

14 *In vitro*, and in comparison with the other compounds (*d*-camphene and geranyl acetate) investigated in this study.

Limonene is a cyclic monoterpene that exist in *d-* and *l-* forms. The *d-* isomer is more common, it has a citrus-lemon odour and is found in citrus oils. The *l-* form occurs in some oils from the Pinaceae, Cupressaceae and Poaceae families, also in star anise, peppermint and spearmint, and lemon-scented ironbark; it has a turpentine-like odour. Limonene often co-occurs with terpinolene and α-terpinene, and it can be difficult to separate these constituents. The naturally occurring racemic mix of the two isomers is sometimes called dipentene. It has been shown that *d*-limonene has significant anti-nociception, and acts without opioid receptor stimulation; Hirota *et al.* (2010) suggested that this might be due to its considerable anti-inflammatory activity – it decreases cell migration and cytokine release, and this is coupled with a 'potent' anti-oxidant effect.

α-Terpineol is a cyclic monoterpene alcohol which has been shown to have anti-nociceptive activity via both central and peripheral pathways; it has anti-inflammatory actions too (Quintans-Junior *et al.* 2011c).

α-Phellandrene is a cyclic monoterpene with anti-nociceptive activity, which appears to involve multiple systems, including the glutamatergic, opioid, nitrergic, cholinergic and adrenergic systems (Lima *et al.* 2012a, cited by Guimarães *et al.* 2013).

1,8-cineole is a bicyclic monoterpene oxide, formerly known as eucalyptol, reflecting its presence in many oils of the *Eucalyptus* genus. It is well known as a skin penetration enhancer, a decongestant and an antitussive, and it is a licenced product for the treatment of bronchitis, sinusitis, respiratory tract infections and rheumatic conditions. 1,8-cineole also has anti-nociceptive activity which does not involve the opioid system. However, high doses (400mg/kg) can have adverse effects on locomotion (Santos and Rao 2000), and a study conducted by Liapi *et al.* (2007) suggested that low doses of 1,8-cineole were almost equivalent to morphine in rats, with nociception at spinal and supraspinal levels. However, in mice the supraspinal effect was poor. Santos and Rao (2000) reported that 1,8-cineole is also a 'potent' anti-inflammatory agent[15] with an 'excellent' peripheral analgesic effect. An anaesthetic property was suggested by Guimarães *et al.* (2013), as it can act directly on sensory nerves and excitability is blocked, related to concentration. Observed 'cooling' sensations may be due to its activation of specific ion channels.

α- and **β-pinene** have been the subject of several studies, which have on occasion thrown up une xpected results. Guimarães *et al.* (2013) note that α-pinene displayed weak anti-nociceptive activity, but that anti-inflammatory activity has been observed, which could explain its analgesic effect. β-Pinene, however, actually reversed the anti-nociceptive effects of morphine (Liapi *et al.* 2008); it too appears to have anti-inflammatory activity, which might explain possible analgesic activity.

---

15 1,8-cineole is a COX inhibitor and suppressor of arachidonic acid metabolism and cytokine production.

l-Fenchone is a bicyclic monoterpenoid ketone; it has anti-nociceptive activity (Him *et al.* 2008, cited by Guimarães *et al.* 2013).

Rotundifolone is a monoterpenoid with an α,β-unsaturated ketone and an epoxide group.[16] It displays anti-nociceptive activity, with the epoxide group contributing as much as the ketone group to this activity; it is thought that the position of the epoxide group influenced the anti-nociceptive activity (de Sousa *et al.* 2007). Its analgesic effect can be blocked by naloxone pretreatment, suggesting an opioid mechanism (Almeida, Hiruma and Barbosa-Filho 1996, cited by de Sousa *et al.* 2007).

It is indisputable that the monoterpenes and their derivatives have enormous potential as analgesics, and very likely that it is not simply functional group influence which is important, but the position of the functional groups on the carbon framework.

Some phenylpropanoids are also noted for their pain-relieving actions. These include the phenol **eugenol**, which has a well-established temporary anaesthetic action; it is an analgesic and anti-inflammatory agent (Daniel *et al.* 2008). **Methyl salicylate** is an ester, and it too has analgesic and anti-inflammatory actions (Bowles 2003). In many of these examples we can see how the pain-relieving effects might be inextricably linked with anti-inflammatory actions.

Inflammation

Inflammation is a protective reaction to any harmful stimuli, such as invasion of pathogens, or injury and damaged cells; acute inflammation is the first stage of the healing process, triggered by the innate immune system. Inflammatory mediators include tumour necrosis factor-α (TNF-α), a range of interleukins and prostaglandin E_2 (PGE_2), and vasoactive amines such as histamine; other factors are enzymes such as COX-2 (cyclooxygenase 2), 5-LOX (5-lipoxygenase), specific kinases and phospholipases. For example, phospholipase A_2 is an enzyme involved in the conversion of phospholipids in the cell membrane into arachidonic acid, which is a reactive metabolite that is rapidly metabolised by cyclooxygenases into prostaglandins. Some inflammatory mediators, such as interleukin-1β and TNF, can stimulate additional pathways of inflammation which result in prostaglandin, leukotriene and nitric oxide production, adhesion molecules and further cytokines. However, prolonged 'chronic' inflammation is a dysregulated response to persistent stimuli, and can lead to diseases such as autoimmune disease, allergy, arthritis, cancers and atherosclerosis.

Most of the recent studies regarding the anti-inflammatory ('antiphlogistic') activities of essential oils and their components have suggested that they either increase or decrease the formation of inflammatory mediators, or suppress

16   It is significant in many *Mentha* species, particularily *M. × villosa* and also *M. rotundifolia, M. suaveolens, M. spicata* and *M. longifolia* (Guedes *et al.* 2004a).

the activity of specific enzymes such as COX-2, 5-LOX and phospholipase A$_2$ (Adorjan and Buchbauer 2010; Baylac and Racine 2003; de Cássia da Silveira e Sá *et al.* 2014; Kumar *et al.* 2009). Some essential oils and their components – for example, tea tree and terpinen-4-ol – can alleviate allergy by suppressing histamine release and cytokine production (Edris 2007).

In addition to the anti-inflammatory monoterpenes already discussed under 'Pain' above, other constituents in essential oils that have been shown to have anti-inflammatory activity include the following.

Monoterpenes and their derivatives

Sabinene is a bicyclic monoterpene that has anti-inflammatory action. It is present in significant amounts in nutmeg (*Myristica fragrans*), yarrow (*Achillea millefolium*) and plai (*Zingiber cassumunar*), and can occur at over 10% in aromatic ravensare leaf (*Ravensara aromatica*), bergamot (*Citrus bergamia*), black pepper (*Piper nigrum*), blackcurrant bud (*Ribes nigrum*), combava peel (*Citrus hystrix*), juniperberry (*Juniperus communis*), laurel leaf (*Laurus nobilis*), ravintsara (*Cinnamomum camphora* CT cineole), and lesser-known essential oils such as hallabong flower [(*Citrus unshiu* × *Citrus sinensis*) × *Citrus reticulata*]. Isolated sabinene displayed strong anti-inflammatory activity, working through nitric oxide scavenging and inhibition (Kim *et al.* 2013a; Valente *et al.* 2013).

Citronellol and **geraniol** have anti-inflammatory actions, acting via inhibition of NO and PGE2 in macrophages (Su *et al.* 2010).

Terpinen-4-ol can alleviate allergy by supressing histamine release (Edris 2007).

Bornyl acetate, an ester derived from the bicyclic monoterpene *d*-camphene, has anti-inflammatory action. Wu *et al.* (2004) investigated the effects of bornyl acetate in the essential oil of *Amomum villosum*[17] on induced pain and inflammation in mice, concluding that bornyl acetate had both analgesic and anti-inflammatory actions. Matsubara *et al.* (2011a) cite a 2008 study which explored the anti-inflammatory effects of bornyl acetate from an indigenous species – *Cinnamomum osmopheloeum*[18] – again confirming its anti-inflammatory activity.

Sesquiterpenes and their derivatives

α-**Bisabolol**, β-**caryophyllene**, *trans*-**nerolidol** and **farnesol** inhibit 5-LOX (Baylac and Racine 2003).

---

17 *Amomum villosum* is a plant belonging to the Zingiberaceae family, cultivated in Southeast Asia and south China for its fruits, which are dried and used as a culinary spice, in a similar way to cardamom. It also has traditional medicinal applications.

18 *Cinnamomum osmopheloeum* is also known as 'pseudocinnamon' or indigenous cinnamon; in Taiwan it is used in the treatment of gout.

Phenylpropanoids

Cinnamaldehyde, **cinnamyl acetate**, **cinnamic acid**, **eugenol**, **myristicin**, **elemicin**, **trans-anethole** and **phenylethanol** display anti-inflammatory activity. The polarity[19] of these molecules might be implicated in their actions, and studies have indicated that their anti-inflammatory activity is via many different mechanisms of action. Cinnamaldehyde has marked anti-inflammatory activity, which could suggest that it could be used in chronic inflammatory diseases, and also anti-neuro-inflammatory activity, making it a candidate for the management of neurodegenerative diseases (de Cássia da Silveira e Sá *et al.* 2014).

Butadienes

Trans-1-(3,4- dimethoxyphenyl) butadiene, abbreviated to **DMPBD**, is present in plai essential oil from 1–16%. This compound has potent anti-inflammatory action (Jeenapongsa *et al.* 2003). It is a COX-2 inhibitor, and also inhibits PGE_2.

Curcuminoids

It has also been reported that phenolic compounds named **cassumunins A**, **B** and **C** are found in plai (*Zingiber cassumunar* rhizome) extracts. These belong to the group known as curcuminoids, and many of the pharmacological actions of the rhizome – anti-oxidant, anti-inflammatory and anti-allergic activities – have been attributed to their presence (Bua-in and Paisooksantivatana 2009).

---

19   The more polar a molecule is, the more able it is to dissolve in water. Even the more polar essential oil constituents, however, are relatively insoluble in water, but do dissolve readily in alcohol.

Table 7.1 Pain and inflammation: analgesic, anti-nociceptive, anti-inflammatory and related actions

Essential oil	Actions	Evidence
African bluegrass (*Cymbopogon validus*)	Anti-inflammatory Analgesic	Anti-inflammatory and analgesic potential due to dominance of β-myrcene (15–20%) – see text above.
Alpinia calcarata rhizome	Anti-nociceptive Anti-inflammatory Analgesic	*Alpinia calcarata* rhizomes are used in traditional medicine (Sri Lanka, India and Malaysia) for the treatment of arthritis; aqueous and ethanolic extracts have anti-oxidant and anti-nociceptive actions (Arambewela, Arawwawala and Ratnasooriya 2004), and possess anti-inflammatory actions, possibly via inhibition of histamine and prostaglandin synthesis (Arawwawala, Arambewela and Ratnasooriya 2012). The essential oil displays anti-inflammatory and analgesic actions (Rahman *et al.* 2012).
Basil, African (*Ocimum gratissimum*)	Analgesic Anti-inflammatory	Highlighted in a review (Prabhu *et al.* 2009); contains methyl chavicol, which has carcinogenic potential, but also the anticarcinogenic *d*-limonene and α-caryophyllene; Tisserand and Young (2014) recommend a maximum dermal use of 0.2%.
Basil, CT linalool (*Ocimum basilicum*)	Analgesic Anti-inflammatory	The linalool CT contains around 53–58% linalool and 9–15% eugenol; based on the known anti-nociceptive (Batista *et al.* 2008; Daniel *et al.* 2008) and anti-inflammatory (Daniel *et al.* 2008; Rivot *et al.* 2002) actions of these principal constituents, it is highly likely that this essential oil will share these properties. Studies (Behrendt *et al.* 2004; Batista *et al.* 2011) have also revealed some of the molecular mechanisms[1] behind linalool's anti-nociceptive effects.
Basil, holy (*Ocimum sanctum*)	Analgesic Anti-inflammatory	The main constituent, eugenol (30–50%) (Prakash and Gupta 2005), has analgesic and anti-inflammatory actions (Dusan *et al.* 2006). The extract and eugenol can reduce uric acid levels and could play a role in the management of rheumatoid arthritis (Sarkar *et al.* 1994; Sen 1993).
Bay laurel (*Laurus nobilis*)	Analgesic Anti-nociceptive Anti-inflammatory	An animal study (Sayyah *et al.* 2003) indicated that the leaf oil had analgesic (anti-nociceptive) and anti-inflammatory actions which were comparable with conventional analgesic and non-steroidal anti-inflammatory medications.

Bergamot (*Citrus aurantium* var. *bergamia* fruct., *C. bergamia*)	Analgesic Anti-nociceptive	Bergamot had anti-nociceptive activity in induced pain/irritation in mice (Sakurada *et al.* 2009). The same study confirmed the importance of linalool as a TRPA1 agonist and linalyl acetate as an anti-nociceptive agent (see text above).
		Bergamot essential oil released exocytotic and carrier-mediated discrete amino acids, with neurotransmitter functions, in the hippocampus, and there was evidence of neuroprotection in the case of ischaemia and pain. This supported the use of bergamot in treating the symptoms of cancer pain, mood disorders and stress-induced anxiety (Bagetta *et al.* 2010).
Black cumin (*Nigella sativa*)	Anti-nociceptive Anti-inflammatory	The essential oil and its component thymoquinone have anti-nociceptive activity (Abdel-Fattah, Matsumoto and Watanabe 2000); properties shared by two other significant components, *para*-cymene and γ-terpinene.
		Thymoquinone from *Nigella sativa* supressed induced rheumatoid arthritis in rats (Adorjan and Buchbauer 2010).
Black pepper (*Piper nigrum*)	Analgesic Anti-nociceptive	Based on its dominant constituents (β-caryophyllene, *d*-limonene, α- and β-pinene) the essential oil, which is often said to be rubefacient and warming, is very likely to have analgesic, anti-nociceptive and anti-inflammatory actions.
		In a randomised controlled study, black pepper essential oil combined with marjoram, lavender and peppermint (a 3% cream formulation, applied daily) was significantly more effective in reducing neck pain in comparison with the control group; effectiveness was assessed by a visual analogue scale, pressure pain threshold and motion analysis (Ou *et al.* 2014).
Camphor, CT nerolidol (*Cinnamomum camphora*)	Anti-inflammatory	The nerolidol chemotype contains 40–60% nerolidol, with 20% each of monoterpenoids and sesquiterpenoids (Behra, Rakotoarison and Harris 2001; Baylac and Racine (2003) suggest that nerolidol inhibits 5-LOX, and that the oil might have anti-inflammatory effects.
Cassie absolute (*Acacia farnesiana*)	Anti-inflammatory	The presence of both farnesol and methyl salicylate suggests the potential for anti-inflammatory actions; farnesol is an inhibitor of 5-LOX (Baylac and Racine 2003).
Cedar, Himalayan (*Cedrus deodara*)	Anti-inflammatory Analgesic	Inhibition of 5-LOX (Baylac and Racine 2003) suggests anti-inflammatory potential. Himachalol and other sesquiterpenes from *C. deodora* were shown to have spasmolytic activity (Kar *et al.* 1975; Patnaik *et al.* 1977, cited by Burfield 2002), and *C. deodora* was shown to have analgesic and anti-inflammatory activity in animal studies (Schinde *et al.* 1999a and 1999b, cited by Burfield 2002).

Chamomile, German (*Matricaria recutita*)	Anti-inflammatory	Contains α-bisabolol, which inhibits 5-LOX (Baylac and Racine 2003) and chamazulene. Bowles (2003) states that the essential oil is anti-inflammatory *in vivo*, citing the work of Safayhi *et al.* (1994), who suggest that this effect is due to the blocking of formation of leukotriene B4, an inflammatory mediator, produced by neutrophils at sites of inflammation.
Cinnamon leaf (*Cinnamomum verum* or *C. zeylanicum*)	Anti-inflammatory Analgesic	Potential anti-inflammatory effects will be due, in part, to the dominant eugenol content, and cinnamaldehyde, possibly in synergy with minor constituents linalool and β-caryophyllene. Potential in the management of nerve pain; see text above.
Citrus species (80%+ *d*-limonene)	Anti-nociceptive Anti-inflammatory	Hirota *et al.* (2010) and other studies cited by Guimarães *et al.* (2013) suggest that *d*-limonene has significant anti-nociceptive, anti-inflammatory and anti-oxidant actions; it is possible that citrus oils with a high *d*-limonene content might share these. However, in an animal study (Sakurada *et al.* 2009), *C. sinensis* did *not* display any anti-nociceptive activity, so such actions cannot be taken for granted.
Clary sage (*Salvia sclarea*)	Analgesic Anti-nociceptive	Sakurada *et al.* (2009) demonstrated that clary sage oil had an anti-nociceptive effect on induced pain in mice. In a randomised, double-blind trial, a blend of lavender, clary sage and marjoram (2:1:1 ratio, 3% in a cream base for abdominal massage²) provided pain relief and reduced the duration of pain in outpatients with primary dysmenorrhoea (Ou *et al.* 2012).
Clove bud (*Syzygium aromaticum*)	Analgesic Anti-inflammatory	Dominated by eugenol, which has anti-inflammatory activity.
Combava peel (*Citrus hystrix* peel)	Anti-nociceptive Anti-inflammatory	Combava peel oil contains α-terpineol, and this has been shown to have anti-nociceptive activity via both central and peripheral pathways; it has anti-inflammatory actions too (Quintans-Júnior *et al.* 2011c).
Combava petitgrain (*Citrus hystrix* leaf)	Anti-nociceptive Anti-inflammatory	The main component, citronellal, has anti-nociceptive and anti-inflammatory actions (Melo *et al.* 2010a; Quintans-Júnior *et al.* 2010; Quintans-Júnior 2011a; see text above).
Coriander seed (*Coriandrum sativum*)	Analgesic	The presence of *d*-linalool, α- and β-pinene, γ-terpinene, *para*-cymene and others would suggest that the essential oil has analgesic potential. In aromatherapy, the essential oil is indicated as an analgesic for osteoarthritis and rheumatic pain (Price and Price 2007).

Cypress (*Cupressus sempervirens*)	Analgesic Anti-inflammatory	The Mediterranean cypress is traditionally used to treat pain and inflammation; the essential oil is a good scavenger of NO (Aazza *et al.* 2014).
Eucalyptus species (1,8-cineole types)	Analgesic Anti-nociceptive Anti-inflammatory	Santos and Rao (2000), Liapi *et al.* (2007) and Guimarães *et al.* (2013) – activities related related to 1,8-cineole.
Eucalyptus camadulensis	Anti-nociceptive	An animal study indicated anti-nociceptive potential possibly due to 1,8-cineole (Liapi *et al.* 2008).
Eucalyptus globulus	Analgesic Anti-nociceptive Anti-inflammatory	An animal study (Silva *et al.* 2003) indicated that it has dose-related central analgesic activity, peripheral anti-nociceptive activity, and anti-inflammatory effects.
Fennel, sweet (*Foeniculum vulgare* var. *dulce*)	Anti-inflammatory Analgesic (antispasmodic)	*Trans*-anethole has spasmolytic effects on skeletal muscle, and this could help explain its analgesic effects (Albuquerque, Sorenson and Leal-Cardoso 1995). The *trans*-anethole content of the essential oil might confer anti-inflammatory properties (de Cássia da Silveira e Sá *et al.* 2014).
Fir, Korean (*Abies koreana*)	Anti-inflammatory	Yoon *et al.* (2009a) demonstrated that the essential oil (bornyl acetate, limonene and α-pinene) inhibited pro-inflammatory mediators, related to the modulation of enzyme expression (including that of COX-2).
Frankincense (*Boswellia carterii* and others, including *B. sacra* and *B. serrata*)	Anti-inflammatory Anti-arthritic	Used in traditional medicine for its anti-inflammatory and anti-arthritic effects (Hussain *et al.* 2013).

Geranium (*Pelargonium* × *asperum*, or *P. roseum* [a hybrid of *P. capitatum* × *P. radens*], *P. capitatum*, *P. radens*, *P. odoratissimum*)	Analgesic Anti-inflammatory	Maruyama *et al.* (2006) investigated the effects of the oil, via injection, on induced oedema and arthritis in mice; geranium reduced swelling and inflammation in both the early and later phases of the inflammatory response, and neutrophil accumulation decreased. The intraperitoneal injections had toxic effects. They suggested that cutaneous application of geranium might be used in the treatment of rheumatoid arthritis. A multi-centre, double-blind crossover study (Greenway *et al.* 2003) showed that geranium (at various concentrations from 100% to 10% in mineral oil) could relieve pain due to postherpetic neuralgia in 'minutes' and that 25% of the patients had 'dramatic relief of spontaneous pain'. The oil was well-tolerated, with only a few cases of minor skin irritation even at 100%.
Ginger (*Zingiber officinale*)	Analgesic Anti-inflammatory	Used in traditional medicine for relief of pain and inflammation (Carrasco *et al.* 2009). Oral administration of ginger oil elicited a significant reduction in paw and joint swelling in rats with severe chronic adjuvant arthritis (Sharma, Srivastava and Gan 1994). Ginger supreses/inhibits synthesis of pro-inflammatory cytokines; inhibitor of COX and 5-lipoxygenase (Rahmani, Al Shabrmi and Aly 2014). Therapeutic importance in the treatment of osteoarthritis (Rahmani, Al Shabrmi and Aly 2014).
Hemlock (*Tsuga canadensis*)	Analgesic Anti-inflammatory	Contains 41–43% bornyl acetate; a component noted for its analgesic and anti-inflammatory properties (Wu *et al.* 2004).
Hemp (*Cannabis sativa*)	Analgesic Anti-inflammatory	Analgesic and anti-inflammatory potential (Tubaro *et al.* 2010); Baylac and Racine (2004) demonstrated that, *in vitro*, it could inhibit 5-LOX.
Immortelle (*Helichrysum angustifolia*)	Analgesic Anti-inflammatory	Voinchet and Giraud-Robert (2007) investigated the therapeutic effects and potential clinical applications of *Helichrysum italicum* var. *serotinum* and a macerated oil of musk rose (*Rosa rubiginosa*) after cosmetic and reconstructive surgery. This combination reduced inflammation, oedema and bruising; they attributed these effects to italidiones, and commented that neryl acetate, a principal constituent, contributed to a pain-relieving effect.
Jasmine absolute (*Jasminum grandiflorum*)	Analgesic	Analgesic properties noted by Holmes (1998/1999, 2001); traditionally used to relax muscles. In Ayurvedic medicine it is used as a mild analgesic (Shukla 2013).

Essential oil	Actions	Notes
Juniperberry (*Juniperus communis*)	Analgesic Anti-nociceptive Anti-inflammatory	The dominant constituents of the essential oil (including α-pinene, β-myrcene, sabinene, terpinen-4-ol) and others (including *l*-limonene, β-pinene, γ-terpinene, *para*-cymene) are noted for their analgesic, anti-nociceptive and anti-inflammatory actions, supporting the use of juniperberry essential oil for alleviating pain and inflammation. Juniperberry oil displayed remarkable anti-inflammatory and anti-nociceptive activities in an animal study (Akkol, Güvenc and Yesilada 2009).[3]
Kewda (*Pandanus odoratissimus*, *P. fascicularis*)	Anti-nociceptive Anti-inflammatory (potential)	Kewda essential oil is dominated by phenylethyl methyl ether; it contains up to 22% terpinen-4-ol, with *para*-cymene and α-terpineol, which is all suggestive of anti-inflammatory, analgesic and anti-nociceptive actions (see text above).
Lavender, true (*Lavandula angustifolia*)	Analgesic	Lavender displayed anti-nociceptive actions in an animal study (Sakurada *et al.* 2009). Lavender, administered via oxygen face masks, can reduce the application of analgesic opioids immediately post-surgery (Kim *et al.* 2007). In a randomised, double-blind trial, a blend of lavender, clary sage and marjoram (2:1:1 ratio, 3% in a cream base for abdominal massage) provided pain relief and reduced the duration of pain in outpatients with primary dysmenorrhoea (Ou *et al.* 2012). In a randomised controlled study, lavender essential oil, combined with marjoram, black pepper and peppermint (a 3% cream formulation, applied daily) was significantly more effective in reducing neck pain in comparison with the control group; effectiveness was assessed by a visual analogue scale, pressure pain threshold and motion analysis (Ou *et al.* 2014).
Lavandin (*Lavandula hybrid*)	Anti-nociceptive	Lavandin displayed anti-nociceptive actions in an animal study (Sakurada *et al.* 2009).
Lemon (*Citrus limon*)	Anti-inflammatory	Inhibitor of 5-LOX (Baylac and Racine 2003).
Lemon balm (*Melissa officinalis*)	Anti-inflammatory Analgesic	Bounihi *et al.* (2013) demonstrated that oral administration of a Moroccan-grown *M. officinalis* essential oil to rats with carrageenan and trauma-induced paw oedema has anti-inflammatory actions, and has the potential to treat diseases associated with inflammation and pain. They suggested that this action was in part due to the presence of citral (27%). The principal component of the Moroccan oil in this study was nerol (30.44%); *iso*-pulegol was present at 22%.

Lemongrass (*Cymbopogon citratus*)	Analgesic Anti-nociceptive	Dominated by citral, noted for its role in the management of pain that involves superficial sensory nerves and the skin, such as allodynia or itching. Quintans-Júnior et al. (2011b) demonstrated that it has anti-nociceptive activity, and can also reduce induced oedema and inflammation. Therefore, citral-rich oils such as lemongrass are indicated in the treatment of pain with accompanying oedema and inflammation.
Linden blossom absolute (*Tilea vulgaris*)	Anti-inflammatory	Dominated by farnesol, which is a 5-LOX inhibitor (Baylac and Racine 2003).
Long pepper (*Piper longum*)	Anti-inflammatory Analgesic Reduces oedema related to inflammation	In Ayurvedic medicine, it is used as a counter-irritant and analgesic, applied topically for muscular pain and inflammation. The essential oil had significant anti-inflammatory activity in carrageenan-induced paw oedema (rats) – this was dose dependent, and 1ml/kg (oral) was more effective than ibuprofen in reducing oedema (Kumar et al. 2009). Zaveri et al. (2010) noted that long pepper had weak opioid but potent NSAID type of analgesic activity.
Mandarin (*Citrus reticulata*)	Anti-inflammatory	Inhibitor of 5-LOX (Baylac and Racine 2003).
Marjoram, sweet (*Origanum majorana*)	Analgesic	Many of the key major and minor constituents of the essential oil are known to have analgesic, anti-nociceptive and anti-inflammatory actions (terpinen-4-ol, linalyl acetate, γ-terpinene, *para*-cymene), supporting its uses for pain and inflammation. In a randomised, double-blind trial, a blend of lavender, clary sage and marjoram (2:1:1 ratio, 3% in a cream base for abdominal massage) provided pain relief and reduced the duration of pain in outpatients with primary dysmenorrhoea (Ou et al. 2012). In a randomised controlled study, sweet marjoram essential oil combined with black pepper, lavender and peppermint (a 3% cream formulation, applied daily) was significantly more effective in reducing neck pain in comparison with the control group; effectiveness was assessed by a visual analogue scale, pressure pain threshold and motion analysis (Ou et al. 2014).
'Mojito' mint (*Mentha* × *villosa*,[4] Cuba)	Anti-nociceptive	Both the essential oil and a major constituent, piperitone oxide, have anti-nociceptive activity, probably an indirect effect of anti-inflammatory action, not involving the CNS. Neither displayed analgesic activity in an animal study (Sousa et al. 2009).

Myrrh (*Commiphora myrrha*)	Anti-inflammatory Analgesic	Inhibitor of 5-LOX (Baylac and Racine 2003). Analgesic and anti-inflammatory activity (Su *et al.* 2011). Used in Chinese medicine for arthritis and in Ayurveda for inflammatory diseases (Shen *et al.* 2012).
Nagarmotha (*Cyperus scariosus*)	Analgesic Anti-nociceptive	In a review of the potential of the species and its essential oil, Bhwang *et al.* (2013) noted that the essential oil has analgesic and anti-nociceptive actions.
Neroli (*Citrus aurantium* var. *amara* flos.)	Antinociceptive Anti-inflammatory	Khodabakhsh *et al.* (2015) investigated the analgesic and anti-inflammatory actions of neroli essential oil on induced pain and inflammation in both mice and rats; neroli has a central analgesic effect and peripheral antinociception effect, and good anti-inflammatory action, comparable to that of diclofenac sodium (at 50mg/kg), supporting the traditional ethnomedical use of neroli in the management of both acute and chronic inflammation and pain.
Nutmeg (*Myristica fragrans*)	Anti-inflammatory	Myristicin has anti-inflammatory actions (de Cássia da Silveira e Sá *et al.* 2014). Many of nutmeg's other constituents (α- and β-pinene, terpinen-4-ol, γ-terpinene, linalool, β-myrcene, *para*-cymene, sabinene) are also noted for their analgesic, anti-nociceptive and/or anti-inflammatory actions.
Orange blossom absolute (*Citrus aurantium* var. *amara* flos.)	Analgesic Anti-nociceptive Anti-inflammatory	Chemically, it is dominated by *l*-linalool (32%) and linalyl acetate (16.8%), nerolidol and farnesol at around 7%, and phenylethanol at 4.5%; these constituents suggest that the absolute should have analgesic, anti-nociceptive and anti-inflammatory actions.
Orange, sweet (*Citrus sinensis*)	Anti-inflammatory	Inhibition of 5-LOX (Baylac and Racine 2003) suggests anti-inflammatory potential.
Palmarosa (*Cymbopogon martinii*)	Anti-inflammatory Anti-nociceptive (potential)	Dominated by geraniol (75–80%) which has anti-inflammatory action, via inhibition of NO and PGE_2 in macrophages (Su *et al.* 2010); also geranyl acetate (10%) which is analgesic and has anti-nociceptive action; it does not impair motor activity (Quintans-Júnior *et al.* 2013).
Patchouli (*Pogostemon. cablin, P. herba*)	Anti-inflammatory	Using computational docking technology, which allows the visualisation of molecular-level interactions, Raharjo and Fatchiyah (2013) screened patchouli oil constituents for their ability to inhibit COX-1. It was suggested that of the major constituents, α-patchouli alcohol was a potential COX-1 inhibitor and thus anti-inflammatory agent.

Peppermint (*Mentha × piperita*)	Analgesic	Gobel, Schmidt and Soyka (1994) and Davies, Harding and Baranowski (2002) state that menthol has analgesic action (see text above). In a randomised controlled study, peppermint essential oil, combined with marjoram, lavender and black pepper (a 3% cream formulation, applied daily), was significantly more effective in reducing neck pain in comparison with the control group; effectiveness was assessed by a visual analogue scale, pressure pain threshold and motion analysis (Ou et al. 2014).
Pine (*Pinus sylvestris*)	Analgesic Anti-inflammatory	In traditional Turkish medicine, a decoction of pine resin, *Juniperus* species and *Sambucus ebulus* is used in bathing to treat rheumatism (Süntar et al. 2012). The essential oil is dominated by α- and β-pinene; α-pinene has anti-inflammatory actions and weak anti-nociceptive activity (Guimarães, Quintans and Quintans-Júnior 2013); β-pinene has anti-inflammatory activity, which might explain possible analgesic activity (Liapi 2008).
Pink pepper (*Schinus molle*)	Anti-inflammatory	The essential oil has been shown to have anti-oxidant and anti-inflammatory properties (Marongiu et al. 2004).
Plai (*Zingiber cassumunar*)	Analgesic Anti-inflammatory	Contains several anti-inflammatory constituents including sabinene and DMPBD; the oil has high anti-oxidant activity and anti-inflammatory actions (Leelarungrayub and Suttagrit 2009). Evidence of efficacy in human inflammatory joint conditions (Chiranthanut, Hanpraserpong and Teekachunhatean 2014; Loupattarakasem et al. 1993; Niempoog, Siriarchavatana and Kaisongkram 2012). In rheumatoid arthritis, pro-inflammatory cytokines and matrix metalloproteinases are upregulated, and this results in joint inflammation, cartilage degradation and erosion. Chaiwongsa et al. (2013) conducted an *in vitro* study with a human synovial fibroblast cell line, to evaluate the inhibitory effects of DMPBD against cytokine-induced upregulation of the catabolic genes involved in cartilage degradation. They demonstrated that DMPBD acts as an up-stream inhibitor of this catabolic cascade of reactions, concluding that it has joint protective properties, and that the results fully support the use of *Z. cassumunar* in the treatment of chronic inflammatory joint diseases.
Rose absolute (*Rosa damascena*)	Anti-inflammatory Analgesic	Contains phenylethanol, which has anti-inflammatory actions (de Cássia da Silveira e Sá et al. 2014), and farnesol, which is an inhibitor of 5-LOX (Baylac and Racine 2003); this suggests that the absolute has anti-inflammatory potential.

Rose essential oil (*Rosa damascena*)	Analgesic Anti-inflammatory	*R. damascena* oil has analgesic actions (Hosseini *et al.* 2003, cited by Boskabady, Kiani and Rakhshandah 2006). The main constituent, citronellol, has anti-inflammatory actions, and analgesic properties are possibly mediated by inhibition in peripheral and central systems (Brito, Guimarães and Quintans 2012).
Rosemary (*Rosmarinus officinalis*)	Analgesic Anti-nociceptive Anti-inflammatory	Animal studies have indicated that rosemary has peripheral anti-nociceptive activity and anti-inflammatory activity, probably by inhibiting leukocyte chemotaxis (Takaki *et al.* 2008). Rosemary essential oil alleviated arthritic pain in rats, and had a dose-dependent anti-nociceptive effect involving the opioid and serotonergic systems, and the camphor content might act as a TRP modulator (Martinez *et al.* 2009).
Sage, Dalmatian (*Salvia officinalis*)	Analgesic Anti-inflammatory	The essential oil can contain over 50% camphor, a TRP modulator (Martinez *et al.* 2009); other dominant constituents also share these properties, including α-thujone, borneol and 1,8-cineole.
Sandalwood (*Santalum album*)	Anti-inflammatory	Inhibition of 5-LOX (Baylac and Racine 2003) suggests anti-inflammatory potential.
Spearmint (*Mentha spicata*)	Anti-nociceptive	*l*-Carvone, present in spearmint oil, has anti-nociceptive activity that does not involve the opioid system; it is believed to modulate Na⁺ ion channels (de Sousa *et al.* 2007).
Star anise (*Illicium verum*)	Anti-inflammatory	Star anise contains around 70% *trans*-anethole, a compound with anti-inflammatory actions (de Cássia da Silveira e Sá *et al.* 2014).
Tea tree (*Melaleuca alternifolia*)	Anti-inflammatory Analgesic Anti-nociceptive	The essential oil and its constituent terpinen-4-ol can suppress histamine release, and cytokine production, which causes allergic symptoms (Brand *et al.* 2002; Koh *et al.* 2002). It also contains α-terpineol which is anti-nociceptive and anti-inflammatory, and 1,8-cineole, which has anti-nociceptive, anti-inflammatory and peripheral analgesic actions. Tea tree oil, and terpinen-4-ol, can reduce the expression of the inflammatory mediator interleukin-8 (Ramage *et al.* 2012).
Thyme (*Thymus vulgaris*)	Analgesic Anti-nociceptive	*T. vulgaris* CT linalool had an anti-nociceptive effect on induced pain in mice (Sakurada *et al.* 2009). Thymol and its isomer carvacrol are also noted for their anti-nociceptive actions.

Turmeric (*Curcuma longa*)	Analgesic Anti-nociceptive Anti-inflammatory Anti-arthritic	Turmeric has significant anti-oxidant and anti-inflammatory activity in both acute and chronic models of inflammation (Liju, Jeena and Kuttan 2011). Funk *et al.* (2010) demonstrated that although turmeric essential oil could reduce inflammation and joint swelling in an animal model of rheumatoid arthritis, if administered via intraperitoneal injection, this effect was accompanied by a significant morbidity and mortality. Oral administration of a much higher dose was not toxic, but was only mildly protective of the joints (20%). This highlights the relatively high dose required to exert beneficial effects, and safety concerns. Jacob and Badyal (2014) evaluated the anti-inflammatory and analgesic actions of oral doses of turmeric oil and fish oil in comparison with aspirin. Turmeric oil had greater anti-inflammatory activity than aspirin and fish oil, and the combination of turmeric and fish oils was equivalent to aspirin. The combination of the two decreased analgesic activity.
Yarrow (*Achillea millefolium*)	Anti-inflammatory	Yarrow essential oil is often cited as having anti-inflammatory action (Price and Price 2007); this might be due to some of its constituents such as chamazulene, sabinene and 1,8-cineole (see notes above).
Yuzu (*Citrus × junos*)	Analgesic Anti-inflammatory	Analgesic and anti-inflammatory actions were demonstrated (Hirota *et al.* 2010).

1. *l*-Linalool inhibits TRPA1 (transient receptor potential A1) and N-methyl-D-aspartate (NMDA) channels, this reducing induced nociception (Batista *et al.* 2011). Behrendt *et al.* (2004) and Proudfoot *et al.* (2006) suggested that chronic nerve pain might be controlled via its activation of TRPM8 (transient receptor potential cation channel 8).

2. The blended essential oils contained 79.29% of four key analgesic constituents, namely linalyl acetate, linalool, 1,8-cineole and β-caryophyllene.

3. In this study, *Juniperus communis* var. *saxatilis* was used; *J. oxycedrus* subsp. *oxycedrus* also displayed notable anti-inflammatory and anti-nociceptive actions.

4. Also known as 'hortelã-da-folha-miúda', cultivated extensively in northeastern Brazil, widely used in phytotherapy for its anti-parasitic, tranquillising actions and for treating stomach complaints and menstrual pain (Guedes *et al.* 2004a).

Chapter 8

Smooth Functioning

Antispasmodic and Anticonvulsant Actions

Essential oils with antispasmodic (spasmolytic or relaxant) action have therapeutic potential to counteract spasm and pain in voluntary (skeletal) muscle and involuntary (visceral) muscle. However, these relaxant actions also extend to the blood vessels (vasorelaxant, vasodilation) – hence the impact on the cardiovascular system, and so here we shall include essential oils that may have a role to play in the treatment or prevention of cardiovascular disease. (LDL anti-oxidants and atherosclerosis will be addressed in Chapter 9.) We shall also consider oils with anticonvulsant action in this chapter.

Antispasmodic activity

Contraction and relaxation of smooth muscle are regulated by changes in cytoplasmic calcium ion (Ca^{2+}) concentration and signalling mechanisms generated by this (known as Ca^{2+} sensitisation). An increase in Ca^{2+} causes contraction via the activation of myosin light chain kinase, mediated by Ca^{2+} sensitisation. Some essential oils and their constituents have been shown to have antispasmodic (spasmolytic) activity; that is, they can prevent muscle contraction by inhibiting the flow of calcium ions through the cell membrane and into cells. This happens via Ca^{2+} channels in neurons, heart muscle and smooth muscle. It is possible, in some cases, that there may also be inhibition of intracellular Ca^{2+} release (Guedes *et al.* 2004a).

Peppermint essential oil, for example, has antispasmodic activity; this has been established using a series of *in vitro* models. Peppermint is noted particularly for this effect on the gastrointestinal tract, partially due to Ca^{2+} antagonism (Heinrich *et al.* 2004). Some essential oil constituents such as *trans*-anethole, methyl chavicol[1] and eugenol can have spasmolytic effects on skeletal muscle *in vitro* (Albuquerque, Sorenson and Leal-Cardoso 1995, cited by Bowles 2003).

De Sousa *et al.* (2008) investigated the relationship between molecular structure and spasmolytic activity in monoterpenes, finding that functional groups and their position on the molecule contributed to spasmolytic activity, and that the absence of an oxygen-containing functional group is not a requirement for activity.

---

1   Also known as estragole.

Cardiovascular effects

Edris (2007) mentions some studies which indicate that essential oils may have a role to play in the treatment of cardiovascular disease. For example, the oral administration of some essential oils such as oregano, cinnamon and cumin exerted hypotensive effects, decreasing systolic blood pressure in rats (Talpur *et al.* 2005), and Guedes *et al.* (2004b) investigated the effects of intravenous administration of the essential oil of *Mentha × villosa*. In the latter study, it was postulated that the effect was due to piperitone oxide (present at 55.4% of the oil), possibly because it has direct cardiodepressant actions and causes peripheral vasodilation. It has also been found that intravenous administration of *Ocimum gratissimum* induced hypotension and bradycardia, due to vasodilatory effects by acting on the smooth vascular muscle. In this case, eugenol was suggested as being partially responsible (Lahlou *et al.* 2004). Intravenous administration of terpinen-4-ol, present in essential oils of tea tree and sweet marjoram, was also shown to induce smooth muscle relaxation, resulting in hypotensive effects (Lahlou, Leal-Cardoso and Duarte 2003).

Citronellol, which is found in significant amounts in rose (up to 45% in *Rosa damascena, R. centifolia*), geranium (from 20% to 48% in *Pelargonium × asperum*) and citronella (up to 22% in *Cymbopogon nardus*), was the subject of an investigation into its potential hypotensive and vasorelaxant effects; Bastos *et al.* (2010) determined that citronellol could lower blood pressure by a direct vasodilatory effect on vascular smooth muscle.

Linalyl acetate, a major component of bergamot, bergamot mint, clary sage and lavender essential oils, can induce relaxation of smooth muscle, probably (and at least partially) via endothelial-dependent pathways.[2] Kang *et al.* (2013) investigated the effects of bergamot (*Citrus bergamia* Risso) essential oil on intracellular Ca^{2+} in human umbilical endothelial cells. The results suggested that the oil can mobilise Ca^{2+} from intracellular stores and affect the promotion of Ca^{2+} influx, thus having a vasorelaxant effect.

Silva *et al.* (2011) investigated the pharmacology of the hypotensive, bradycardic and vasorelaxant effects of rotundifolone, the major component of *Mentha × villosa* Hudson. They established that vasodilation involved the inhibition of Ca^{2+} influx through L-type[3] voltage-dependent calcium channels; it also inhibited L-type Ca^{2+} currents which affected voltage-dependent activation of these currents and a steady state inactivation. The study also revealed that these two complementary mechanisms are dose dependent. Lima *et al.* (2012b) explored the structural relationships and vasorelaxant effects of monoterpenes, including rotundifolone, *d*-limonene epoxide, pulegone epoxide, carvone epoxide,

---

2   In endothelial cells, an increase in Ca^{2+} is involved in the synthesis and release of NO and prostaglandins; this alters Ca^{2+} sensitisation (a signalling mechanism in the contraction/relaxation mechanism) in smooth muscle cells.

3   The 'L' designates 'long lasting'; L-type currents and channels are responsible for excitation contraction of skeletal, smooth and cardiac muscle.

d-pulegone and the non-oxygenated *d*-limonene. They found that both the oxygenated and non-oxygenated constituents have vasorelaxant activity, that the presence of an oxygenated functional group was not a critical requirement, and that the position of ketone and oxide groups influenced vasoactive potency and efficacy. It was also suggested that the mechanisms of action should also be related to their metabolites; for example, *d*-limonene is metabolised and transformed into *d*-limonene epoxide, *d*-carvone and perillyl alcohol, and perillyl alcohol has hypotensive actions (Miyazawa, Shindo and Shimada 2002, cited by Lima *et al.* 2012b).

In 2012 Yvon *et al.* published the results of their investigation into the relationships between the chemical composition, anti-oxidant activity and anti-hypertensive activity of six essential oils (*Juniperus phoenicea* leaves and berries, *Thymus capitatus*, *Laurus nobilis*, *Melaleuca armillaris* and *Eucalyptus gracilis*). The anti-hypertensive action was due to vasorelaxant actions (on precontracted rat aortas) and they found that there was a good correlation between anti-oxidant ability and anti-hypertensive action; it was concluded that anti-oxidant activity can contribute to the prevention of an increase in blood pressure. It was also reported that *para*-cymene, β-elemene and β-myrcene showed significant correlation with anti-hypertensive action. In contrast, other essential oils, notably rosemary, have been investigated with regard to potential hypertensive activity, which could be harnessed to improve the quality of life in primary hypotensive patients (Fernández, Palomino and Frutos 2014).

Anti-thrombotic activity

There is evidence of interactions between some essential oils and blood coagulation. Tisserand and Young (2014) list these, and caution against oral administration of these in individuals taking anticoagulant medication. However, the therapeutic angle – where essential oils with antiplatelet activity might prevent clot formation – was the subject of two studies. In 2006 Tognolini *et al.* screened 24 essential oils for their antiplatelet activity and ability to inhibit clot retraction.[4] It was identified that there was a significant positive correlation between these actions and the phenylpropanoid content of the oils, and it was suggested that a phenylpropanoid content of 54–86% was indicative of a key role for this group of compounds. The three essential oils that were identified as having the highest antiplatelet action and ability to inhibit clot retraction were *Ocotea quixos*, *Foeniculum vulgare* and *Artemisia dracunculus*. Subsequently, Tognolini *et al.* (2007) reported their observations regarding the protective effect of *Foeniculum vulgare* essential oil and *trans*-anethole in an experimental model of thrombosis.[5] It was concluded that the

---

4   Screened in guinea pig and rat plasma.

5   Here, anethole was tested in guinea pig plasma, where it prevented thrombin-induced clot retraction, and the essential oil and anethole were tested in rat aorta (with and without endothelium), and displaying NO-independent vasorelaxant activity at concentrations which were not cytotoxic.

essential oil and *trans*-anethole have a broad spectrum antiplatelet activity, a clot destabilising effect and vasorelaxant action, resulting in what was described as 'safe antithrombotic activity'.

Anticonvulsant activity

Epilepsy is a group of disorders where spontaneous seizures result from central nervous system neurotransmitter processes. The neurotransmitters involved include the glutamatergic, cholinergic and GABAergic neuromodulation systems. In their 2011 review, de Almeida *et al.* highlighted the anticonvulsant activity of 30 essential oils, established using several experimental models of seizure – the same models are used to identify synthetic anticonvulsant drugs. Although we cannot offer treatment for epilepsy, in the light of this research we can identify essential oils that are most likely safe for use on clients with epilepsy. Conversely, until now, most aromatherapy texts have identified aromatics that are to be avoided.

Table 8.1 Antispasmodic, digestive, cardiovascular and anticonvulsant effects

Essential oil	Actions	Evidence
Angelica (*Angelica archangelica*)	Antispasmodic	The essential oil can inhibit contraction of the uterus via several mechanisms and is indicated for dysmenorrhea (Du *et al.* 2005).
Basil (*Ocimum basilicum*)	Anticonvulsant	Higher doses showed anticonvulsant activity in mice (Ismail 2006); anticonvulsant activity also identified by Oliveira *et al.* (2009).
Basil, African (*Ocimum gratissimum*)	Anticonvulsant	The essential oil obtained from the spring crop was protective against seizures (Freire, Marques and Costa 2006).
Basil, CT methyl chavicol (*Ocimum basilicum*)	Antispasmodic	By virtue of its methyl chavicol (estragole) content (Albuquerque, Sorenson and Leal-Cardoso 1995, cited by Bowles 2003).
Basil, holy (*Ocimum sanctum*)	Anticonvulsant Cardioprotective Vasodilator Anti-oxidant Antihyperlipidemic	The essential oil (and eugenol) has been shown to have membrane-stabilising properties on synaptosomes, erythrocytes and mast cells, supporting its therapeutic potential for convulsions, epilepsy, as well as inflammatory and allergic disorders (Prakash and Gupta 2005). The oil also has potential as a cardioprotective and hypolipidemic agent, and its main constituent, eugenol, has vasorelaxant actions (Prakash and Gupta 2005). Anti-oxidant activity protected rats from damage to cardiac (and liver) tissues due to stress-induced oxidation (Suanarunsawat *et al.* 2010).
Bay laurel (*Laurus nobilis*)	Anticonvulsant Anti-hypertensive	Sayyah, Valizadeh and Kamalinejad (2002) demonstrated that the essential oil had anticonvulsant activity, and at effective doses sedation and motor impairment were also observed. Yvon *et al.* (2012) demonstrated that the essential oil had notable anti-hypertensive activity.
Bergamot (*Citrus aurantium* var. *bergamia* fruct.; *C. bergamia* Risso)	Vasorelaxant	Vasorelaxant action was identified by Kang *et al.* (2013).

Oil	Properties	Notes
Black cumin (*Nigella sativa*)	Anticonvulsant (anti-oxidant) Hypotensive	The essential oil prevented seizures in one model, while significantly decreasing oxidative injury to the mouse brain (Ilhan *et al.* 2005). Huseini *et al.* (2013) conducted a double blind, block randomised study which demonstrated that a daily dose of 5ml *N. sativa* seed oil in healthy volunteers, for eight weeks, lowered systolic (by average of 8.17%) and diastolic blood pressure (by 12.46%) without adverse effects on hepatic and renal functions. It was suggested that this was due to the anti-oxidant actions of thymoquinone, and the cardiovascular depressant action of the oil, which is centrally mediated in the brain.
Cedar, Himalayan (*Cedrus deodara*)	Antispasmodic	Himachalol and other sesquiterpenes from *C. deodara* were shown to have spasmolytic activity (Kar *et al.* 1975; Patnaik *et al.* 1977, cited by Burfield 2002).
Chamomile, German (*Matricaria recutita*)	Antispasmodic	Mills (1991) suggested that chamazulene and α-bisabolol have antispasmodic actions. Price and Price (2007) state that chamazulene (and α-bisabolol) are not only anti-inflammatory but also antispasmodic.
Chamomile, Roman (*Anthemis nobilis*)	Antispasmodic	Bowles (2003) cites Franchomme and Pénoël (1990), who stated that the esters in Roman chamomile, such as isobutyl angelate, have antispasmodic activity.
Citronella, Java (*Cymbopogon winterianus*)	Anticonvulsant Vasorelaxant Hypotensive	Used by traditional medicine practitioners in Brazil to treat epilepsy; Silva *et al.* (2010) demonstrated that the essential oil has a CNS depressant activity and anticonvulsant properties. Anticonvulsant activity also reported by Quintans-Júnior *et al.* (2008). Bastos *et al.* (2010) investigated one of its components, citronellol, which displayed hypotensive and vasorelaxant effects in an animal study.
Clove bud (*Syzygium aromaticum*)	Vasorelaxant	By virtue of eugenol, its main constituent, clove bud may have a role in preventing atherosclerosis, and its anti-oxidant activity may protect cardiac (and liver) tissues from stress-induced oxidation.
Coriander seed (*Coriandrum sativum*)	Antispasmodic	Used in aromatherapy for its spasmolytic actions and support of the digestive tract (Price and Price 2007).
Cumin seed (*Cuminum cyminum*)	Anticonvulsive	The essential oil protected against induced epileptic activity (Janahmadi *et al.* 2006).
Fennel, sweet (*Foeniculum vulgare* var. *dulce*)	Antispasmodic Antithrombotic Vasorelaxant	One of its main constituents, *trans*-anethole, has spasmolytic effects on skeletal muscle (Albuquerque, Sorenson and Leal-Cardoso 1995). Sweet fennel oil has a direct, relaxing effect on the uterine muscle (Ostad *et al.* 2001). An *in vitro* study by Tognolini *et al.* (2007) showed that the essential oil and anethole had antiplatelet activity, a clot destabilising effect, and vasorelaxant action.

Geranium (*Pelargonium × asperum*, or *P. roseum* [a hybrid of *P. capitatum* × *P. radens*], *P. capitatum, P. radens, P. odoratissimum*)	Hypotensive Vasorelaxant	The oil contains significant quantities of citronellol (up to 48%); this constituent has vasorelaxant and hypotensive properties (Bastos *et al.* 2010); see text above.
Ginger (*Zingiber officinale*)	Anti-emetic Antispasmodic	Geiger (2005) demonstrated that a 5% solution of ginger in grapeseed oil, applied naso-cutaneously, benefited patients who have a high risk of post-operative nausea and vomiting. A study conducted by de Pradier (2006) looked at the efficacy of the topical application of a mixture of equal parts of essential oils of ginger, cardamom and tarragon on 86 post-operative patients. Overall, 75% had a favourable response – especially those who has also received one single dose of a pro-emetic drug. If more than one drug had been administered, there was still a positive response in 50% of the patients, i.e. a complete blocking of nausea and vomiting within 30 minutes. A negative response was recorded in 19 patients. It was not established if the results were due to percutaneous effects or inhalation. It is thought that gingerols, shogaols, galanolactone and diterpenoids are implicated in ginger's anti-emetic effect; animal studies have demonstrated that ginger extract has antiserotoninergic and 5-HT3 receptor agonism effects that are important in post-operative nausea and vomiting; the flavour may also play a role (Rahmani, Al Shabrmi and Aly 2014).[1] Riyazi *et al.* (2007) established that the essential oil and some components (terpinolene, β-pinene and α-phellandrene) acted via the serotoninergic system and the 5-HT3 receptor complex to elicit spasmolytic effects in the ileum.
Jasmine absolute (*Jasminum grandiflorum, J. sambac*)	Antispasmodic	Traditionally used as a uterine tonic and relaxant (Potterton 1983). In Ayurvedic medicine it is used as an antispasmodic, parturient and uterine tonic (Shukla 2013).
Lavandin (*Lavandula hybrid* Reverchon 'Grosso')	Gastrointestinal effects	Inhaled and orally administered lavender essential oil had anti-nociceptive and gastroprotective effects, possibly by activation of the vagus nerve, which enhances food intake (Barocelli *et al.* 2004).

Plant	Action	Description
Lavender, French (*Lavandula stoechas*)	Anticonvulsant	Inhalation of the oil has anticonvulsive action, and complementary activity possibly related to modulation of Ca^{2+} channels (Yamada, Mimaki and Sashida 1994).
Lemon balm (*Melissa officinalis*)	Antispasmodic	In traditional Moroccan medicine, *M. officinalis* is used as an antispasmodic with calming actions (Bounihi *et al.* 2013).
Lemongrass (*Cymbopogon citratus*)	Anticonvulsant	Anticonvulsant activity observed (Blanco *et al.* 2009). Used in Brazilian folk medicine as a sedative; Silva *et al.* (2010) postulate that the essential oil has the ability to alter the course of convulsive episodes, interfere with the seizure threshold and/or block the seizure propagation; its components citral and myrcene do not have this activity, so the results are due to synergism between other components in the oil.
Lime (Key lime, *Citrus aurantifolia*)	Antispasmodic	Spadaro *et al.* (2012) demonstrated that the distilled essential oil has important spasmolytic properties (*in vitro*, on isolated rabbit jejenum, aorta and uterus), possibly due to its constituents limonene (58.4%), β-pinene (15.4%), γ-terpinene (8.5%) and citral (4.4%).
Marjoram, sweet (*Origanum majorana*)	Smooth muscle relaxation Vasodilator	Intravenous administration of terpinen-4-ol, present in sweet marjoram essential oil, can induce smooth muscle relaxation resulting in hypotensive effects (Lahlou, Leal-Cardoso and Duarte 2003). This supports the use of sweet marjoram as a relaxing essential oil, and possible vasodilatory actions.
'Mojito' mint (*Mentha × villosa*)	Hypotensive Vasodilator Vasorelaxor Antispasmodic	Sousa *et al.* (2009) note that the herb is used in folk medicine for its antispasmodic actions (amongst others). Lahlou *et al.* (2001) investigated the intravenous administration of the essential oil in anaesthetised rats, to establish any cardiovascular effects; it induced hypotension, probably because it has vasodilatory effects on smooth vascular muscle. Guedes *et al.* (2004a) explored the vasorelaxing activity of rotundifolone (63.4% in the essential oil), establishing that it was a calcium agonist which produced vasorelaxation in rat aortas *in vitro* and *in vivo*. De Sousa *et al.* (2008) demonstrated that rotundifolone, isolated from the essential oil, had a potent spasmolytic effect on isolated guinea pig ileum.
Nagarmotha (*Cyperus scariosus*)	Antispasmodic	In a review of the potential of the herb and essential oil Bhwang *et al.* (2013) noted that the essential oil has antispasmodic action.

Essential oil	Properties	Notes
Neroli (*Citrus aurantium* var. *amara* flos.)	Anticonvulsant Anti-hypertensive Reduces menopausal symptoms	In Iran, neroli is used to prevent seizures. The essential oil protects against induced convulsions in mice, and the GABAergic system may be involved (Azanchi *et al.* 2014). Inhalation of a blend of lavender, ylang ylang, marjoram and neroli had immediate and continuous effects on systolic blood pressure; it decreased daytime ambulatory BP in prehypertensive and hypertensive patients; there was also a decrease in salivary cortisol. It was suggested that this might be a helpful 'relaxation' intervention that could prevent the progression of hypertension (Kim *et al.* 2012). Choi *et al.* (2014) conducted a randomised controlled trial investigating the effects of inhalation of neroli essential oil on menopausal symptoms, stress and oestrogen in healthy postmenopausal women. Neroli relieved many symptoms, especially in relation to physical factors such as hot flushes and low libido; also improved systolic blood pressure was noted. Hot flushes are a complex phenomenon – with the vasomotor element being significant. This study demonstrated that vasomotor symptoms improved significantly, perhaps by modulation of 5-HT, which is involved in regulating body temperature.
Nutmeg (*Myristica fragrans*)	Anticonvulsant	Nutmeg essential oil displayed significant anticonvulsant activity in some experimental models, even at low doses. In one model, higher doses produced weak proconvulsant actions. It was suggested that the oil had potential to treat grand mal and partial seizures, but should not be used for myoclonic or absence seizures (Wahab *et al.* 2009).
Orange, bitter (*Citrus* × *aurantium* subsp. *amara* peel)	Anticonvulsant	Anticonvulsant activity demonstrated by Carvalho-Freitas and Costa (2002).
Patchouli (*Pogostemon cablin*)	Antiplatelet activity	The essential oil has antiplatelet activity due to the presence of α-bulnesene (Hsu *et al.* 2006; Tsai *et al.* 2007, cited by Tisserand and Young 2014).
Peppermint (*Mentha × piperita*)	Antispasmodic	Noted for its spasmolytic action on the gastrointestinal tract (Heinrich *et al.* 2004).
Pink pepper (*Schinus molle*)	Antispasmodic	The essential oil has been shown to have anti-inflammatory and antispasmodic properties (Marongiu *et al.* 2004).
Plai (*Zingiber cassumunar*)	Antispasmodic Inhibitor of COX-2 and PGE2	Plai is used in a traditional Thai formula (along with black cumin and other aromatic herbs and spices), known as *Prasaplai*, in the treatment of primary dysmenorrhea and regulation of the menstrual cycle. Dysmenorrhea is characterised by higher than normal levels of prostaglandins; plai essential oil is a COX-2 inhibitor and consequently also inhibits PGE2 (Aupaphong, Ayudhya and Koontongkaew 2013). Plai aqueous extract is a smooth muscle relaxant (Aupaphong Ayudhya and Koontongkaew 2013); it is possible that the essential oil has spasmolytic activity.

Plant	Activity	Notes
Rose (*Rosa damascena, R. centifolia*)	Vasorelaxant Hypotensive Anticonvulsive	Rose essential oil may have vasorelaxant and hypotensive qualities, based on its *l*-citronellol content, which can be up to 43%, depending on species and source (Bastos *et al.* 2010). *R. damascena* had relaxant effects on guinea pig trachea that were comparable to that of theophylline (Boskabady, Kiani and Rakhshandah 2006). Anticonvulsive and hypnotic effects of *R. damascena* essential oil are due to its affinity with the GABA$_A$ system (Rakhshandah, Hosseini and Dolati 2004).
Rosemary (*Rosmarinus officinalis*)	Antispasmodic Anti-hypotensive	Takaki *et al.* (2008) noted that rosemary essential oil is used in folk medicine for its antispasmodic effects. Fernández, Palomino and Frutos (2014) conducted a study that demonstrated that rosemary essential oil has a significant anti-hypotensive effect that can improve patients' quality of life.
Spanish oreganum (*Thymus capitatus*)	Anti-oxidant Anti-hypertensive	Yvon *et al.* (2012) demonstrated that the essential oil had notable anti-hypertensive activity, which is correlated with its anti-oxidant activity.
Spearmint (*Mentha spicata*)	Antispasmodic	Souza *et al.* (2013) reported that *l*-carvone, found in *M. spicata* var. *crispa*, had a more potent intestinal antispasmodic effect than *d*-carvone; their study[2] revealed that this action (*l*-carvone and spearmint oil) was due to a calcium channel blocker-like action.
Spikenard (*Nardostachys jatamansi*)	Anticonvulsant	Anticonvulsant activity observed, but the constituent jatamansone was more effective than the essential oil (Arora, Sharma and Kapila 1958).
Szechuan (Japanese) pepper (*Zanthoxylum piperitum*)	Prokinetic	An ingredient in the traditional Japanese medicine Daikenchuto (which also contains ginger and ginseng) used to treat various gastrointestinal disorders; *X. piperitum* is thought to accelerate intestinal transit via contraction and relaxation of smooth muscle of intestines (Munekage *et al.* 2011).
Tarragon (*Artemisia dracunculus*)	Anticonvulsant Antiplatelet activity	Identified in a review of anticonvulsant activity (de Almeida *et al.* 2011). Showed the highest antiplatelet activity and also ability to prevent clot formation in a study conducted by Tognolini *et al.* (2006).
Thyme (*Thymus vulgaris*)	Antispasmodic	Antispasmodic activity on gastrointestinal tract tissues, demonstrated in an *in vitro* study (Meister *et al.* 1999).

1. Flavour and aroma are inextricably linked; so if flavour is significant, it could be argued that the scent of ginger is too.
2. This study was an investigation into its pharmacological effects on guinea pig ileum.

Chapter 9

Health Maintenance and Enhancement

Anti-oxidant and Anti-cancer Actions

Anti-oxidant activity is at the foundation of many of the therapeutic properties attributed to essential oils and their constituents, including a range of 'anti-cancer' effects. Although the treatment of cancer does not form part of aromatherapy practice, several investigations have highlighted this potential of essential oils. These oils might be used in prescriptions with a preventative intention, or when maintenance or enhancement of general wellbeing is the main goal.

Anti-oxidant activity

From the therapeutic viewpoint, anti-oxidant activity is possibly one of the most important biological actions attributed to essential oils. Anti-oxidants scavenge ('mop up') free radicals (and other reactive oxygen species) which damage proteins, amino acids, lipids and DNA. Miguel (2010) argues that if essential oils are free radical scavengers, they are also anti-inflammatory agents, because one of the inflammatory responses is an 'oxidative burst' that occurs in cells of the immune system, including monocytes, neutrophils, eosinophils and macrophages. Macrophages are involved in the phagocytosis of bacterial pathogens, which results in a large increase in oxygen consumption and the formation of superoxide anion radicals, which are rapidly converted to hydrogen peroxide and then hydroxyl radicals. These radicals are very damaging – setting off a chain of reactions resulting in the formation of further toxic radicals known as 'reactive oxygen species' and also 'reactive nitrogen species' such as nitric oxide. Reactive oxygen species are thought to be one of the most powerful stimuli for the inflammatory response. These radicals are produced to neutralise the pathogens and signal messenger molecules, but if produced in sufficient quantities they also damage cells at sites of inflammation.

This type of damage could be viewed as the root cause of inflammation, ageing and many degenerative diseases such as cancer, liver disease, arthritis, diabetes,[1] Parkinson's disease and atherosclerosis. Although we have intrinsic defence systems that can quench free radicals, if there is an imbalance between free radical production and removal, we have a situation known as 'oxidative stress' that can only be remedied by an external source of anti-oxidants (Edris 2007). Shaaban, El-Ghorab and Shibamoto (2012) conducted a review of recent *in vitro* and *in vivo* studies which investigated the biological actions of essential oils, including their anti-oxidant activity, and concluded that they could be used to replace some of the synthetic anti-oxidants in the treatment of degenerative diseases. Some of the components highlighted were:

- α-terpinene, β-terpinene and β-terpinolene in tea tree essential oil

- 1,8-cineole in *Mentha aquatica*, *M. longifolia* and *M. piperita* essential oils

- menthone and *iso*-menthone in *M. longifolia* and *M. piperita* essential oils

- thymol, eugenol and linalool in black cumin, cinnamon bark and ginger essential oils

- thymol and eugenol in thyme and clove leaf essential oils

- linalool and 1,8-cineole in thyme essential oils (*Thymus caespititius*, *T. camphorates* and *T. mastichina*)

- citral, citronellal, *iso*-menthone and menthone in lemon balm (*Melissa officinalis*) essential oil.

Adorjan and Buchbauer (2010) commented that phenolic compounds, such as thymol, carvacrol and eugenol, and the 'nearly non-volatile flavonoids' in aromatic plant extracts are more responsible for anti-oxidant activity than the monoterpenes and sesquiterpenes. Shaaban, El-Ghorab and Shibamoto (2012) cite several studies that identified essential oils with notable activity; Wei and Shibamato (2010a, b) studied the anti-oxidant activity of 25 essential oils; thyme had the greatest effect, followed by clove leaf, cinnamon leaf, basil, eucalyptus and chamomile; other studies concluded that coriander, eucalyptus, juniper, cumin, basil, cinnamon, clove and thyme possessed 'appreciable' anti-oxidant activity (the botanical names were not given in this review).

---

1   Type-2 diabetes is associated with an increased generation of free radicals and a defective anti-oxidant defence system. The alternative/natural management of type-2 diabetes (and hypertension) is via the use of dietary anti-oxidants (free radical scavengers) and the inhibition of α-amylase and α-glucosidase (key enzymes involved in starch digestion), and in the case of hypertension, angiotensin-I converting enzyme (which leads to the formation of angiotensin II – a potent vasoconstrictor). Inhibition of α-amylase and α-glucosidase delays the absorption of glucose. Some essential oils could be used to manage these conditions; for example, *Piper guineense* inhibits α-amylase and α-glucosidase and angiotensin-I converting enzyme in a dose-dependent manner (Oboh *et al.* 2013).

LDL anti-oxidants

Atherosclerosis, where plaque deposits build up in the innermost layer of arteries, leads to reduced blood flow and serious cardiovascular disease. Atherosclerosis is initiated by an increase in oxidized low density lipoproteins (LDL) in cholesterol, and this can be reduced by administration of anti-oxidants. However, statins are more often used to lower LDL cholesterol but, although there has been some success, some individuals do not tolerate statins and they are not always effective. There have been efforts to develop more effective and better tolerated plant-derived drugs, and so Vallianou *et al.* (2011) investigated the potential of Chios mastic gum (*Pistacia lentiscus* var. *chia*) and camphene as alternative lipid-lowering agents, finding that both had a strong hypolipidemic action, and that the mechanism of action was different from that of statins.[2]

Essential oils could have a role to play in the prevention of atherosclerosis due to their anti-oxidant activity against LDL. Edris (2007) cites studies which highlight several essential oil constituents that have therapeutic potential in this respect – but as dietary supplements, not in the context of aromatherapy. These are terpinolene, γ-terpinene, eugenol and thymol. Other essential oils and constituents have been shown to lower plasma cholesterol and triglyceride levels, notably black cumin[3] (*Nigella sativa*) and its main constituent, thymoquinone. However, it has also been demonstrated that inhalation of lavender and monarda (species not identified) essential oils (0.1–0.2mg/m^3 of air) can reduce the cholesterol content in the aorta and atherosclerotic plaques, but without affecting blood cholesterol (Nikolaevskii *et al.* 1990, cited by Shaaban, El-Ghorab and Shibamato 2012). Given that essential oils are inhaled and absorbed during aromatherapy treatment, it is therefore not unreasonable to suggest that they might have a preventative role in atherosclerosis. Other than lavender and monarda, essential oils that are characterised by the identified LDL anti-oxidants include tea tree (terpinolene, γ-terpinene), *Pinus mugo* (terpinolene), thyme species (thymol), clove (eugenol), narcissus absolute, mandarin petitgrain, and the citrus peel oils yuzu, mandarin, bergamot, lemon and lime (γ-terpinene).

2　Statins inhibit HMG-CoA reductase, the enzyme that catalyses the rate-determining step of cholesterol biosynthesis in the liver.

3　Black cumin essential oil is not always dominated by thymoquinone; it can also be dominated by *para*-cymene; Wajs, Bonikowski and Kalembar (2008) give a figure of 60.2%, followed by γ-terpinene (12.9%), with only traces of thymoquinone and hydrothymoquinone.

Anti-cancer activity

Most chemotherapeutic drugs kill cancer cells by apoptosis,[4] a process mediated by enzymes known as caspases. It is believed that drugs which produce selective activation of caspases, or lower their activation level, can stimulate apoptosis in cancer cells (Itani *et al.* 2008). Other than induction of apoptosis, some other distinct anti-cancer mechanisms have been identified – anti-oxidant, antimutagenic,[5] antiproliferative, enhancement of immune function and surveillance, enzyme induction and enhancing detoxification,[6] and modulation of multidrug resistance – which can result in chemoprevention[7] and cancer suppression.[8]

Edris (2007) highlighted several constituents that had been investigated with regard to their cancer suppression activities, namely α-bisabolol (German chamomile, *Matricaria recutita*), geraniol (palmarosa, *Cymbopogon martinii*), *d*-limonene (many *Citrus* species), diallyl suphide (garlic, *Allium sativum*), perillyl alcohol (*Perilla frutescens*) and 1,8-cineole (many *Eucalyptus* species). Chen *et al.* (2013) cite studies which have shown that cadinol (a rarely occurring bicyclic sesquiterpene alcohol), *d*-limonene, *n*-octanol (an aliphatic alcohol found in small amounts in a few essential oils such as spearmint), δ-elemene (a monocyclic sesquiterpenoid alcohol present at around 9% in myrrh, amd small amounts in some *Boswellia* species), aromadendrene (also known as viridiflorene, a tricyclic sesquiterpene present in minor quantities in a few oils such as patchouli, tea tree and rosalina) and *l*-spathulenol have anti-tumour activity. Their own study revealed that β-elemene was significant in the anti-cancer activities of myrrh and frankincense – in fact, they demonstrated that β-elemene was more active than either essential oil. This is in stark contrast with the philosophy that underpins phytotherapy and aromatherapy; however, this was an *in vitro* study using human

---

4   Apoptosis is programmed cell death; a normal physiological process in maintaining homeostasis and tissue development in multicellular organisms. Cancer is characterised by the uncontrolled growth of cells, with no normal cell death, invasion and perhaps metastasis – so anti-cancer activity includes the ability of essential oils to induce apoptosis in cancer cells. For example, Verma *et al.* (2008) demonstrated that *Tanacetum gracile* (an alpine aromatic herb) essential oil could induce apoptosis via the mitochondrial pathway.

5   Bhalla, Gupta and Jaitak (2013) suggested an antimutagenic mechanism where the essential oil can inhibit the metabolic conversion by P450 of promutagens into mutagens, inactivate mutagens due to scavenging activity, activate the detoxification of mutagens, and modulate by metabolic inhibition the activation of promutagens.

6   Some essential oil constituents increase the rate of synthesis of glutathione S-transferase in the liver. This is an important enzyme in detoxification pathways; it offers protection from mutagenesis. Constituents that induce glutathione S-transferase include *d*-carvone, β-caryophyllene, citral, eugenol, geraniol, *d*-limonene and myristicin; some essential oils include angelica root, holy basil, basil CT linalool, caraway, cardamom, coriander seed, sweet fennel, ginger, grapefruit, lemon, lemongrass, nutmeg, orange, oregano, sandalwood (*S. album*), spearmint, tangerine and thyme (Tisserand and Young 2014).

7   Via the induction of drug metabolising enzymes which can protect against chemical carcinogenesis.

8   This includes anti-angiogenic activity, where aberrant angiogenesis is arrested; perillyl alcohol is notable in this respect.

cancer cell lines,[9] and although this type of research is valuable and can reveal much about biological activities and mechanisms of action, it cannot be expected to consider the wider effects of essential oils within the holistic context.

In a review article, Adorjan and Buchbauer (2010) also cite several studies that have highlighted anti-cancer activities of monoterpene alcohols and sesquiterpene hydrocarbons, including evidence of synergistic interactions. For example, β-caryophyllene potentiated the anti-cancer effects of α-humulene, *iso-caryophyllene* and paclitaxel, a drug used to treat cancer (Legault and Pichette 2007), and it was suggested that there may be a synergistic relationship between thymol, piperitone and methyl eugenol in *Anemopsis californica* essential oil (Verma *et al.* 2008). In 2013 Russo *et al.* investigated the anti-cancer effects of bergamot essential oil and its components on human neuroblastoma cells. They found that *d*-limonene, linalyl acetate, linalool, γ-terpinene, β-pinene and bergapten when administered alone did not elicit cell death, but that co-treatment with limonene and linalyl acetate caused morphological and biochemical changes, similar to those of bergamot oil, such as capsase-3 activation, DNA fragmentation, cell shrinkage, and cytoskeletal changes resulting in necrotic and apoptotic cell death.

It has also been postulated that some essential oils or their components could complement conventional cancer treatments. Adorjan and Buchbauer's review highlights some studies that support this; for example, linalool improved the activity of anthracyclines against breast cancer cells (Ravizza *et al.* 2008). An *in vitro* study using human tumour cell lines indicated that some essential oil constituents potentiate the effects of anti-cancer drugs by stimulating accumulation and crossing of the cell membrane (Legault and Pichette 2007). Finally, an *in vivo* animal study indicated that the toxic effects of some anti-cancer drugs on the male reproductive system are in part due to the formation of free radicals, and that the anti-oxidant potential of essential oils could offer protection (Rezvanfar *et al.* 2008).

In their 2013 review Bhalla, Gupta and Jaitak concluded that essential oils (and indeed aromatherapy) have a positive effect on the immune system, at a chemical level, over and above their direct effects on tumour cells. Although they acknowledge that major components have effects, these are modulated by minor components, and 'for biological purposes, it is more important to study an entire essential oil rather than some of its components, because the theory of synergism appears to be more significant' (p.3649).

---

9   MCF-7 (breast), HS-1 (human epithelial carcinoma), HepG2 (hepatocellular carcinoma), HeLa (cervical) and A549 (lung).

Table 9.1 Anti-oxidant and anti-cancer actions

Essential oil	Actions	Evidence
Anemopsis californica	Antiproliferative	The ethnobotanical use of Anemopsis californica root to treat uterine cancer led to a study of its essential oil with lung, breast, prostate and colon cancer lines, which demonstrated its ability to inhibit the proliferation of these cell lines (Medina-Holguin et al. 2008).
Angelica root (Angelica archangelica)	Anti-cancer	Induces glutathione S-transferase (Lam and Zeng 1991, cited by Tisserand and Young 2014).
Basil (Ocimum basilicum)	Anti-oxidant Anti-cancer Antiproliferative	Basil essential oil displayed appreciable anti-oxidant activity, comparable to that of α-tocopherol (Wei and Shibamoto 2010a). However, another study conducted by Wei and Shibamoto (2010b) suggested that basil is only able to prevent the primary oxidation of lipids. A basil essential oil which contained trans-nerolidol as a major component had in vitro cytotoxicity against HeLa and Hep-2 human cancer cell lines and NIH 3T3 mouse embryonic fibroblasts (Kathirvel and Ravi 2012). Basil oil, with the major component eugenol, had antiproliferative activity (apoptosis-induced) against a range of cancer cell lines and animal models (Jaganthan and Supriyanto 2012).
Basil, holy (Ocimum sanctum)	Anti-oxidant Chemopreventative Hypolipidemic	Anti-oxidant activity protected rats from damage to cardiac and liver tissues due to stress-induced oxidation (Suanarunsawat et al. 2010). Significant chemopreventative activity was demonstrated by Manosroi, Dhumtanom and Manosroi (2006). The oil has potential as a cardioprotective and hypolipidemic agent, and its main constituent, eugenol, has vasorelaxant actions (Prakash and Gupta 2005).
Bay laurel (Laurus nobilis)	Anti-oxidant Antiproliferative	A component, eugenol, has antiproliferative activity (apoptosis-induced) against a range of cancer cell lines and animal models (Jaganthan and Supriyanto 2012). Saab et al. (2012) demonstrated that bay laurel (leaf) oil has anti-oxidant and antiproliferative activity against K562 human chronic myelogenous leukaemia cells.

Bergamot (*Citrus aurantium* var. *bergamia* fruct., *C. bergamia* Risso et Poiteau)	Anti-oxidant Cancer suppression Necrotic (cancer cells) Apoptosis-inducing LDL-anti-oxidant Anti-atherosclerosis	Contains *l*-linalool (anti-oxidant) and *d*-limonene (cancer suppression). The essential oil activates multiple death pathways in cancer cells, and significant cytotoxicity (necrotic and apoptotic cell death) in neuroblastoma cultures is observed when *d*-limonene and linalyl acetate are co-administered (Russo *et al.* 2013). Contains up to 12% *γ*-terpinene, an LDL anti-oxidant. It is possible that the essential oil might play a preventative role in the development of atherosclerosis (Takahashi *et al.* 2003).
Black cumin (*Nigella sativa*)	Anti-oxidant Chemopreventative Anti-atherosclerosis	The essential oil has anti-oxidant activity (Edris 2009). The oil is an anti-oxidant, improves the body's defence system, induces apoptosis; the constituent thymoquinone is a 'potent' anti-oxidant, anticarcinogenic and antimutagenic agent; oral administration of the oil is considered a promising natural radioprotective agent against the immunosuppressive and oxidative effects of ionising radiation (Khan *et al.* 2011). Alenzi, El-Bolkini and Salem (2010) investigated the essential oil and its major constituent thymoquinone and concluded that it had anti-oxidant activity and protected against toxicity induced by cyclophosphamide.[1] Hepatoprotective activity, partly due to thymoquinone (Mansour *et al.* 2001). The oil and thymoquinone have a role in cancer prevention through the activation or inactivation of molecular cell signalling pathways. The enzyme COX-2 is overexpressed in a wide range of cancers; this plays a role in the upregulation of angiogenesis by prostaglandin, and increases resistance to apoptosis. COX-2 inhibition is critical in cancer prevention; thymoquinone showed a critical effect in the inhibition of COX-2 and prostaglandin production (Rahmani, Al-Shabrmi and Aly 2014). The essential oil can decrease plasma cholesterol and triglycerides, due to thymoquinone content (Ali and Blunden 2003). The essential oil prevented seizures in one model, while significantly decreasing oxidative injury to the mouse brain (Ilhan *et al.* 2005).
Black pepper (*Piper nigrum*)	Free radical scavenger Cancer suppression potential	Contains β-caryophyllene, which can potentiate the anti-cancer effects of other compounds, and *d*-limonene which is noted for its cancer suppression actions; both compounds have been shown also to induce glutathione-S-transferase. Free radical scavenging activity might be helpful in chemoprevention and suppressing tumour growth (Butt *et al.* 2013).

Caraway (*Carum carvi*)	Anti-oxidant	Samojlik *et al.* (2010) demonstrated that caraway essential oil strongly inhibited lipid peroxidation in both test systems, and was hepatoprotective (in comparison with coriander oil, which exhibited pro-oxidant activity).
Chamomile, German (*Matricaria recutita*)	Anti-oxidant Antiproliferative Cytotoxic	A significant component of the oil, α-bisabolol, has a marked cytotoxic effect on human and rat malignant glioma cell lines (Cavalieri *et al.* 2004), leading to their conclusion that α-bisabolol may have potential use in clinical treatment of glioma, a highly malignant brain tumour. α-Bisabolol has been identified as having cancer suppression action (Edris 2007). Anti-oxidant and antiproliferative actions were identified in a review of the bioactivity of the tea made from the dried herb (McKay and Blumberg 2006).
Cinnamon leaf (*Cinnamomum zeylanicum*)	Anti-oxidant	Wei and Shibamoto (2010b) identified anti-oxidant activity; see text above.
Citronella (*Cymbopogon nardus*)	Anti-oxidant Cancer suppression potential	Contains up to 30% geraniol, which has cancer suppression potential (Edris 2007), and citronellal (up to 50%), which has anti-oxidant action (Shaaban, El-Ghorab and Shibamoto 2012).
Clove bud (*Syzygium aromaticum*)	Anti-oxidant Antiproliferative Anti-atherosclerosis	Clove essential oil has appreciable anti-oxidant activity, comparable to α-tocopherol (Wei and Shibamoto 2010a, b). A major component, eugenol, has antiproliferative activity (apoptosis-induced) against a range of cancer cell lines and animal models (Jaganthan and Supriyanto 2012). By virtue of eugenol, its main constituent, clove bud may have a role in preventing atherosclerosis, and its anti-oxidant activity may protect cardiac (and liver) tissues from stress-induced oxidation.
Coriander seed (*Coriandrum sativum*)	Anti-oxidant	Alenzi, El-Bolkini and Salem (2010) and Shaaban, El-Ghorab and Shibamoto (2012) mention the essential oil's anti-oxidant potential.
Cumin (*Cuminum cyminum*)	Anti-oxidant	Free radical scavenging and also ferric reducing power noted by Miguel 2010. Anti-oxidant activity noted by Shaaban, El-Ghorab and Shibamoto (2012).
Cypress (*Cupressus sempervirens, C. sempervirens* var. *horizontalis*)	Anti-oxidant NO scavenger Antiproliferative Antiglycation	Cypress essential oil is a good scavenger of NO, and has antiproliferative action (Aazza *et al.* 2014). *C. sempervirens* var. *horizontalis* essential oils (obtained from both branchlets and fruits) have anti-oxidant and antiglycation[2] properties, which may find a role in the prevention of cardiovascular complications such as hardening of the arteries, and also Alzheimer's disease, cancers, peripheral neuropathy (Asgary *et al.* 2013).

Eucalyptus blue gum (*Eucalyptus globulus*)	Anti-oxidant	Wei and Shibamoto (2010b) identified anti-oxidant activity (see text above).
Eucalyptus camadulensis (wild, Sardinia)	Anti-oxidant	Displayed high anti-oxidant activity, but this varied according to harvesting place, season and chemical composition (Barra *et al.* 2010).
Fennel, sweet (*Foeniculum vulgare* var. *dulce*)	Anti-oxidant Chemopreventative	Anti-oxidant activity identified by Mohamad *et al.* (2011). Miguel (2010) noted that for higher concentrations of oils (leaf 750mg/l, and seed > 1000mg/l), the anti-oxidant activity decreases, and higher concentrations display a pro-oxidant activity, independent of their *trans*-anethole (leaf) or methyl chavicol[3] (seed) content. Hepatoprotective actions due to presence of *d*-limonene and β-myrcene (Ozbek *et al.* 2003).
Frankincense (*Boswellia carterii*, *B. sacra*)	Anti-oxidant Antiproliferative Apoptosis-inducing	Yang *et al.* (2010) reported that in their study, along with peppermint, frankincense oil had the best free radical (ABTS) scavenging ability. Frank *et al.* (2009) investigated the effects of *B. carterii* oil on bladder cancer J82 cells and normal bladder urothelial cells; at a range of concentrations the oil suppressed viability in cancer cells, but not normal cells – apparently distinguishing between the cells. The frankincense activated genes that were responsible for cell cycle arrest, cell growth suppression and apoptosis in J82 cells, but it did not cause DNA fragmentation (which is normal in apoptosis). Dozmorov *et al.* (2014) demonstrated that *B. carterii* essential oil elicited selective bladder cancer cell death via NRF-2-mediated oxidative stress. *B. sacra* essential oil induced breast cancer cell-specific cytotoxicity – it suppressed signalling pathways and cell cycle regulators – and shows promise as a therapeutic agent for treating breast cancer[4] (Suhail *et al.* 2011).
Ginger (*Zingiber officinale*)	Anti-oxidant Anti-tumour	Free radical scavenging and also ferric-reducing power noted by Miguel 2010; potent anti-oxidant capacity also noted by Shaaban, El-Ghorab and Shibamoto 2012, Rahmani, Al Shabrmi and Aly 2014. Inhibits tumour development via various mechanisms, including upregulation of tumour suppression gene, cell cycle arrest, induction of apoptosis, and inhibition of angiogenesis. A constituent, 6-gingerol, is significant in these activities (Rahmani, Al Shabrmi and Aly 2014). The essential oil contains 7.2–7.3% β-sesquiphellandrene, which has anti-oxidant and *in vitro* anti-tumoural actions (Tisserand and Young 2014).
Juniperberry (*Juniperus communis*)	Anti-oxidant	Anti-oxidant activity highlighted by Shaaban, El-Ghorab and Shibamoto (2012).

Lavender, true (*Lavandula angustifolia*)	Anti-oxidant Anti-atherosclerosis	Inhaled lavender reduced cholesterol in the aorta and atherosclerotic plaques (Nikolaevskii *et al.* 1990). Yang *et al.* (2010) reported that lavender (from Australia) was significantly more effective against lipid peroxidation that the five other oils studied. Also, in an assay determining free radical scavenging ability (DPPH), lavender exhibited the strongest performance, similar to that of *d*-limonene. (However, lemon oil did not perform as well as *d*-limonene alone.)
Lemon (*Citrus limon*)	LDL anti-oxidant Anti-atherosclerosis	Contains up to 13% γ-terpinene, an LDL anti-oxidant. It is possible that the essential oil might play a preventative role in the development of atherosclerosis (Takahashi *et al.* 2003).
Lemon balm (*Melissa officinalis*)	Anti-cancer	Anti-cancer activity against several human and a mouse cancer cell lines, *in vitro* (de Sousa *et al.* 2004).
Lemongrass (*Cymbopogon citratus*, *C. flexuosus*)	Anti-cancer Apoptosis-inducing Antiproliferative Chemopreventative	*C. flexuosus* essential oil showed anti-cancer activity by activating apoptosis and reducing tumour cell viability *in vitro* and *in vivo*, via injection (Sharma *et al.* 2009). Citral, a major component of lemongrass, has a chemopreventative effect. Chaouki *et al.* (2009, cited by Guimarães, Quintans and Quintans-Júnior 2013) showed that it can inhibit cell proliferation and induce apoptosis in the MCF-7 (breast cancer) cell line.
Ginger (*Zingiber officinale*)	Anti-oxidant Anti-cancer Chemopreventative	In a review of the cancer-preventative properties of ginger, Shukla and Sing (2007) attributed the anti-cancer properties of ginger to its pungent components gingerol and paradol.
Lime (*Citrus aurantifolium*)	Antiproliferative LDL anti-oxidant Anti-atherosclerosis	The essential oil caused apoptosis-mediated inhibition of proliferation of human colon cancer cell lines (Patil *et al.* 2009). Contains up to 15% (expressed) and 12% (distilled) γ-terpinene, an LDL anti-oxidant; it is possible that the essential oil might play a preventative role in the development of atherosclerosis (Takahashi *et al.* 2003).
Long pepper (*Piper longum*)	Anti-oxidant Apoptosis-inducing Antiproliferative	The oil and piperine displayed anti-oxidant, apoptotic and restorative actions against the proliferative and mutagenic responses and phenotypic alterations; it could be used in immunocompromised conditions (Zaveri *et al.* 2010).
Mandarin (peel) (*Citrus reticulata*)	LDL anti-oxidant Anti-atherosclerosis	Contains up to 22% γ-terpinene, an LDL anti-oxidant. It is possible that the essential oil might play a preventative role in the development of atherosclerosis (Takahashi *et al.* 2003).
Mandarin petitgrain (leaves) (*Citrus reticulata*)	LDL anti-oxidant Anti-atherosclerosis	Contains up to 29% γ-terpinene, an LDL anti-oxidant. It is possible that the essential oil might play a preventative role in the development of atherosclerosis (Takahashi *et al.* 2003).

Marjoram, wild (*Majorana hortensis*)	Anti-oxidant	Activity might be due to synergism between carvacrol and other components (Martino *et al.* 2010).
Mastic (*Pistacia lentiscus*)	Hypolipidemic	*Pistacia lentiscus* var. *chia* gum (the essential oil contains α-pinene, β-myrcene, *d*-limonene, terpinen-4-ol, and others) displayed strong lipid-lowering action (Vallianou *et al.* 2011).
Monarda species	Anti-atherosclerosis	Inhaled monarda reduced cholesterol in the aorta and atherosclerotic plaques (Nikolaevskii *et al.* 1990).
Myrrh (*Commiphora myrrha*)	Anti-cancer Apoptosis-inducing Hypolipidemic (potential)	Chen *et al.* (2013) investigated the anti-cancer activities of both myrrh and frankincense against a range of human cancer cell lines. They found that a significant inhibitory effect was observed with myrrh essential oil in comparison with frankincense and a mixture of the two oils, and they suggested that apoptosis-induction was a major factor in its biological activity (especially in relation to MCF-7 cells – a breast cancer line). They also found that β-elemene was more active than frankincense and myrrh. The resins of *C. mukul* (India) and *C. molmol* (Egypt) have been developed as anti-hyperlipidemia (and also anti-schistosomal) agents (Shen *et al.* 2012).
Narcissus absolute (*Narcissus poeticus*)	LDL anti-oxidant Anti-atherosclerosis	Contains up to 28% γ-terpinene, an LDL anti-oxidant; it is possible that the essential oil might play a preventative role in the development of atherosclerosis (Takahashi *et al.* 2003).
Neroli (*Citrus aurantium* var. *amara* flos.)	Antimicrobial	Neroli oil displayed marked antibacterial activity, notably against *Pseudomonas aeruginosa*, and very strong antifungal (anti-*Candida*) activity in comparison with Nystatin (Ammar *et al.* 2012).
Nutmeg (*Myristica fragrans*)	Antiproliferative Chemopreventative	Eugenol in nutmeg oil had antiproliferative activity (apoptosis-induced) against a range of cancer cell lines and animal models (Jaganthan and Supriyanto 2012). The essential oil has hepatoprotective activity, probably related to its major constituent myristicin, and the likely mechanisms are: 1. Inhibition of TNF-α release from macrophages and suppression of apoptosis (Morita *et al.* 2003). 2. Induction of a detoxifying enzyme glutathione-S transferase (Ahmad, Tijerina and Tobola 1997). 3. Induction of cytotoxicity in human neuroblastoma cells by inducing apoptosis (Lee *et al.* 2005).
Orange, sweet (*Citrus sinensis*)	Chemopreventative Anti-oxidant	Hepatoprotective activity, due to *d*-limonene (Bodake *et al.* 2002). Singh *et al.* (2010) reported that the essential oil, characterised by *d*-limonene, has considerable anti-oxidant activity.
Palmarosa (*Cymbopogon martini* var. *martini*)	Cancer suppression (potential)	Geraniol, which occurs in the essential oil at high levels of 59–84%, displayed cancer suppression activity via several mechanisms (Edris 2007).

Plant	Properties	Description
Patchouli (*Pogostemon cablin*)	Antiproliferative; Apoptosis-inducing	Jeong et al. (2013) demonstrated that patchouli alcohol, a major constituent of the essential oil (up to 33%), has anti-cancer activity in human colo-rectal cancer cells; it decreased cell growth and increased apoptosis.
Pepper, West African (*Piper guineese*)	Anti-oxidant; Inhibitor of α-amylase, α-glucosidase, and angiotensin-I converting enzyme	*Piper guineese* essential oil[5] is a potent free radical scavenger that inhibits α-amylase, α-glucosidase and angiotensin-I converting enzyme in a dose dependent manner; potential use in the management of type-2 diabetes and hypertension (Oboh et al. 2013).
Peppermint (*Mentha × piperita*)	Anti-oxidant	Peppermint displayed good free radical-scavenging ability in the ABTS test method (Yang et al. 2010). The anti-oxidant activity is perhaps due to its 1,8-cineole, menthone and *iso*-menthone content (Shaaban, El-Ghorab and Shibamoto 2012).
Perilla (*Perilla frutescens*)	Cancer suppression (potential)	The perillyl alcohol content would imply that it might be a promising antiproliferative agent (interfering with angiogenesis, and other anti-tumour activities) but it has not been shown to be a chemopreventative agent for various human cancers (Edris 2007).
Pine (*Pinus mugo*)	LDL anti-oxidant	Terpinolene in *P. mugo* has LDL antioxididative activity (Grassmann et al. 2003, 2005); therefore it is possible that the oil might play a preventative role in the development of atherosclerosis.
Pink pepper (*Schinus molle*)	Anti-oxidant; Apoptosis-inducing	The essential oil has been shown to have anti-inflammatory and anti-tumoural properties (Marongiu et al. 2004). Díaz et al. (2008) demonstrated that the essential oil[6] was a weak anti-oxidant that induced cytotoxicity in several cell lines via an apoptosis-like mechanism, concluding that it might have anti-tumoural effects. Martins et al. (2014) demonstrated that the essential oil has significant anti-oxidant activity with a low level of toxicity, and this warrants further studies in human tumour cell lines to assess its effects on cellular proliferation, viability and apoptosis, and potential as a therapeutic agent.
Plai (*Zingiber cassumunar*)	Anti-oxidant; Chemopreventative; Antiproliferative	Vimala, Norhanom and Yadav (1999) noted that *Z. cassumunar* (and *Z. officinale*) have strong tumour-inhibitory activity (no cytotoxicity) in human lymphoblastoid Raji cells. It was suggested that the rhizomes and their extracts could be used to prevent cancer at the tumour-promoting stage. Significant chemopreventative activity, where the essential oil was more effective than three out of the four control drugs,[7] and antiproliferative activity of the essential oil were demonstrated in an *in vitro* study with cancer cell lines[8] – suggesting the potential for cancer treatment (Manosroi, Dhumtanom and Manosroi 2006).

Plant	Properties	Description
Pomelo (*Citrus maxima* peel)	Anti-oxidant	Singh et al. (2010) reported that the essential oil, characterised by *d*-limonene, citral and 3,3-dimethyl-1-hexene, had considerable anti-oxidant activity.
Poplar bud (*Populus balsamifera*)	Anti-cancer Apoptosis-inducing	Poplar bud essential oil, and a main component *d*-α-bisabolol (isolated from spring buds), was assessed for cytotoxic activity against human lung carcinoma and colo-rectal carcinoma cell lines. Both displayed pronounced activity, the oil more than the isolated bisabolol – but both were more active than the *l*-form of α-bisabolol, which is well known for its apoptosis-inducing effects against glioma cells (Piochon-Gauthier et al. 2014).
Rosemary (*Rosmarinus officinalis*)	Anti-oxidant Hepatoprotective	Rosemary essential oil has anti-oxidant activity (it is a free radical scavenger) and has hepatoprotective effects. The liver is very susceptible to chemical-induced toxicity, and it is believed that xenobiotics are converted into reactive oxygen species that induce oxidative stress and damage the macromolecules. Rosemary essential oil is hepatoprotective and (at 5 and 10mg/kg) can reverse the activities of anti-oxidant enzymes catalase, peroxidase, glutathione peroxidase and glutathione reductase in the liver (Rašković et al. 2014).
Sage, Lebanese (*Salvia libanotica*)	Apoptosis-inducing Antiproliferative	*S. libanotica* essential oil inhibited cancer cell growth, cell cycle arrest and apoptosis in HCT116 human colon cancer cells, but not in normal intestinal cells. The effects were thought to be due to synergistic interactions between linalyl acetate, terpineol and camphor, and the mechanism of action was proposed (Itani et al. 2008).
Sandalwood (*Santalum album*)	Antiproliferative Apoptosis-inducing	Used in traditional Chinese medicine for cancer prevention and therapy, Dozmorov et al. (2014) found that sandalwood essential oil induced non-selective cancer cell[9] death via DNA damage and cell cycle arrest.
Szechuan (Japanese) pepper (*Zanthoxylum piperitum*)	Anti-oxidant	Of 100 plant extracts screened for anti-oxidant activity and free radical scavenging ability, *X. piperitum* was one of 14 identified as a good source of natural anti-oxidants (Kim et al. 1997).
Tagetes (*Tagetes minuta*)	Anti-oxidant Anti-inflammatory	Karimian, Kavoosi and Amirghofran (2014) demonstrated that tagetes essential oil is a good anti-oxidant: it scavenges superoxide, H_2O_2 and NO radicals, and reduces oxidative stress. This activity was attributed to phenolic groups and/or due to an inhibition of iNOS and NOX gene expressions. It also decreased the expression of genes for the pro-inflammatory cytokine TNF-α. Based on these results, it was suggested that the essential oil could be used in therapy against oxidative damage, and in the management of some inflammatory diseases.

Tea tree (*Melaleuca alternifolia*)	LDL anti-oxidant Anti-atherosclerosis Anti-cancer Anti-oxidant	The constituents γ-terpinene (Takahashi *et al.* 2003) and terpinolene (Grassmann *et al.* 2003, 2005) are LDL anti-oxidants, therefore it is possible that tea tree oil might play a preventative role in the development of atherosclerosis. Calcabrini *et al.* (2004) demonstrated that the essential oil and terpinen-4-ol induced apoptosis in human melanoma cells, probably by interacting with plasma membranes. Kim *et al.* (2004) identified anti-oxidant activity in the essential oil, possibly due to α-terpinene, β-terpinene and β-terpinolene (Shaaban, El-Ghorab and Shibamoto 2012).
Thyme (*Thymus vulgaris* and other species)	Anti-oxidant	*Thymus vulgaris* essential oil has appreciable anti-oxidant activity, comparable to α-tocopherol (Wei and Shibamoto 2010a, b). *Thymus zygis* and *T. zygis* subsp. *sylvestris* from Portugal have good anti-oxidant activities (Dandlen *et al.* 2010).
Turmeric (*Curcuma longa*)	Anti-cancer Anti-oxidant	Cheng, Chang and Wu (2001) demonstrated that a hepatic arterial infusion had a positive effect in treating primary liver cancer (comparable effect to chemical drugs). Tisserand and Young (2014) noted that turmeric displayed significant anti-oxidant and anticarcinogenic activity; this may be, in part, due to the presence of β-sesquiphellandrene (8.8–9.5%).[10]
Yuzu (*Citrus × junos*)	LDL anti-oxidant Anti-atherosclerosis	The essential oil contains 12–13% γ-terpinene, an LDL anti-oxidant; the essential oil might play a preventative role in the development of atherosclerosis (Takahashi *et al.* 2003).

1. Cyclophosphamide is an anti-cancer drug.

2. Glycation is the binding of sugars such as fructose and glucose with proteins or lipids, leading to the formation of advanced glycation products (AGEs), which, in the presence of free radicals, are involved in further cross-linking with proteins. This causes hardening of the tissue (e.g. cardiovascular structures and also collagen in the skin). AGEs are implicated in many diseases such as cancers, cardiovascular disease, Alzheimer's and peripheral neuropathy. Causes can be exogenous, for example where sugars are cooked with fats at high temperatures, forming carcinogenic and inflammatory acrylamides, or endogenous, where if there is a high blood sugar level, absorbed simple sugars form AGEs. It is interesting to note that dried cypress needles are used in traditional medicine for the treatment of diabetes (Selim *et al.* 2014).

3. Methyl chavicol; often called estragole.

4. Hussain *et al.* (2013), commenting on this and other studies, noted that tumour cell plasticity allows malignant tumour cells to express endothelial cell-specific markers and form multicellular spheroid aggregates that afford protection for cancer cells against some chemotherapeutic drugs. These spheroids have been used in screening tests for anti-cancer drugs; *B. sacra* can disrupt these aggregates and spheroids, and might be considered for the treatment of invasive breast cancer.

5. Oboh *et al.* (2013) state that the main constituents of the essential oil are α-pinene, β-pinene, *cis*-ocimene, myrcene, *allo*-ocimene and 1,8-cineole.

6. This essential oil had β-pinene and α-pinene as major constituents.

7. These were 1% DMSO 5-FU, MTX and vincristine.
8. In both studies, these were human mouth epidermal carcinoma (KB) and murine leukaemia cell lines P388.
9. Human bladder cancer cells J82 and immortalised normal bladder urothelial UROtsa cells were used in this study.
10. β-Sesquiphellandrene is a monocyclic sesquiterpenoid polyalkene; also found in ginger (Tisserand and Young 2014).

Chapter 10

Infection and Immunity

Antimicrobial and Immunomodulant Actions

Essential oils display a broad spectrum of antimicrobial activity, evidenced in numerous publications. However, they may also have a role to play in combating antibiotic resistance and stimulating the immune system. In this chapter we will examine antimicrobial activity and immunomodulation to establish potential aromatherapeutic applications.

Antimicrobial activity and antibiotic resistance

Saad, Muller and Lobstein (2013), in their review of the major bioactivities of essential oils, noted that the significant divergence in results could be due to differing compositions as a result of natural variations, also the methods of analysis, and not least the solubility of the oil or its components, and the use of emulsifiers to overcome solubility problems. However, activity is also dependent on the target micro-organisms, and some are more resilient than others.

The 'Gram stain' is a staining technique that differentiates bacteria into two large groups based on the properties of their cell walls. It is often noted that the antimicrobial actions of essential oils are more pronounced against Gram-positive than Gram-negative bacteria. It has been suggested that this is because the Gram-negative bacteria have an outer phospholipidic membrane which renders them virtually impermeable to the lipophilic constituents in essential oils. This barrier is not present in Gram-positive bacteria – and so the hydrophobic constituents can act on the cell membrane, causing damage, altered ion-permeability, leakage, and enzyme impairment (Selim *et al.* 2014).

In modern medicine, antibiotic therapy has been commonplace, and indiscriminate use and indeed overuse has led to antibiotic resistance, which is now a major public health concern. Since the 1990s there has been a search for new antimicrobial agents, but despite the developments in molecular biology and screening technologies, 'new' antibiotics have not been found.

Yap *et al.* (2014) suggest that the reason for this failure is that 'too much emphasis has been placed on identifying targets and molecules that interact, while too little placed on the actual ability of these molecules to permeate the bacterial cell wall, evade influx and avoid mutational resistance' (p.6). They also suggest that antibiotics with a single target are especially vulnerable to mutational resistance. In their comprehensive review they discuss the modes of action of antibiotics and how bacteria have developed resistance. Several themes emerge that highlight the potential future role of essential oils as 'phytopharmaceuticals'. First, essential oils are distinct and versatile, because their chemical and structural variance, the activity of major and minor constituents, and the capacity for synergistic interactions ensure that they are not 'single target' agents. Spontaneous bacterial resistance is less likely to occur because of their complex composition; however, there is limited evidence to suggest that resistance is indeed possible, and would certainly be more likely if essential oils were to become routinely applied in the clinical arena. Second, essential oils are capable of cell wall and membrane disturbance,[1] they can inhibit the bacterial efflux pump,[2] and inhibit quorum sensing[3] – and so they have huge potential as natural alternatives to synthetic antibiotics. Third, combination therapy, where essential oils and antibiotics are used together, is on the horizon; there is evidence of synergistic interactions,[4] and essential oils could be used as resistance-modifying agents. For example, geraniol reduced chloramphenicol[5] resistance in *Enterobacter aerogenes*[6] via efflux pump inhibition, and modulated the intrinsic resistance of the wild-type control strain and other Gram-negative bacteria. Geraniol was identified as a potent inhibitor of efflux mechanisms; it is synergistic with β-lactams and the fluoroquinolone norfloraxin, and the combination could be used to combat multidrug-resistant Gram-negative bacteria such as *Enterobacter aerogenes* (Lorenzi *et al.* 2009).

Perhaps the best known example of bacterial antibiotic resistance is *Staphylococcus aureus* – a highly adaptive, Gram-positive bacterium that can cause superficial skin infections, infected, deep abcesses and life-threatening infections. Methicillin-resistant (and vancomycin-resistant) strains are now a real cause for concern – they are a major cause of skin and soft tissue infections, and hospitalised patients are at considerable risk.[7] Muthaiyan *et al.* (2012a) noted the recent increase

---

1   Essential oils are lipophilic and can bind to proteins and glycoproteins; they can permeate bacterial cell walls and have an affinity for cell membranes, leading to the leakage of cell contents.

2   This is a bacterial mechanism that enables cells to 'pump out' a large range of compounds, including synthetic antibiotics.

3   Quorum sensing (QS) is an important part of bacterial ecology; QS is a form of 'signalling' – where QS bacteria accumulate signalling molecules that stimulate bacterial motility and swarming, biofilm formation and stress resistance.

4   For example, rosewood and gentamicin, geranium and gentamicin, coriander with chloramphenicol, ciprofloxacin, gentamicin and tetracyclin, eugenol with vancomycin (Yap *et al.* 2014, p.9).

5   Chloramphenicol is not currently used as an antibiotic against Gram-negative bacteria – β-lactams such as ampicillin and penicillin, and quinolones such as norfloxacin, are preferred, although resistance to these is a major problem. Geraniol is synergistic with β-lactams and norfloxacin.

6   *Enterobacter aerogenes* is a Gram-negative bacterium that is found in the GI tract. It is an opportunistic pathogen, and a risk to hospitalised individuals; it can cause bacteremia, lower respiratory tract infections, skin and soft tissue infections and endocarditis; it is multidrug resistant, and particularly resistant to β-lactams.

7   Patients admitted to hospital with burn wounds are at high risk from MRSA infection. Normally, dressings and topical antimicrobial agents are used as a preventative in burn and wound care; Muthaiyan *et al.* (2012b) evaluated the effects of CPV as a potential anti-staphylococcal agent on wound dressings; their *in vitro* study showed that it had promise, and that further studies to establish safety and efficacy would be recommended.

in infections due to MRSA – now a worldwide public health concern – and the increasing incidence of antibiotic therapy failure. They tested a range of aromatic products derived from cold-pressed Valencia orange (*Citrus sinensis*)[8] against a range of methicillin-resistant and susceptible, and methicillin and vancomycin intermediate-resistant strains of *Staphylococcus aureus*. Of the eight aromatics, it was found that the terpeneless, cold-pressed Valencia orange oil (CPV) and cold-pressed citronellal had the highest level of inhibition agains all test strains. In order to clarify the mode of action against MRSA, they identified the effect of CPV on the bacterial cell lysis related gene expression, confirming that it potentially acts on cell walls as well as membranes, and that CPV may also repress the 'SOS' system that the bacterium uses to survive adverse conditions. Muthaiyan *et al.* (2012a) concluded that CPV has potential as an 'alternative natural therapeutic antimicrobial agent against MRSA.

Notable antibacterial constituents

Phenolic constituents such as carvacrol, thymol and eugenol are very active against a broad spectrum of micro-organisms, possibly due to their phenol ring structure. The isomers thymol and carvacrol display different activities against Gram-positive and Gram-negative bacteria,[9] suggesting that the position of the hydroxy group on the phenol ring also has significance. Other types of isomers show varying activities. In general, α-isomers are more active than β-isomers, which are relatively inactive, and *trans*-isomers are more active than *cis*-isomers. It would appear that esters are more active than their parent alcohols – for example, the ester group in geranyl acetate and bornyl acetate increases antimicrobial activity in comparison with geraniol and borneol. However, alcohols tend to be bactericidal rather than bacteriostatic, and some are very effective, possibly because they denature proteins in the cell walls. The carbonyl functional group, found in ketones and aldehydes, also increases antimicrobial activity. Possibly the most active antimicrobial components are terpinolene, α-terpineol and terpinen-4-ol – all constituents with unsaturated ring structures (Saad, Muller and Lobstein 2013).

Lang and Buchbauer (2012) reviewed the recent (2008–2010) research on essential oils as antimicrobial agents. They concluded that although many essential oils have strong antimicrobial activity across a range of micro-organisms, the prevailing constituents were thymol and carvacrol, cinnamaldehyde, eugenol, camphor, limonene, linalool, α-pinene, terpinen-4-ol and 1,8-cineole. They also noted that, even with the chemical complexity of essential oils, microbes could

---

8   These were the cold-pressed essential oil, terpeneless essential oil, cold-pressed orange terpenes, high purity orange terpenes, *d*-limonene, and terpenes from orange essence. All products are commercially available.

9   Gram-negative bacteria (such as *E. coli*) are generally more resistant to essential oils, partly because of the lipopolysaccharide in the outer membranes (Gulfraz *et al.* 2008).

develop tolerance by habituation – especially if sub-optimal concentrations are used.

Notable antifungal constituents

In 2007 Abad, Ansuategui and Bermejo suggested that fungi are among the 'most neglected pathogens', and that the current antimycotic drug – amphotericin B – was actually discovered in 1956! In reality, serious systemic fungal infections are on the rise, and difficult to treat, and resistant strains are appearing. Aromatic plants are the source of many natural antimycotics – often from the Lamiaceae and Asteraceae families. For example, *Thymus vulgaris* CT thymol was highly effective against the yeast *Candida albicans* (Giordani *et al.* 2004), and linalool isolated from *Lavandula angustifolia* was more active against clinical *Candida albicans* strains than the essential oil, while linalyl acetate was ineffective. In the Asteraceae, *Artemisia absinthium*, *A. santonicum* and *A. spicigera* have potent, broad spectrum antifungal activity; camphor and 1,8-cineole are their common constituents that display comparable activity (Kordali *et al.* 2005).

The dermatophytic fungi – the ones that infect human skin, hair and nails – comprise *Epidermophyton*, *Microsporum* and *Trichophyton* species. In their review, Lang and Buchbauer (2012) noted that the constituents which were prevalent in the most active essential oils were phenylpropanoids such as methyl chavicol and eugenol, and the monocyclic sesquiterpene alcohol α-bisabolol. It was also observed that camphor could increase activity against some dermatophytes. There is a strong possibility that the monoterpene sabinene, found in substantial amounts in plai (*Zingiber cassumunar*), yarrow (*Achillea millefolium*) and nutmeg (*Myristica fragrans*) essential oil, has anti-dermatophytic activity (Valente *et al.* 2013).

Although *Candida* species are part of our normal flora, inhabiting the gut, genito-urinary tract and the skin, some are opportunistic pathogens, and can cause local and systemic infections. The most common yeasts that cause candidiasis are *Candida albicans* and, to a lesser extent, *C. glabrata* and *C. tropicalis*. This can be a serious problem for immunosuppressed individuals. In a few cases the mode of action of anti-candida essential oils has been investigated; for example, the main components of *Ocimum sanctum* essential oil were able to exert a synergistic effect in inhibiting essential proton pumps (Khan *et al.* 2010, cited by Lang and Buchbauer 2012). The most active component of clove essential oil, eugenol, can impair ergosterol synthesis and cause cell wall rupture, and impair germ tube development (Pinto *et al.* 2009).

Lang and Buchbauer (2012) noted that the constituents most active against yeasts were eugenol, thymol and carvacrol; however, other notable constituents were geraniol, citral, α-pinene, γ-terpinene, *para*-cymene, terpinen-4-ol, methyl eugenol, methyl chavicol and 1,8-cineole. The antifungal activity of citral was the subject of a study conducted by Tao, OuYang and Jia (2014); however, it was *Penicillium italicum* – a problematic citrus fruit post-harvest decay fungus, not a dermatophyte – that was investigated. However, the research did reveal the antifungal mechanism. Citral caused morphological alterations to the mycelia[10] (the vegetative growth structure) due to a loss of cytoplasm. Increased exposure to citral caused increased membrane permeability, with release of cell constituents, increased extracellular pH and leakage of potassium ions, and a decrease in cellular lipids and ergosterol. This is all indicative of the disruption of membrane integrity and permeability.

Antiviral potential

Viruses are very small, infectious particles that consist of genetic material and a protein 'coat'; some are also surrounded by an 'envelope'. They infect cells of another organism, where they can replicate – most viruses cannot survive for long, or reproduce, outside a host cell. Viral infection instigates an immune response in the host. Essential oils have potential to treat some of the common human viral infections such as *Herpes simplex* types I and II (cold sores are caused by HSVI and genital herpes by HSVII), and they have very low toxicity in comparison with many antiviral drugs such as acyclovir. Studies cited by Adorjan and Buchbauer (2010) have identified several essential oils with activity against the debilitating HSVII, including anise (*Pimpinella anisum*), hyssop (*Hyssopus officinalis*), thyme (*Thymus vulgaris*), ginger (*Zingiber officinale*), German chamomile (*Matricaria recutita*) and sandalwood (*Santalum album*). It transpired that often the results are dose dependent, and depend on the stage in the viral infection cycle at which they are introduced; some are less active during the pre-incubation period and after the adsorption period. They suggested that the oils tested interact with the viral envelope.

Edris (2007) reviewed a small range of *in vitro* studies that confirmed the antiviral potential of essential oils, but did not find any literature concerning the antiviral activity of essential oils against epidemic viruses such as HIV or hepatitis C. However, it has been demonstrated that greater mugwort (*Artemisia arborescens*) essential oil, when incorporated in liposomes and delivered into infected cells, was active against HSV1;[11] lemon balm (*Melissa officinalis*) could inhibit the replication of HSVII,[12] probably because of citral and citronellal; and lemongrass (botanical name not given) at a low concentration of 0.1%, has potent HSVI activity, completely inhibiting viral replication for 24 hours. Other essential oils mentioned in Edris' review with regard to their antiviral activity (preceding adsorption and penetration into cells) were peppermint (*Mentha × piperita*), tea tree (*Melaleuca alternifolia*), and to a lesser extent eucalyptus (*Eucalyptus globulus*). Adorjan and Buchbauer (2010) noted that studies had revealed that the whole oils of *Eucalyptus globulus*, *Melaleuca alternifolia*, *Illicium verum* and *Thymus* spp. are

10 This can be witnessed with other secondary metabolites including some mycotoxins.
11 It is thought that it inactivates the virus and inhibits cell-to-cell virus diffusion.
12 Possibly by affecting the virus before adsorption but not after penetration.

more effective than their component monoterpenes and monoterpenoids, and act in a dose-dependent manner, during the adsorption phase.

It is clear that more studies are required to elucidate the antiviral activity of essential oils and their therapeutic potential; however, in the context of aromatherapy, it is strongly advised that treatment of some viral infections such as HSVII is not attempted.

Immunomodulation

Immunomodulation is, literally, a procedure that alters the immune system of an organism by interfering with its functions; if this enhances the system it is called immunostimulation, and refers to non-specific stimulation of, for example, granulocytes, lymphocytes and natural killer cells, and also to the production of mediators. This is called '*para*-immunity'. It has been noted that many plants and their isolated constituents can enhance normal cellular and humoral immunity, and some can also restore suppressed immunity. Stress, autoimmune disease and nutritional deficiency can suppress immunity, and so plants and their extracts, including essential oils, could be valuable therapeutic agents in such instances (Carrasco 2009).

Saad, Muller and Lobstein (2013) note that the immunomodulatory actions of essential oils such as tea tree (*Melaleuca alternifolia*), clove (*Syzygium aromaticum*) and lemongrass (*Cymbopogon citratus*) can be related to their anti-inflammatory effects and their impact on interleukins. As one example they cite Ramage *et al.* (2012) who demonstrated that tea tree oil, well known for its antimicrobial and antifungal actions, and its principal active component terpinen-4-ol, reduced the expression of interleukin-8, a major inflammatory mediator in oropharyngeal candidiasis. They also discuss possible modes of action for eugenol and clove essential oil, suggesting that a synergistic effect between eugenol and terpinen-4-ol might be worthy of investigation. In relation to the mode of action of lemongrass and its major components neral and geranial (citral), they ask 'is there a difference between the molecular mechanism of the preventative and the therapeutic activity?' (p.277).

However, it might be wrong to assume that essential oils can exert only positive effects on immunity. Cosentino *et al.* (2014) investigated the effects of bergamot (*Citrus aurantium* L. subsp. *bergamia*) essential oil on reactive oxygen species (ROS) in human polymorphonuclear leukocytes and the role of Ca^{2+} in the responses. Bergamot essential oil increased the intracellular production of ROS, a process that required the presence of both extracellular and intracellular Ca^{2+}; it also significantly increased induced ROS production. It was suggested that this might be why bergamot has antimicrobial and tissue healing activity – because it has pro-inflammatory potential – and that as a result of these findings, the clinical uses of the oil require 'careful consideration'.

Olfaction and immune function

Trellakis *et al.* (2012) explored the hypothesis that olfactory cues could have immunomodulatory effects. Animal studies had revealed that, for example, long-term inhalation of lemon counteracted stress-induced immunosuppression (Fujiwara *et al.* 1998), and that inhaled linalool repressed stress and changed the gene expression of neutrophils and lymphocytes (Nakamura *et al.* 2009). However, Trellakis *et al.*'s *human* study investigated short-term (30 minutes) exposure in blindfolded male and female subjects. A selection of stimulant (grapefruit, fennel and pepper) and relaxing (lavender, patchouli and rose) oils were used; there was also a no-odour control. Outcomes were measured by psychological questionnaires and physiological parameters, namely the activity of neutrophil granulocytes and the peripheral blood concentrations of neutrophil-related immunological markers. It was shown that short-term subconscious odour exposure did not affect human immune functions. However, the discussion highlighted a few important factors that could have influenced this result – namely the choice of odours, whether the participants were conscious of the odours, human–animal differences, and perhaps wrong assumptions in relation to the mechanism of odour-to-immune effects. There may well be a difference in subconscious and conscious exposure, as well as short- and long-term exposure. Indeed, stimulant and relaxing odours may elicit different effects on the immune system as well as the central nervous system. Trellakis *et al.* also make the point that 'the effects of essential oils depend on the way of application and their concentration' (p.1914) – something that is of real relevance for aromatherapy, especially regarding the research and evidence base that underpins our practice. In this, as well as so many other areas, aromatherapy may have far-reaching therapeutic potential, but further studies are needed.

Table 10.1 Antimicrobial and immunomodulant actions

Essential oil	Actions	Evidence
Basil, African (*Ocimum gratissimum*)	Antifungal (dermatophytes and *Candida* species)	Active against *Microsporum canis*, *M. gypseum*, *Trichophyton rubrum*, *T. mentagrophytes* and *Cryptococcus neoformans*, *in vitro* (Silva *et al.* 2005, cited by Abad, Ansuategui and Bermejo 2007). Active against *Candida albicans*, *C. krusei*, *C. parapsilosis* and *C. tropicalis*; alters the cell wall structure and the morphology of some subcellular organelles (Nakamura *et al.* 2004, cited by Abad, Ansuategui and Bermejo 2007).
Basil, holy (*Ocimum sanctum*)	Immunostimulant Antifungal (active against *Candida* species)	Therapeutic potential in immunological disorders associated with immunosuppression (Prakash and Gupta 2005). Traditionally used in Ayurvedic medicine as an antimicrobial; Amber *et al.* (2010) demonstrated that the essential oil had activity against several pathogenic *Candida* strains, including fluconazole/ketoconazole resistant and sensitive strains.
Bay laurel (*Laurus nobilis*)	Antiviral	Out of seven Lebanese essential oils studied, bay laurel, containing β-ocimene, 1,8-cineole, α-pinene and β-pinene, showed most promising activity against SARS-CoV (Loizzo *et al.* 2008a).
Bergamot (*Citrus aurantium* var. *bergamia* fruct., *C. bergamia*)	Antimicrobial Antifungal (active against yeasts and dermatophytes)	Used in folk medicine for the treatment of infections (Bagetta *et al.* 2010). *In vitro* activity against clinically relevant *Candida* species (Romano *et al.* 2005). *In vitro* activity against common dermatophytes (Sanguinetti *et al.* 2007).
Carrot seed (*Daucus carota* subsp. *carota*)	Antifungal (active against dermatophytes)	The essential oil was very active against several dermatophytic species. The Portuguese oil was dominated by geranyl acetate and α-pinene; the more active Sardinian oil was dominated by β-bisabolene and 11-α-(h)-himachal-4-en-1-β-ol (Maxia *et al.* 2009).
Cedar, Lebanese (*Cedrus libani*)	Antiviral	This species is used in Lebanese traditional medicine to treat infections; the essential oil, containing himachalol (22.5%), β-himachalene (21.9%) and α-himachalene (10.5%), displayed activity against HSV1 (Loizzo *et al.* 2008b).
Chamomile, German (*Matricaria recutita*)	Antifungal	A study conducted by Pauli (2006) investigated the antifungal activity of α-bisabolol, a major component in the essential oil, concluding that it is a potential selective, non-toxic inhibitor of ergosterol biosynthesis.[1]
Cinnamon leaf (*Cinnamomum zeylanicum*)	Antibacterial Antifungal	The essential oil contains substantial amounts of eugenol (69–87%), which has substantial, broad spectrum antibacterial actions (Lang and Buchbauer 2012) and antifungal actions – particularly against yeasts, including *Candida* species (Saad, Muller and Lobstein 2013).

Plant	Properties	Details
Clove bud (*Syzygium aromaticum*)	Immunostimulant (cellular and humoral) Antifungal (*Candida* species) Antiviral	Clove essential oil increased the total white blood cell count and enhanced the delayed-type hypersensitivity response in mice, and also restored both cellular and humoral immune responses in immunosuppressed mice in a dose-dependent manner (Carrasco *et al.* 2009). The essential oil is highly active against several strains of *Candida*, impairing ergosterol synthesis and causing cell membrane rupture, and germ tube development was impaired (Pinto *et al.* 2009). Tragoolpua and Jatisatienr (2007) demonstrated that the essential oil has activity against HSVI and HSVII.
Combava petitgrain and peel (*Citrus hystrix*)	Antimicrobial (respiratory pathogens)	Srisukh *et al.* (2012) investigated the bioactivity of both the peel and leaf oils against 411 clinical isolates.[2] Combava peel and leaf oils were described as having 'excellent' activity against many respiratory pathogens, and indeed all of the isolated multidrug-resistant pathogens were 'highly sensitive'. One component in particular was highlighted for its activity – α-terpineol. This study certainly highlighted the potential of combava in this specific clinical area where drug resistance is a major problem, and some clinical uses were suggested.
Coriander seed (*Coriandrum sativum*)	Antibacterial	The essential oil displayed strong activity against *S. pyogenes*, *S. aureus* and MRSA, with excellent skin tolerance, and has potential as an antiseptic for the prevention and treatment of Gram-positive infections (Casetti *et al.* 2012).
Cypress (*Cupressus sempervirens*)	Antibacterial Antibiofilm	The essential oil displayed good antimicrobial activity against Gram-positive and Gram-negative bacteria, and *Klebsiella pneumoniae*[3] in particular. It was suggested that the activity was due in part to the major constituents α-pinene and cedrol. The essential oil and methanol extract both efficiently reduced biofilms of *K. pneumoniae* on biomaterial surfaces – and could be an option for controlling colonisation and microbial infections in the clinical environment (Selim *et al.* 2014).
Eucalyptus blue gum (*Eucalyptus globulus*)	Antibacterial	Cermelli *et al.* (2008) investigated the effects of *E. globulus* essential oil on a range of bacterial respiratory pathogens and two viruses (adenovirus and mumps virus). Its strongest activity was against *Haemophilus influenzae*, *H. parainfluenzae*, *Stenotrophomonas maltophilia* and *Streptococcus pneumoniae*. Antiviral activity was minimal.
Fennel seed (*Foeniculum vulgare*)	Antimicrobial	Fennel oil is active against a wide range of organisms, including Gram-positive and Gram-negative bacteria and yeasts. The essential oil was notably active against *Candida albicans*, *P. putida* and *Escherichia coli*; *trans*-anethole was named as an active constituent (Gulfraz *et al.* 2008).

Plant	Activity	Notes
Fennel, sweet (*Foeniculum vulgare* var. *dulce*)	Antifungal	Sweet fennel oil has antifungal activity, and could be used in the treatment of fungal nail infections (Patra *et al.* 2002).
Fir, Korean (*Abies koreana*)	Antimicrobial	The essential oil inhibited drug-resistant skin pathogen growth, notably *P. acnes* and *S. epidermidis*, which can be resistant to erythromycin and clindamycin (Yoon *et al.* 2009a).
Fir, silver (*Abies alba*)	Anti-oxidant	Yang *et al.* (2009) demonstrated that the essential oil, rich in bornyl acetate (30.31%), had strong radical scavenging activity but no activity against the bacterial strains tested, except mild activity against *S. aureus*.
Frankincense (*Boswellia carterii* and other species)	Antibacterial Antifungal	The essential oil of *B. carterii* was active against *E. coli*, *P. aeruginosa* and some strains of *S. aureus*, but not MRSA; the essential oils of another four limonene-containing *Boswellia* species had significant antifungal activity against *Candida albicans* and *C. tropicalis* (Camarda *et al.* 2007, cited by Hussain *et al.* 2013).
Geranium (*Pelargonium* × *asperum*, or *P. roseum* [a hybrid of *P. capitatum* × *P. radens*], *P. capitatum*, *P. radens*, *P. odoratissimum*)	Antifungal (*Candida* and *Trichophyton* species)	The essential oil (47% citronellol) was active against several *Candida* strains (Rosato *et al.* 2008). Maruyama, Takizawa and Ishibashi (2008) reported that the vaginal application of rose geranium essential oil (and its main component geraniol) suppressed *Candida* growth when combined with vaginal washing (an *in vivo* study with mice). The essential oil was active against *Trichophyton* species (Shin and Lim 2004, cited by Abad, Ansuategui and Bermejo 2007).
Ginger (*Zingiber officinale*)	Immunostimulant (humoral)	Ginger essential oil restored the humoral response in immunosuppressed mice (Carrasco *et al.* 2009).
Hemp, industrial (*Cannabis sativa*)	Antimicrobial	Industrial hemp contains very small amounts of the psychotropic delta-tetrahydrocannabinol (0.2%). The essential oil has very good activity against some Gram-positive bacteria, including GI pathogens such as *Enterococcus* species and *Clostridium* species, and some Gram-negative bacteria such as *Pseudomonas* species (Nissen *et al.* 2010).

Immortelle (*Helichrysum italicum*)	Bacterial resistance modification	The essential oil, used at a 2.5% concentration, significantly reduced the multidrug resistance of the Gram-negative *Enterobacter aerogenes*, *E. coli*, *Pseudomonas aeruginosa* and *Acetobacter baumanni* (Lorenzi *et al.* 2009). Immortelle was also included in a study investigating the antimicrobial activities of essential oils whose principal constituents have floral-rosy aromas (Jirovetz *et al.* 2006). All of the oils and most of the principal aroma compounds showed medium to high antimicrobial activities against both Gram-positive bacteria (including *Staphylococcus aureus* and *Enterococcus faecalis*) and Gram-negative bacteria (including *Escherichia coli* and *Salmonella* species) and also the yeast *Candida albicans*.
Juniperberry (*Juniperus communis*)	Antimicrobial	Glišić *et al.* (2007) investigated the antimicrobial activity of Siberian juniper essential oil and its fractions; the essential oil showed weak activity, but the fractions with a high α-pinene, or high α-pinene with sabinene content displayed good antimicrobial (and particularly antifungal) activity, and showed a wider spectrum of inhibition than antibiotics, including gentamycin, clindamycin, streptomycin, tetracycline, erythromycin, vancomycin, ampicillin and penicillin.
Lavender, true (*Lavandula angustifolia*)	Antimicrobial	De Rapper *et al.* (2013) explored the interactive *in vitro* antimicrobial properties of 45 essential oils when combined in various ratios with lavender (*Lavandula angustifolia*). They reported a 26.7% incidence of synergism, and 48.9% incidence of additive effects. There was only one instance of antagonism – a combination of lemongrass (*Cymbopogon citratus*) and lavender (*L. angustifolia*).
Lemon balm (*Melissa officinalis*)	Antiviral potential	Active against genital herpes (HSVII) *in vitro* (Allahverdiyev *et al.* 2004).
Lemon myrtle (*Backhousia citriodora*)	Antimicrobial	Significant activity against *Staphylococcus aureus*, MRSA, *Escherichia coli*, *Pseudomonas aerugionosa*, *Candida albicans*, *Klebsiella pneumoniae* and *Propionibacterium acnes* (Hayes and Markovic 2002).
Lemongrass (*Cymbopogon citratus* and *C. flexuosus*)	Antiviral potential	Active against cold sores (HSVI) *in vitro* (Minami *et al.* 2003).
Lemongrass (*Cymbopogon citratus*)	Immunostimulant (possibly preventative rather than therapeutic) Antifungal (*Candida* species)	Immunostimulant activity is related to the anti-inflammatory activity of the essential oil and citral, possibly by changing the homeostatic balance of opposing cellular processes (Saad, Muller and Lobstein 2013). Active against several strains of *Candida*, especially *C. albicans*; the essential oil contained 76% citral, which was equally active (Silva *et al.* 2008).

Manuka (*Leptospermum scoparium*)	Antimicrobial Antiviral	Used in traditional Maori medicine, and widely regarded as an antibacterial and antifungal essential oil; *Leptospermum scoparium* also has virucidal activity against HSV1, including drug-resistant isolates (Schnitzler, Wiesenhofer and Reichling 2008).
Myrtle (*Myrtus communis*)	Antifungal (*Aspergillus* and *Candida* infections)	Dominated by 1,8-cineole and α-pinene, the essential oil showed a synergistic effect when combined with amphotericin (Mahboubi and Ghazian Bidgoli 2010).
Nagarmotha (*Cyperus scariosus*)	Antibacterial Antifungal	In a review of the potential of the herb and essential oil, Bhwang *et al.* (2013) noted that the essential oil has antibacterial and antifungal actions.
Palmarosa (*Cymbopogon martinii*)	Antifungal (yeasts) Bacterial resistance modifier (potential)	The main constituent, geraniol (75–82%), is active against yeasts, including *Candida* species (Lang and Buchbauer 2012). Geraniol was identified as a potent inhibitor of efflux mechanisms; it is synergistic with β-lactams and the fluoroquinolone norfloraxin, and the combination could be used to combat multidrug-resistant Gram-negative bacteria (Lorenzi *et al.* 2009).
Patchouli (*Pogostemon cablin*)	Immunostimulant Antibacterial	Hu *et al.* (2006) suggested that the essential oil strengthens immune activity and resistance to bacterial infection. Yang *et al.* (2013) used molecular docking software technology, a procedure used in drug discovery studies, and *in vitro* tests,[4] to evaluate the antibacterial activity of patchouli essential oil. The essential oil itself had strong antimicrobial effects – possibly due to multi-target effects because of its complex composition (26 constituents were assessed). For example, *l*-patchouli alcohol, α-guaiene and *trans*-β-farnesene caused bacterial cell wall defects similar to benzylpenicillin; others such as pogostone, *trans-trans*-farnesol, *trans*-β-caryophyllene, *l*-germacrene and α-humulene hindered bacterial folic acid metabolism, as with sulfadiazine and trimethoprim; while others such as *trans-trans*-α-farnesene and *l*-nerolidol could inhibit bacterial DNA replication, as does ciprofloxacin. However, *l*-patchouli alcohol and pogostone were considered to be the most significant in terms of antibacterial activity because of their multi-target effects. It was concluded that patchouli oil had broad therapeutic prospects in bacterial infection.
Pink pepper (*Schinus molle*)	Antimicrobial Antifungal	Traditionally used in the treatment of infectious diseases, *S. molle* extracts and essential oil are active against a wide range of bacteria, including *Klebsiella pneumoniae*, *Pseudomonas aeruginosa* and *Escherichia coli*, *Listeria monocytogenes*, *Staphylococcus aureus*, *Streptococcus pyogenes*, *Streptococcus pneumoniae*, *Haemophilus influenzae* and *Mycobacterium tuberculosis*, *Bacillus cereus*, *Salmonella enteritidis*; and dermatophytes, including *Microsporum gypseum*, *Trichophyton mentagrophytes*, *T. rubrum* (Perez-López *et al.* 2011).

Plai (*Zingiber cassumunar*)	Antimicrobial Antifungal	The essential oil has antimicrobial and antifungal actions (Lang and Buchbauer 2012; Saad, Muller and Lobstein 2013). The essential oil contains up to 45% terpinen-4-ol, which has antimicrobial actions. Pithayanukul, Tubprasert and Wuthi-Udomlert (2007) evaluated the *in vitro* antimicrobial activity of plai essential oil and a 5% plai oil gel. The oil displayed antimicrobial activity across a wide range of both Gram-positive and Gram-negative bacteria, dermatophytes and yeasts (possibly due to the presence of sabinene); however, bacteria were less susceptible than dermatophytes and yeasts.
Rosemary (*Rosmarinus officinalis*)	Anti-oxidant Antibacterial (including *P. acnes*)	Fu *et al.* (2007) reported that the essential oil was active against *P. acnes*, attributed to 1,8-cineole, α-pinene, camphor and camphene.
Sage (*Salvia* species)	Antimicrobial	Some sage essential oils display strong antimicrobial activity (Lang and Buchbauer 2012). Essential oil of *S. officinalis* did not display immunomodulatory activity, contrary to expectations (Carrasco *et al.* 2009).
Tea tree (*Melaleuca alternifolia*)	Antimicrobial Antiviral	'Outstanding effect against a wide spectrum of micro-organisms', including MRSA, *S. aureus*, *L. pneumophilia* and dermatophytes. Some *Pseudomonas aeruginosa* strains are resistant (Lang and Buchbauer 2012, p.36). Tea tree oil shows promise in the treatment of influenza, having an inhibitory effect on A/PR/8 virus subtype H1N1 replication at non-cytotoxic concentrations (Garozzo *et al.* 2009).
Thyme (*Thymus vulgaris*)	Antifungal (*Candida* species)	Studies cited by Lang and Buchbauer (2012); also showed antagonism with amphotericin B.
Thyme (*Thymus zygis*)	Antimicrobial (MSSA)	A blend of four cultivars of *T. zygis* with a high concentration of thymol (31.1%), linalool (23.6%), and a relatively high concentration of α-terpinene (13.2%) and terpinen-4-ol (11.7%) and also 1.1% carvacrol had 'substantial' anti-staphylococcal activity (against MSSA), compared with a linalool chemotype (Caplin, Allan and Hanlon 2009).

1. Ergosterol synthesis is an important step in the formation of fungal cell walls. This example shows a different mode of action to that of existing antifungal drugs, and this is significant because of emerging problems with resistance – for example in the case of *Candida albicans*.

2. These included *Acinetobacter baumannii*, *Haemophilus influenzae*, methicillin-resistant and methicillin-sensitive *Staphylococcus aureus* (MRSA and MSSA) and *Streptococcus pneumoniae* strains.

3. *K. pneumonia* is a Gram-negative bacterium; it is a normal part of the skin, mouth and gut microflora, but if aspirated, it can cause infection in the lower respiratory tract and lungs, resulting in inflammation and haemorrhage. It is thus an opportunistic pathogen, and commonly implicated in nosocomial (hospital-acquired) infections.

4. The test bacteria were *E. coli*, *P. aeruginosa*, *Bacillus proteus*, *Shigella dystenteriae*, *Typhoid bacillus* and *S. aureus*.

Chapter 11

Respiratory Support

*Expectorant, Mucolytic, Decongestant
and Antitussive Actions*

Aromatic vapours reach the tissues of the respiratory tract easily via inhalation, and therefore the molecules may have direct effects on the cells of the mucous membranes. We witness a range of actions as a consequence.

Expectorant, mucolytic and antitussive actions

Expectorant effects are due to the stimulation of the mucous-producing goblet cells and cilia of the respiratory tract. Some essential oil constituents, such as 1,8-cineole, are noted not only for expectorant action but also anti-inflammatory action, meaning that they are of particular value in problems such as asthma and congestion. For example, inhalation of a product containing 1,8-cineole helped patients with chronic obstructive bronchitis by aiding expectoration, decreasing coughing and lengthening the breath (Ulmer and Schott 1991, cited by Bowles 2003). However, the fact that the cells of the tract are stimulated means that they may also be irritated, so caution must be exercised. Tisserand and Young (2014) state that essential oils that contain significant amounts of 1,8-cineole (including the oils mentioned in Table 11.1) can cause central nervous system and breathing problems in young children, and that such oils must not be applied to (or near) their faces.

Antitussive agents can work in two ways – by acting centrally on the cough centre of the brain, or peripherally on the cough receptors in the respiratory system, via protection and demulcent actions. However, some essential oils are credited with antitussive actions that are of value in conditions where cough is a symptom. Usually antitussive action is combined with expectorant and mucolytic actions, and often with antibacterial action.

Franchomme and Pénoël (1990) suggest that ketones are able to reduce mucosal secretions. This has not been established, but some ketones such as menthone in peppermint (*Mentha piperita*), *l*-carvone in spearmint (*M. spicata*) and camphor in common sage (*Salvia officinalis*), and in the camphor chemotype of rosemary (*Rosmarinus officinalis*) do appear to have this effect.

Thymus species are often credited with broncholytic effects. Begrow *et al.* (2010) investigated the antispasmodic action on the trachea and the effect on ciliary activity of the major components thymol and carvacrol, finding that both compounds were active. However, since even low levels of thymol in extracts were active, other constituents may be contributing to the antispasmodic activity and stimulation of ciliary activity.

Although it is useful to be able to identify active constituents, especially when presented with the chemical profile of an essential oil with yet to be established properties, we should bear in mind that, more often than not, it will be the interactions between the constituents that determine its overall activity.

Bronchodilatory actions

Histamine, a vasoactive amine that is produced in mast cells, initiates the inflammatory response. There are histamine receptors in bronchial and visceral (smooth) muscle, known as H_1 receptors. When histamine binds to these, there is an influx of Ca^{2+} ions which has two effects – bronchoconstriction and vasodilation. It is thought that some essential oil constituents might act as histamine antagonists (Bowles 2003). Essential oils such as tea tree, plai, sweet marjoram, kewda and juniperberry, which contain substantial amounts of the histamine agonist terpinen-4-ol[1] (Brand *et al.* 2002; Koh *et al.* 2002), might be of value in allergic responses that manifest in the respiratory tract; they might also be able to alleviate bronchoconstriction that is a consequence of histamine release.

Anti-inflammatory action

Chen *et al.* (2014) conducted a study that aimed to establish the mechanisms that underlie bornyl acetate's anti-inflammatory property – in this case by investigating its actions *in vitro* and *in vivo* in mice with induced acute lung injury. They found that bornyl acetate downregulated the levels of pro-inflammatory cytokines, reduced the number of total cells, neutrophils and macrophages in bronchoalveolar lavage fluid, attenuated the histological alterations in the lung, and suppressed the activity of a range of kinases. This led to the conclusion that bornyl acetate could be developed as a preventative agent for inflammatory lung diseases. A few essential oils contain substantial amounts of *l*-bornyl acetate, notably inula, hemlock, black, red and white spruce, and Siberian, Japanese, balsam and silver fir; valerian can contain traces up to 33.5%, and golden rod up to 20% (Tisserand and Young 2014).

---

1   Terpinen-4-ol is also an anti-inflammatory and smooth muscle relaxant – and so essential oils that contain substantial amounts of this constituent may be of particular value in allergic responses and bronchoconstriction.

Asthma

Individuals with asthma, which has no cure and can only be managed, are often anxious about exposure to odours, including those of essential oils. Asthma is characterised by chronic inflammation in the lungs, and can be triggered by exposure to irritating chemicals, fragrances and allergens, and also by emotions and stress. However, with asthma, we can see a powerful example of the placebo/expectation mechanism at work. Jaén and Dalton (2014) conducted a study in which individuals with 'moderate-persistent' asthma were exposed to the odour of phenylethanol – a predominant constituent of rose absolute (see Table 11.1), which is not associated with any irritating qualities – but were informed it was either asthmogenic or therapeutic. Those who had been told it was asthmogenic reported elevated irritation and annoyance ratings, and displayed a rapid and persistent increase in airway inflammation. This somatic response reflected the perceived risk of the odour.

Obviously this has implications for aromatherapy practice. Many essential oils and their constituents can be of benefit in asthma; however, if a client expresses any negative reactions about specific essential oils, or indeed fragrance, their expectation must be respected, and the potential for a placebo mechanism taken into account. In some circumstances it might be prudent to avoid using any particularily pungent/diffusive essential oils, and those that might cause respiratory irritation.

Table 11.1 Expectorant, mucolytic, bronchodilatory, decongestant and antitussive actions

Essential oil	Actions	Evidence
Alpinia calcarata	Expectorant Decongestant Anti-inflammatory	*Alpinia calcarata* rhizomes are used in traditional medicine (Sri Lanka, India and Malaysia) for the treatment of bronchitis, cough and respiratory ailments; 1,8-cineole is the major component of the oil from the rhizomes (Arawwawala, Arambewela and Ratnasooriya 2012).
Anthopogon (*Rhododendron anthopogon*)	Antimicrobial (*Mycobacterium tuberculosis*) Decongestant Anti-inflammatory	Traditional use (Nepal) and Tibetan medicine; the essential oil was shown to have anti-inflammatory activity, and was active against *M. tuberculosis* (Innocenti *et al.* 2010).
Basil, holy (*Ocimum sanctum*)	Antimicrobial (*Mycobacterium tuberculosis*)	The essential oil is active (*in vitro*) against *M. tuberculosis*, and in Ayurveda the herb is used to treat bronchitis and asthma (Prakash and Gupta 2005).
Bay laurel (*Laurus nobilis*)	Expectorant Antimicrobial	Based on its significant 1,8-cineole content (up to 40–45%), and minor bornyl acetate content, bay laurel may have beneficial effects on the respiratory system, including an expectorant effect. It might also be useful for infections.
Black cumin (*Nigella sativa*)	Antispasmodic	Used in folk medicine to treat and prevent asthma, the oil decreases blood pressure and increases respiration (Ali and Blunden 2003). Inhaled thymoquinone aerosol protected against histamine-induced bronchospasm (Marozzi, Kocialski and Malone 1970, cited by Tisserand and Young 2014). Has a strong antihistaminic effect on airways of asthmatic patients (Boskabady, Mohsenpoor and Takaloo 2010).
Cajuput (*Melaleuca cajuputi*)	Expectorant Antimicrobial	Used in traditional Vietnamese and Indonesian medicine for respiratory tract infections, cajuput oil has a 1,8-cineole content in the region of 40–70% (see 1,8-cineole in text above).
Cardamom (*Elettaria cardamomum*)	Expectorant	Contains up to 50% 1,8-cineole, which suggests expectorant action; see text above.
Chamomile, German (*Matricaria recutita*)	Histamine suppression	Mills (1991) suggested that the major constituents, chamazulene and α-bisabolol, are anti-inflammatory and can reduce histamine-induced reactions; this may help prevent histamine-induced bronchoconstriction.

Plant	Actions	Notes
Eucalyptus, 1,8-cineole-rich (*E. globulus, E. polybractea, E. camadulensis, E. smithii* and others)	Expectorant Anti-inflammatory Antibacterial (respiratory pathogens)	1,8-cineole has an expectorant effect (Ulmer and Schott 1991, cited by Bowles 2003). Cermelli *et al.* (2008) investigated the effects of *E. globulus* essential oil on a range of bacterial respiratory pathogens. Its strongest activity was against *Haemophilus influenzae, H. parainfluenzae, Stenotrophomonas maltophilia* and *Streptococcus pneumoniae*.
Fennel, sweet (*Foeniculum vulgare* var. *dulce*)	Antispasmodic	Contains substantial amounts of *trans*-anethole, credited with antispasmodic actions (Albuquerque, Sorensen and Leal-Cardoso *et al.* 1995, cited by Bowles 2003); this may possibly alleviate bronchial spasm.
Fir, Siberian, Japanese, balsam and silver (*Abies sibirica, A. sachalinensis, A. balsamea* and *A. alba*)	Anti-inflammatory Antitussive Expectorant	All contain bornyl acetate, which has anti-inflammatory, antitussive and expectorant actions; see text above. Siberian fir contains 31%, Japanese fir 28%, and silver fir 30%. Balsam fir has less bornyl acetate (15%) but contains up to 56% β-pinene, which has anti-inflammatory action.
Fragonia (*Agonis fragrans*)	Antimicrobial Expectorant Anti-inflammatory	The essential oil contains roughly equal proportions of 1,8-cineole (26–33%, see text above), α-pinene (22–27%) and monoterpene alcohols such as α-terpineol (5–8%), linalool, geraniol and terpinen-4-ol. This is considered to be the ideal ratio of these compounds for the treatment of respiratory infections (Pénoël 2005, cited by Turnock 2006).
Ginger (*Zingiber officinale*)	Anti-inflammatory Decongestant Bronchodilator	Used in traditional medicine for cold/moist conditions such as excess mucus; Franchomme and Pénoël (1990) suggested that it is anti-inflammatory, and a bronchodilator that is useful for chronic bronchitis.
Hemlock (*Tsuga canadensis*)	Anti-inflammatory Antitussive Expectorant	Contains 41–43% bornyl acetate (Lagalante and Montgomery 2003); see text above.
Inula (*Inula graveolens*)	Anti-inflammatory Mucolytic	The essential oil contains around 46% bornyl acetate, which is anti-inflammatory, and has potential in the treatment of inflammatory lung diseases (Chen *et al.* 2014). Schnaubelt (1995) states that it is a strong mucolytic agent.

Plant	Actions	Notes
Jasmine (*Jasminum officinale*)	Anti-inflammatory Expectorant	In Ayurvedic medicine *J. officinale* is used as an anti-inflammatory and expectorant (Shukla 2013).
Juniperberry (*Juniperus communis*)	Histamine suppression Anti-inflammatory Antispasmodic (potential)	Contains up to 18% terpinen-4-ol, which is anti-inflammatory and acts as a histamine agonist (Brand *et al.* 2002; Koh *et al.* 2002). It is also a smooth muscle relaxant (Lahlou, Leal-Cardoso and Duarte 2003); this may help prevent histamine-induced bronchoconstriction and spasm.
Kewda (*Pandanus odoratissimus, P. fascicularis*)	Histamine suppression Bronchodilatory Anti-inflammatory Antispasmodic (potential)	Contains up to 22% terpinen-4-ol, which is anti-inflammatory and acts as a histamine agonist (Brand *et al.* 2002; Koh *et al.* 2002). It is also a smooth muscle relaxant (Lahlou, Leal-Cardoso and Duarte 2003); this may help prevent histamine-induced bronchoconstriction and spasm.
Lavender, spike (*Lavandula latifolia, L. spica*)	Anti-inflammatory Expectorant	Contains up to 35% 1,8-cineole which has anti-inflammatory and expectorant actions. See text above.
Long pepper (*Piper longum*)	Expectorant Anti-asthmatic Antitussive	Used in Ayurvedic medicine as an expectorant, in the treatment of respiratory diseases such as cough, bronchitis and asthma (Chauhan *et al.* 2011; Kumar *et al.* 2009); can prevent induced bronchospasm (Zaveri *et al.* 2010).
Marjoram, sweet (*Origanum majorana*)	Histamine suppression Bronchodilatory Anti-inflammatory Antispasmodic (potential)	Contains up to 30% terpinen-4-ol, which is anti-inflammatory and acts as a histamine agonist (Brand *et al.* 2002; Koh *et al.* 2002); it is also a smooth muscle relaxant (Lahlou, Leal-Cardoso and Duarte 2003); this may help prevent histamine-induced bronchoconstriction and spasm.
Marjoram, wild Spanish (*Thymus mastichina*)	Expectorant Mucolytic?	Contains 45–59% 1,8-cineole and 5–9% camphor, suggesting expectorant and mucolytic actions. See text above.

Myrtle (*Myrtus communis*)	Anti-inflammatory Expectorant	Contains around 30% 1,8-cineole which suggests anti-inflammatory and expectorant actions. See text above.
Niaouli (*Melaleuca quinquenervia* CT cineole, CT viridiflorol)	Anti-allergic Expectorant	Contains up to 60% 1,8-cineole which suggests expectorant action. See text above. Schnaubelt (2011) mentions that topical niaouli CT viridiflorol, which contains up to 45% viridiflorol (aromadendrene) and 35% 1,8-cineole, can also be used to relieve allergy.
Peppermint (*Mentha × piperita*)	Decongestant Mucolytic	Contains menthol at around 42%, and menthone at 20%, which have decongestant and mucolytic actions. See text above.
Pink pepper (*Schinus molle*)	Antibacterial (respiratory infections)	Traditionally used in Mexico against coughs, colds, tuberculosis, bronchitis and fever; Pérez-López *et al.* (2011) demonstrated that it was active against *Streptococcus pneumoniae* (a causal agent for respiratory tract diseases), and noted its activity against *Haemophilus influenzae* and *Mycobacterium tuberculosis*. They suggested that δ-cadinene (present at 1.6% in *S. molle* essential oil) was the principal compound responsible for the activity against *S. pneumoniae*, but that all the constituents should be present for the essential oil to be active, either because of synergy or because the minor constituents enhance the antimicrobial activity.
Plai (*Zingiber officinale*)	Anti-allergic Anti-asthmatic Anti-inflammatory Antispasmodic	Early studies indicated that Plai had anti-asthmatic effects (Aupaphong, Ayudhya and Koontongkaeu 2013), and Piromrat *et al.* (1986, cited by Bhuiyan, Chowdhury and Begum 2008) demonstrated that it exerted antihistaminic effects on the skin of children who suffer from asthma. More recently, Twetrakul and Subhadhirasakul (2007) confirmed that it has anti-allergic actions. One of plai essential oil's main constituents, terpinen-4-ol (present around 40%), can alleviate allergy by suppressing histamine release and cytokine production (Edris 2007); terpinen-4-ol also has anti-inflammatory and spasmolytic actions (Lahlou, Leal-Cardoso and Duarte 2003).
Rosalina (*Melaleuca ericifolia*)	Expectorant Anti-inflammatory	Oils from the north of Australia give rise to the type 1 essential oil, which is linalool-rich and cineole-poor; type 2 oils come from the far south and are cineole-rich and linalool-poor (Brophy and Doran 2004). Type 2 rosalina is likely to have expectorant and anti-inflammatory qualities.
Rose absolute (*Rosa damascena*)	Anti-asthmatic Bronchodilator Antitussive	The main constituent, phenylethanol, also a major component of the Chinese formula *Wuhu*, can prevent histamine-induced bronchoconstriction (*in vitro*), hence its value as an anti-asthmatic agent (Chi *et al.* 2009, cited by de Casia da Silveira e Sá *et al.* 2014). Antitussive effect (in guinea pigs) of *R. damascena* identified by Shafei, Rakhshande and Boskabady (2003).

Plant	Properties	Description
Rosemary (*Rosmarinus officinalis* CT cineole, CT bornyl acetate)	Expectorant Anti-inflammatory	It might be expected that the cineole and bornyl acetate chemotypes will have expectorant and anti-inflammatory actions, based on the known activities of these constituents. See text above.
Sage, Greek, Cretan (*Salvia triloba*)	Expectorant Mucolytic	The main constituents are 1,8-cineole and limonene (around 38%), camphor at 15%, terpineol and borneol at around 7%, thujone at 6–7%, and α- and β-pinenes at 5–6% (Harvala, Menounos and Argyriadou 1987); this profile would suggest expectorant and mucolytic qualities.
Spearmint (*Mentha spicata*)	Decongestant Mucolytic	Contains the ketone *l*-carvone at around 50–70% which suggests decongestant and mucolytic actions. See text above.
Spruce, black, red and white (*Picea mariana, P. rubens* and *P. glauca*)	Decongestant Anti-inflammatory	All contain bornyl acetate, which has decongestant and anti-inflammatory actions (see text above); black spruce (37%), red spruce (16.4%) and white spruce (14%).
Tagetes (*Tagetes minuta*)	Anti-oxidant Anti-inflammatory	Tagetes is used in folk medicine for many purposes, notably as an anti-inflammatory, antispasmodic, decongestant and bronchodilatory for chest infections, cough and catarrh. It has radical scavenging actions and anti-inflammatory activity (Karimian, Kavoosi and Amirghofran 2014). The essential oil is phototoxic, and requires caution for skin applications; inhalation would not carry this risk.
Tea tree (*Melaleuca alternifolia*)	Anti-allergic Bronchodilator Antispasmodic	The essential oil and its constituent terpinen-4-ol can suppress histamine release, and cytokine production, which causes allergic symptoms (Brand *et al.* 2002; Koh *et al.* 2002). This may in turn help prevent bronchoconstriction in cases of allergy. Terpinen-4-ol is anti-inflammatory, and also antispasmodic (Lahlou, Leal-Cardoso and Duarte 2003).
Thyme (*Thymus vulgaris*)	Broncholytic Antispasmodic (trachea) Stimulates ciliary clearance	The broncholytic effects of thyme essential oil can be partly attributed to thymol (Begrow *et al.* 2010).
Yuzu (*Citrus × junos* Tanaka)	Anti-inflammatory Broncholytic	Hirota *et al.* (2010) suggested that limonene isolated from yuzu peel had potential anti-inflammatory efficacy for the treatment of bronchial asthma (it inhibited cytokine production, inhibited the formation of reactive oxygen species, and inactivated eosinophil migration).

Chapter 12

The Skin and Soft Tissues

Wound-healing, Regenerating, Anti-allergic and Antipruritic Actions

In aromatherapy there are two main routes by which essential oils enter the body: inhalation and transdermal absorption. Therefore we might expect to see essential oils directly acting on the skin itself. It is known that essential oils have several properties that can be of importance in skin health; for example, skin barrier function, texture and hydration levels can be maintained or indeed restored, inflammation can be reduced, cell regeneration stimulated, wound healing enhanced, infections can be controlled or prevented, and even allergic responses and itching can be alleviated.

Skin barrier function and keratinocyte differentiation

In the epidermis, keratinocytes are important in the formation and maintenance of structure; this is achieved via differentiation. Keratinocytes provide a barrier, but they also control levels of hydration, wrinkles and pigmentation. When keratinocyte differentiation is disturbed, the barrier function is affected, and several problems such as excessive skin dryness and disorders such as atopic dermatitis and psoriasis can manifest.[1] It is also believed that strengthening and improving the texture of the skin by enhancing keratinocyte differentiation can have a positive impact on wrinkle formation, pigmentation and regeneration, and wound healing. Some essential oils and absolutes, notably rose absolute, can enhance keratinocyte differentiation and inhibit hyperproliferation, thus improving skin texture (Kim *et al.* 2010).

It is the texture – the appearance and feel of the surface of the skin – that is of concern to the majority of individuals; it is seen as a reflection of health and age. Therefore, there is a market for surface-rejuvenating phytocosmeceuticals[2] that improve the appearance of wrinkes and pores. In normal skin, ageing is associated with a decrease in receptors for adrenocorticotrophic hormone (a neuropeptide) and β-endorphin. These are synthesised in the epidermis from the precursor

---

1　An abnormal inflammatory immune reaction is also associated with these conditions.
2　Many botanicals have been used in folk medicine to treat skin disorders; by 2005, over 60 different botanical extracts were formulated into cosmeceuticals (Thornfeldt 2005) and by 2010 this had increased to over 70 – but only six of these had been the subject of 'rigorous clinical research' (Sachdev and Friedman 2010, p.63).

pro-opiomelanocortin (POMC), and a decline is associated with alterations in the structural and functional properties of the epidermis.[3] Pain *et al.* (2011) conducted an *in vitro* and *in vivo* study to determine the effects of an extract of yarrow (*Achillea millefolium*) in comparison with glycolic acid (an exfoliating, resurfacing agent) on the epidermis. The *in vitro* study was carried out on monolayer cultures of normal, ageing human keratinocytes, using quantitative image analysis. The *in vivo* study involved a two-month period of treatment with a cosmetic formula containing 2% *Achillea millefolium* aqueous extract in comparison with a 3% glycolic acid preparation and a placebo. The *in vitro* results demonstrated that keratinocyte proliferation and differentiation patterns were improved and epidermal thickness was significantly enhanced – by 10% – and comparable to that of younger skin. The *in vivo* results also significantly improved wrinkle and pore appearance and softness in comparison with the baseline and placebo, comparable with glycolic acid. There was also an increase in epidermal cell turnover. However, yarrow extract does not have exfoliating actions, and the perceived softness and increase in epidermal thickness may be related to an improvement in the surface relief and also the hydrating and emollient properties of the water-in-oil cosmetic base. It is possible that some aromatic plant extracts, like yarrow, might act by upregulating the expression of POMC-related receptors.

Tissue damage and healing

Cell migration, angiogenesis, inflammation and extracellular matrix remodelling are the key stages in tissue healing. The inflammatory phase exists to establish homeostasis, and this is followed by a proliferative phase consisting of granulation tissue formation and collagen synthesis,[4] contraction and epithelialisation. It is the remodelling phase that determines the appearance and strength of the scar tissue. Many essential oils can modulate these natural stages.

Anti-oxidant activity is one of the most important biological activities attributed to essential oils, and is at the root of many other properties, including their anti-inflammatory and pain-relieving actions. As already discussed, many essential oils have anti-inflammatory action. When the skin is damaged, a prolonged or exacerbated inflammatory response results in further cell damage and the production of exudates; pro-inflammatory leukotrienes[5] can accumulate in the tissues. This all contributes to delayed resolution, poor healing and the potential for unsightly scar tissue formation. However, when essential oils are applied to the skin, their lipophilic components act on the lipid parts of the cell membranes,

---

3   Age-induced disturbances include an altered responsiveness to growth factors, hormones and cytokines, delayed calcium-induced differentiation, and epidermal thinning.

4   Collagen is the main structural protein of connective tissue. The collagen 'sponge' enhances tissue formation, and increases vascularisation of repaired tissue and thus enhances the healing process.

5   Pro-inflammatory leukotrienes are derived from the metabolism of arachidonic acid; the enzyme 5-lipoxygenase (5-LOX) is the first enzyme involved in its oxidation.

and can directly affect the production of enzymes (stimulation or inhibition), ion channels and receptors; so we can see how some essential oils can reduce skin inflammation, reduce or prevent oedema, inhibit the formation of enzymes such as 5-lipoxygenase (5-LOX) and human leukocyte elastase (HLE),[6] and promote the production of enzymes involved in the formation of, for example, ceramides[7] in keratinocytes – all contributing to skin functions and health.

Therefore, anti-oxidant activity and anti-inflammatory activity are essential in promotion of the wound-healing process, because a prolonged inflammatory phase delays healing and contributes to pain and scarring.

Cicatrisant and wound-healing actions

For many years it has been believed that basal epidermal keratinocytes are responsible for natural wound healing, and there is increasing evidence that skin–nerve interactions also play a part in the process. The skin has many sensory receptors that detect information from the environment, and keratinocytes have receptors too: transient receptor (TRP) channels, ATP receptors and endocrinology receptors. However, there are also olfactory receptors (OR) in keratinocytes, melanocytes and dendritic cells. In the skin,[8] these ORs have non-olfactory physiological functions; however, Busse *et al.* (2014) suggested that some odorants, such as the synthetic sandalwood aromachemical Sandalore, could induce a reciprocal interaction between keratinocytes and olfactory receptors in the skin, thus enhancing healing. The results of their *in vitro* study indicated that an OR in the human basal layer, identified as OR2AT4, can be contacted by aromatics such as Sandalore, which can easily penetrate the skin barrier, and enhance epidermal wound healing. It was postulated that Sandalore could activate kerinatocytes by activating the cAMP pathway[9] (and others), witnessed in the increased cell proliferation and migration that characterises re-epithelialisation. It would appear that OR2AT4 might only respond to 'small numbers of closely related odorants', but other physiologically active ORs have been identified (Busse *et al.* 2014, p.8). Although we do not use Sandalore in aromatherapy, this study does establish that aromatic molecules, such as those found in essential oils, can interact with ORs in the skin, and that this might be part of their wound-healing mechanism.

---

6   HLE is an enzyme that is important in the pathophysiology of inflammation, and is involved in the degradation of the matrix proteins collagen and elastin.

7   Ceramides are skin lipids that are important in the water-holding and barrier functions of the skin.

8   Olfactory receptors have not been found in connective tissue cells such as fibroblasts and adipocytes.

9   Cyclic adenosine monophosphate (cAMP) is a 'messenger' molecule involved in increasing the metabolic rate in cells. However, it also is involved in vasodilation, relaxation of intestinal smooth muscle and contraction of respiratory smooth muscle, reduction of heart rate, and inhibition of acetylcholine and adrenalin release. The cAMP pathway is a metabolic pathway that is mediated by the enzyme adenylate cyclase, which regulates its production, and cAMP itself upregulates kinases, which in turn activate others by phosphorylation. It is believed that some essential oil components stimulate upregulation of cAMP, and hence have physiological effects such as spasmolysis (Bowles 2003).

Some essential oil components have been investigated with regard to their wound-healing actions (Adams and Thrash 2010; Barreto *et al.* 2014; Tumen *et al.* 2010, cited by Süntar *et al.* 2012; Tumen *et al.* 2012). These include:

Limonene: *l*-limonene in *Pinus* species is important in the wound-healing process, and *Pinus* species rich in *l*-limonene, such as *P. pinea*, can promote wound healing.

Perillyl alcohol: found at around 5.5% in *Perilla frutescens*, this is not a commonly occurring essential oil constituent; however, it is a metabolite of limonene. It too has a significant effect on skin repair and pro-inflammatory cytokine levels.

α-Pinene: when co-occuring with sabinene and *l*-limonene in some *Juniperus* and *Cupressus* species, has moderate anti-inflammatory activity and promotes wound healing.

Borneol: this has antimicrobial (against a range of Gram-positive and Gram-negative pathogens and fungi), wound-healing and anti-inflammatory actions. It reduces leukocyte migration and suppresses cytokines, decreases the growth of fibroblasts and stabilises the membranes of mast cells, amongst other activities. Borneol occurs in *Salvia officinalis*, *Thymus* species CT borneol, *Rosmarinus officinale* CT borneol (also CT bornyl acetate), *Inula graveolens*, *Cymbopogon validus* and others.

Thymol: this inhibits prostaglandin synthesis. It has anti-inflammatory and anti-oxidant activity (it is a COX-1 inhibitor and reduces oedema); it can prevent the auto-oxidation of lipids and the formation of toxins via reactive nitrogen species; it is antimicrobial and promotes wound healing via the stimulation of macrophage migration, and modulation of the growth of fibroblasts and elastase activity. Thymol occurs in substantial amounts (up to 74%) in the thymol chemotypes of *Thymus zygis* and *T. vulgaris*, and in lesser amounts in other *Thymus* species (Tisserand and Young 2014).

α-Terpineol: possesses a spectrum of activities that contribute to wound-healing effects; it is anti-inflammatory (a COX-2 inhibitor, it reduces TNF-α and NO) and inhibits the influx of neutrophils, and has strong antimicrobial and antifungal actions. It is formed in the same pathway as terpinen-4-ol, and is found in many oils.

Anti-oxidant and anti-inflammatory actions

As already discussed, many essential oils have anti-oxidant and anti-inflammatory actions, and some appear to have particular significance in relation to the skin – because it is possible that anti-oxidant activity is linked with keratinocyte differentiation, and thus barrier function and texture.

However, anti-oxidant and anti-inflammatory properties are also important in the formulation of phytocosmeceuticals, including those intended for the 'anti-ageing' niche market. Jorge *et al.* (2011) suggested that agents or synergistic mixtures with a high anti-oxidant capacity can not only protect lipids, DNA and proteins but could also delay cell senescence. In the field of cosmetology, it would seem that natural anti-oxidants, including essential oils, have the potential to provide considerable protection against oxidative skin damage. Kim *et al.* (2013b) investigated the whitening and anti-oxidant properties of bornyl acetate isolated from *Cryptomeria japonica*[10] essential oil, with the intention of establishing its uses in phytocosmeceuticals. Within this study, they established that bornyl acetate had 'extremely high' superoxide dismutase-like activity.[11] The essential oil also has anti-inflammatory action, probably via the inhibition of pro-inflammatory cytokines by monocytes and macrophages, and also via the inhibition of lipopolysaccharide-induced NO (Yoon *et al.* 2009b).

Baylac and Racine (2003) conducted an *in vitro* assessment of a wide range of essential oils, absolutes and nature-identical fragrances to establish their ability to inhibit 5-LOX, and thus potential anti-inflammatory activities. Oils highlighted as inhibitors of 5-LOX were myrrh and sandalwood, Himalayan cedar and the citrus oils lemon, sweet orange and mandarin. Their main component, *d*-limonene, also showed good inhibitory activity. The sesquiterpenes β-caryophyllene and α-bisabolol showed strong inhibitory potential, and it was suggested that oils rich in *trans*-nerolidol and farnesol (isomer not specified) will also show the ability to inhibit 5-LOX. The following year (2004) Baylac and Racine investigated the potential for aromatic extracts to inhibit human leukocyte elastase (HLE) *in vitro*. This enzyme is important in the pathophysiology of inflammation, and is involved in the degradation of the matrix proteins collagen and elastin. UV exposure[12] stimulates HLE activity, and so we witness wrinkles and loss of elasticity in response to sun exposure. This study revealed that some absolutes were effective inhibitors of HLE – and thus could be harnessed in anti-ageing formulae. Turmeric (*Curcuma longa*) oleoresin[13] showed the strongest activity (even greater than the reference), and poplar bud absolute, rosemary extract and benzoin resinoid showed very strong inhibitory activity. Also active were the absolutes and resinoids of gentian, linden blossom, violet leaf, myrrh, cocoa, artichoke, fucus, jasmine, blackcurrant bud, rice and tea.

Lavender (*Lavandula angustifolia* and other species) has long been regarded as being very useful for the skin. However, Baumann (2007a) suggested that lavender has a 'dark side', citing a study conducted by Prashar, Locke and Evans (2004), where it was found that lavender had a cytotoxic effect on endothelial cells and

---

10 *Cryptomeria japonica* is the Japanese 'cedar'; its pollen is notorious for causing allergy. In Nepal it is known as the 'tsugi pine', and is used as incense.

11 Superoxide dismutases (SOD) are enzymes that catalyse the dismutation of superoxide (O_2^-) into oxygen and hydrogen peroxide; this is part of the anti-oxidant defence mechanism. SODs are powerful anti-inflammatory agents; they reduce reactive oxygen species and oxidative stress.

12 UV exposure is considered to be the most important extrinsic factor in skin ageing.

13 Turmeric oleoresin contains three curcuminoids – complex diones with anti-oxidant and anti-inflammatory activity – which are not found in the essential oil.

fibroblasts, possibly due to cell membrane damage. This study led Baumann to caution that lavender is perhaps unsuitable in preparations specifically designed to have an anti-ageing effect. In contrast, rose absolute (*Rosa damascena* and other species) enhances keratinocyte differentiation and hyperproliferation; it accelearates the the recovery of a disrupted skin barrier, and improves skin texture via an increase in natural moisturising constituents such as filaggrin. Thinning of the epidermis and wrinkle formation is linked with a reduction in filaggrin. The main constituent, phenylethanol (also found in other abolutes such as orange blossom and golden champaca) has anti-oxidant and antibacterial properties (Ulusoy, Bosgelmez-Tinaz and Secilmis-Canbey 2009, cited by Kim *et al.* 2010), and anti-oxidants have profound effects on keratinocyte differentiation, although the mechanism has not yet been identified (Kim *et al.* 2010). This suggests that rose absolute, and probably other phenylethanol[14] containing oils would be well suited in preparations for dry and damaged skin, and for anti-ageing purposes.

Antibacterial and antidermatophytic actions

Many commensal bacteria are opportunistic pathogens that can cause mild superficial infections as well as life-threatening infections. The case of *Staphylococcus aureus* and antibiotic resistance has already been discussed, but there are several other commensals that are opportunistic pathogens. For example, *Streptococcus pyogenes*, best known for throat infections, can infect the skin, producing a characteristic strawberry-like rash, impetigo, erysipelas or cellulitis, but can also infect deeper layers and the fascia, resulting in the serious condition known as necrotising fasciitis. It also produces toxins. This bacterium is well protected by a capsule of hyaluronic acid, which prevents neutrophils from migrating to infected areas, and so can be difficult to treat by conventional means. *Enterococcus faecalis*, as its name indicates, is found in the gastrointestinal tract; however, it can infect root canal treated teeth, and can cause urinary tract infections, endocarditis and meningitis. *Klebsiella pneumonia* is another opportunistic pathogen which usually affects immunocompromised individuals, commonly infecting the lungs and the upper respiratory tract, but it can also cause wound infections. Given the growing problem of antibiotic resistance, topical treatment with skin antiseptics can be a preventative strategy, and a method of control as well as treatment of superficial skin and mucous membrane infections (Casetti *et al.* 2012).

---

14 Despite limitations on the use of phenylethanol imposed by the fragrance industry, a pharmacokinetics study and safety evaluation comparison in rats, rabbits and humans suggested that a human dermal systemic exposure of 0.3mg/kg per day (via multiple consumer personal care products) is not a developmental toxicity hazard (Politano *et al.* 2013).

Acne vulgaris

The pathology of acne vulgaris[15] is complex, and involves immune responses known as 'pathogen-associated molecular patterns'; these are antigenic, and stimulate macrophages and monocytes to secrtete inflammatory cytokines. Acne is also associated with an increased production of sebum,[16] hyperkeratinisation of pilosebaceous ducts, inflammation and the proliferation of commensal bacteria. For example, at puberty, *Propionibacterium acnes* (an organism found in the gut) and *Staphylococcus epidermidis* can become involved in the pathogenesis of acne vulgaris. *P. acnes*, an obligate anaerobe,[17] releases chemicals which attract neutrophils to the infected area, and these in turn release reactive oxygen species and lysosomal enzymes which damage the follicular epithelium. In response, pro-inflammatory cytokines (TNF-α, IL-8 and IL-β) are produced. *S. epidermidis* is an aerobic bacterium that commonly infects sebaceous glands. Conventional acne treatments usually involve the use of topical benzoyl peroxide and oral retinoids[18] – but these can cause abnormal skin dryness[19] and irritation. Antibiotics are also used; however, the prolonged use of tetracycline, erythromycin, macrolide and clindamycin has led to the emergence of resistant strains (Yoon *et al.* 2009b). Several essential oils are active against *P. acnes* and *S. epidermidis*, and this, coupled with their anti-inflammatory and in some cases antiseborrheic properties, makes them promising candidates for the alternative management of acne. These oils are identified in Table 12.1.

Dermatophytosis

Dermatophytes are fungi that invade the keratinised, non-living layer of the skin, and the nails.

The most common dermatophytes are *Trichophyton rubrum*, which causes *Tinea pedis* ('athlete's foot'), *Tinea cruris* ('jock itch') and *Tinea corporis* (dermatophytosis or 'ringworm'), and *T. mentagrophytes* var. *interdigitale*, which is responsible for

---

15 There are three types of *acne vulgaris*: comedonal (non-inflammatory), nodular and papopustular (inflammatory). Conventional treatments include topical drugs, oral antibiotics, oral retinoids and oral hormonal drugs.

16 This is caused by androgen-mediated stimulation of the sebaceous glands.

17 As the name suggests, obligate anaerobes can only thrive if oxygen is absent or present in low concentrations; they are killed by normal atmospheric concentrations of oxygen. There are, however, degrees of oxygen tolerance, ranging from 0.5% to 8%.

18 Retinoids (vitamin A), such as retinol, when applied topically, can decrease stratum corneum cohesion, normalise the epidermal–dermal junction, increase collagen, elastin, fibronectin and glycoaminoglycans, decrease melanin, collagenases and metalloproteinases, improve angiogenesis and reduce comedones (Fowler *et al.* 2010).

19 Abnormal skin dryness, or 'xerosis cutis', is associated with reduced formation of lipids and proteins, and disturbances in the skin barrier functions. Some botanicals such as *Aloe vera* leaf gel, *Betula alba* extract, *Helianthus annuus* oleodistillate and *Hypericum perforatum* extract can help reduce water loss from the epidermis, increase skin hydration and promote keratinocyte differentiation (Casetti *et al.* 2011).

onychomycosis (finger and toe nail infections). *T. rubrum* is the species responsible for over 75% of cases; *Epidermophyton floccosum*, *Microsporum canis* and other species cause less than 1%. Fungal skin infections can be difficult to treat; some essential oils and constituents such as sabinene are active against dermatophytes; these are also identified in Table 12.1.

Anti-haematomal actions and phlebotonic properties

Anti-haematomal action is the ability to prevent/alleviate bruising after soft tissue trauma – immortelle (*Helichrysum angustifolium* or *H. italicum*) is noted for this, and Bowles (2003) suggests that this could be due to the presence of italidiones (diketones). The anti-haematomal effect might be due to a combination of anti-inflammatory action, vasodilatory effects and prevention of oedema.

However, immortelle essential oil is worthy of closer examination, because it has multiple actions that benefit the skin and soft tissues. Voinchet and Giraud-Robert (2007) investigated the therapeutic effects and potential clinical applications of *H. italicum* var. *serotinum* and a macerated oil of musk rose (*Rosa rubiginosa*) after cosmetic and reconstructive surgery. This was found to reduce inflammation, oedema and bruising, and again these effects were attributed to italidiones. However, wound healing was also enhanced, and post-operative scarring was reduced; they attributed the latter to the musk rose oil.

Anti-allergic and antipruritic actions

The prevalence of allergic disorders such as atopic dermatitis is increasing. Mitoshi *et al.* (2014) summarise the pathophysiology of allergy, and identify that 'immunologically active mast cells and basophils express the high affinity receptor for immunoglobulin E (IgE) on their surface, and play a critical role in the biological processes associated with allergic diseases' (pp.1643–1644). If antigens interact with the bound IgE, pro-inflammatory mediators are secreted from granules in the cytoplasm, and cytokines are synthesised and released, thus activating the migration of neutrophils and macrophages. The result is inflammation.

Sometimes essential oils or their components are associated with allergic reactions and contact dermatitis, where the skin becomes red, irritated and often itchy. Allergies do not develop suddenly – they are the response when the immune system has become sensitised to a substance, and when faced with exposure to that substance an allergic reaction results.

For example, lemongrass (*Cymbopogon citratus*) essential oil has the potential to cause irritation and sensitisation, as does its major constituent, citral (Tisserand and Young 2014). Paradoxically, it has also been identified as a candidate for the treatment of allergic and inflammatory diseases. It has been suggested that the presence of *d*-limonene and α-pinene can reduce its capacity to cause adverse skin reactions (Tisserand and Young 2014). However, Mitoshi *et al.* (2014) identified that out of the 20 essential oils investigated for their *in vitro* anti-allergic and anti-inflammatory activities, *C. citratus* and citral (geranial was present at 40.16% and neral at 34.24%) had the strongest activity; the authors suggested that it could have therapeutic uses in cases of allergy and inflammation, and in this study German chamomile (*Matricaria chamomilla*) and sandalwood (*Santalum album*) also displayed good anti-allergic activity, producing over 40% inhibition of mast cell degranulation. Good anti-inflammatory activity via inhibition of TFN-α was also identified with chamomile, cold-pressed lemon (*Citrus limon*) and sandalwood, but *Eucalyptus globulus*, cold-pressed lime (*Citrus aurantifolia*) and nutmeg (*Myristica fragrans*) showed 0% inhibition.

Some essential oils have been investigated specifically in relation to their anti-allergic activity. For example, Mills (1991) suggested that chamazulene and α-bisabolol (major constituents of German chamomile oil) are anti-inflammatory and can reduce histamine-induced reactions. The cutaneous benefits of German chamomile were investigated by Baumann (2007b) and it was also shown to have antipruritic potential. It has been shown that tea tree essential oil and its constituent terpinen-4-ol can suppress histamine release and cytokine production, which causes allergic symptoms (Brand *et al.* 2002; Koh *et al.* 2002).

True lavender essential oil has been shown to have anti-allergic action. Tisserand and Young (2014) cite a 1999 study conducted by Kim and Cho (1999) where topically applied lavender inhibited immediate-type reactions in rats and mice. The inhibition was concentration dependent, and thought to be via the inhibition of histamine and TNF-α release by mast cells.

Schnaubelt (2011) also mentions that topical niaouli (*Melaleuca quinquenervia viridiflora*) can also be used to relieve allergy, and that *Tanacetum annuum* from Morocco can mediate inflammation and decrease histamine release (possibly due to its sesquiterpene lactones). Finally, he suggests that *Pinus sylvestris* essential oil might have potential in this regard, because French texts suggest that it has cortisone-like qualities, and it could be used in frictions over the kidney area to 'reduce allergic dispositions' (p.147).

Psychodermatology and neurodermatology

These are relatively new disciplines that have emerged in response to the growing awareness of the psychological impact of skin disorders; for example, *acne vulgaris* – which affects around 80% of young adults and adolescents – is allied with emotional distress, depression, anxiety and other mental health disorders, and it has a serious impact on self-confidence and self-esteem (Nguyen and Su 2011; Safizadeh, Shamsi-Meymandy and Naeimi 2012, cited by Sinha *et al.* 2014). Many essential oils have activities that can alleviate symptoms of skin disorders, including acne – see Table 12.1. However, they also have a positive impact on the psyche. When selecting essential oils for clients with acne and other skin problems, this too should be taken into account (see also Table 13.1).

Table 12.1 Wound-healing, regenerating, anti-inflammatory, anti-haematomal, antimicrobial, anti-allergic and antipruritic actions

Essential oil	Actions	Evidence
African bluegrass (*Cymbopogon validus*)	Anti-inflammatory Wound-healing (potential)	The essential oil contains up to 10% borneol, which is notable for its antimicrobial (against a range of Gram-positive and Gram-negative pathogens and fungi), wound-healing and anti-inflammatory actions; see text above.
Anthopogon (*Rhododendron anthopogon*)	Anti-inflammatory (topical) Antimicrobial	The essential oil was shown to have weak topical anti-inflammatory activity, coupled with antimicrobial actions (Innocenti *et al.* 2010).
Basil (*Ocimum basilicum*)	Skin penetration enhancer	Basil essential oil was identified as a skin penetration enhancer (Jain *et al.* 2008, cited by Adorjan and Buchbauer 2010).
Basil, holy (*Ocimum sanctum*)	Anti-oxidant Anti-inflammatory Inhibitor of 5-LOX	A study investigating the *in vitro* activities of essential oils for acne control included holy basil, revealing that it was more effective against *P. acnes* than sweet basil, and that its anti-oxidant activity suggested that it would be useful for the prevention of scar formation (Lertsatitthanakorn *et al.* 2006).
Bergamot (*Citrus aurantium* var. *bergamia* fruct., *C. bergamia*)	Wound-healing Antifungal	Used in folk medicine as an antiseptic and to facilitate wound healing (Bagetta *et al.* 2010). *In vitro* activity against *Trychophyton, Microsporum* and *Epidermophyton* species; potential for topical clinical use (Sanguinetti *et al.* 2007).
Black cumin (*Nigella sativa*)	Antifungal	Extracts are active against dermatophytes – four strains of *Trichophyton rubrum, T. interdigitale, T. mentagrophytes, Epidermophyton floccosum* and *Microsporum canis* (Abad, Ansuategui and Bermejo 2007).
Blackcurrant bud essential oil and absolute (*Ribes nigrum*)	Antibacterial Anti-pathogenic potential Inhibitor of HLE	Oprea *et al.* (2008) demonstrated that blackcurrant bud oil had a large antibacterial spectrum, including *S. aureus*, and even sub-inhibitory concentrations caused a decrease in the ability of the bacteria to colonise – indicative of antipathogenic potential. Baylac and Racine (2004) identified the ability of the absolute to inhibit HLE – it could have a role in protection and regeneration following UV exposure.
Cacao absolute (*Theobroma cacao* seeds)	Inhibitor of HLE	Baylac and Racine (2004) found that the absolute inhibited HLE; it has anti-inflammatory, protective and regenerative potential.

Plant	Properties	Details
Cade (*Juniperus oxycedrus* subsp. *oxycedrus*)	Anti-inflammatory Wound-healing	Tumen *et al.* (2012) conducted an *in vitro* and *in vivo* animal study which investigated the anti-inflammatory and wound-healing actions of the essential oils of several Turkish-grown *Juniperus* and *Cupressus* species[1] in comparison with the reference drug Madecassol[2] and a base ointment. *J. oxycedrus* var. *oxycedrus* and *J. phoenicia* displayed the highest anti-inflammatory activity, and were the only ones that showed a significant wound-healing effect.
Camphor (*Cinnamomum camphora*) CT nerolidol	Inhibitor of 5-LOX (potential)	The nerolidol type contains 40–60% nerolidol with 20% each of monoterpenoids and sesquiterpenoids (Behra, Rakotoarison and Harris 2001). Nerolidol is potentially an inhibitor of 5-LOX, and thus anti-inflammatory.
Carrot seed (*Daucus carota* subsp. *carota*)	Antifungal (active against dermatophytes)	The essential oil was very active against several dermatophytic species. The Portuguese oil was dominated by geranyl acetate and α-pinene; the more active Sardinian oil was dominated by β-bisabolene and 11-α-(h)-himachal-4-en-1-β-ol (Maxia *et al.* 2009). Abad, Ansuategui and Bermejo (2007) cite Jasicka *et al.* (2004), who demonstrated that carotol, the main constituent of a seed oil, inhibited the radial growth of fungi by 65%.
Cedar, Himalayan (*Cedrus deodara*)	Anti-inflammatory	Inhibitor of 5-LOX (Baylac and Racine 2003).
Cedar, Japanese (*Cryptomeria japonica*)	Antioxidant Anti-inflammatory Antimicrobial Active against *P. acnes* and *S. epidermidis*	Yoon *et al.* (2009b) demonstrated that the essential oil[3] had excellent antibacterial activities against *P. acnes* and *S. epidermidis*, including drug-susceptible and drug-resistant strains, and had anti-inflammatory actions; it acts by inhibiting pro-inflammatory cytokines and mediators (NO, PGE2, TNF-α, IL-1β, IL-6). They suggested that it is a potential acne-mitigating candidate for skin health.
Cedar, Lebanese (*Cedrus libani*)	Anti-inflammatory Wound-healing	Tumen *et al.* (2011) investigated essential oils from a range of Pinaceae cones. *C. libani* essential oil demonstrated the highest anti-inflammatory and wound-healing activity, along with *Abies cilicica* subsp. *cilicica*. *Abies nordmanniana* also showed effective wound-healing capacity, but others did not.
Cedar, Virginian (*Juniperus virginiana*)	Anti-inflammatory Wound-healing	An essential oil obtained by supercritical CO_2 extraction had significant wound-healing and anti-inflammatory activities (Tumen *et al.* 2013).[4]

Chamomile, German	Antipruritic Anti-allergic Anti-inflammatory	Mills (1991) suggested that the major constituents chamazulene and α-bisabolol are anti-inflammatory and can reduce histamine-induced reactions. Chamazulene inhibits leukotriene B4 synthesis via inhibition of 5-LOX and COX, lipid peroxidation, leukocyte infiltration and histamine release, while α-bisabolol promotes the formation of granulation tissue (Baumann 2003, cited by Thornfeldt 2005). The cutaneous benefits of German chamomile were investigated by Baumann (2007b) and it was also shown to have antipruritic potential. This would suggest that German chamomile oil has applications in cases of allergic problems. The essential oil displayed some anti-allergic and anti-inflammatory activity in an *in vitro* study (Mitoshi *et al.* 2014).
Champaca, white (*Michelia alba*)	Strong activity against *P. acnes*	Luangnarumitchai, Lamlertthon and Tiyaboonchai (2007) demonstrated that white champaca oil had strong activity against *P. acnes*.
Citronella (*Cymbopogon nardus*)	Antimicrobial Anti-inflammatory Anti-oxidant	Excellent activity against *P. acnes* and good free radical scavenging activity (Lertsatitthanakorn *et al.* 2006).
Citrus species (*Citrus limon, C. sinensis, C. reticulata, Citrus obovoides* and *C. natsudaidai*)	Anti-inflammatory Anti-oxidant Antibacterial	Inhibitors of 5-LOX – as is the main constituent, *d*-limonene (Baylac and Racine 2003). Cold-pressed lemon oil inhibits TFN-α, contributing to an anti-inflammatory effect (Mitoshi *et al.* 2014). Korean citrus essential oils of *Citrus obovoides* and *C. natsudaidai* are active against *P. acnes* and *S. epidermidis*. They are also good anti-oxidants[5] and reduce *P. acnes*-induced secretion of IL-8 and TNF-α (Kim *et al.* 2008), therefore have potential in the management of acne.
Clary sage (*Salvia sclarea*)	Inhibits *S. epidermidis* Anti-inflammatory	In a review, Kanlayavattanakul and Lourith (2011) identified that clary essential oil could inhibit *S. epidermidis* and that it was anti-inflammatory, and proposed that it was used in anti-acne formulations.

Combava petitgrain (*Citrus hystrix*)	Active against *P. acnes* Anti-inflammatory	Lertsatitthanakorn et al. (2006) investigated the bioactivities of several Thai herbal essential oils, including combava leaf, with regard to their potential for acne control.[6] It was found that combava leaf was an inhibitor of 5-LOX, second in this activity to holy basil (*Ocimum sanctum*). The essential oil did not perform so well as an anti-oxidant, being surpassed by holy basil, citronella and several others. However, combava leaf is useful for reducing inflammation and this might help reduce the potential for post-acne scar formation. Luangnarumitchai, Lamlertthon and Tiyaboonchai (2007) showed that combava leaf oil had strong activity against *P. acnes*.
Coriander seed (*Coriandrum sativum*)	Anti-inflammatory Antibacterial Active against *P. acnes*, *S. epidermidis*, *S. pyogenes*, *S. aureus*, MRSA	Anti-inflammatory potential of the essential oil identified by Reuter et al. (2008), cited by Casetti et al. (2012). The essential oil was active against *P. acnes* and *S. epidermidis*, thus has potential in the management of acne (Vats and Sharma 2012). The essential oil displayed strong activity against *S. pyogenes*, *S. aureus* and MRSA, with excellent skin tolerance, and has potential as an antiseptic for the prevention and treatment of Gram-positive infections, including oozing dermatitis, and for eradicating MRSA in asymptomatically colonised individuals (Casetti et al. 2012).
Cypress (*Cupressus sempervirens*, *C. sempervirens* var. *horizontalis*)	Anti-oxidant NO scavenger Antiglycation	Cypress essential oil is a good anti-oxidant and NO scavenger (Aazza et al. 2014). *C. sempervirens* var. *horizontalis* essential oils (obtained from both branchlets and fruits) have anti-oxidant and antiglycation properties (Asgary et al. 2013); this might mean that the essential oil has a role in anti-ageing formulae, perhaps by preventing the formation of AGEs that cause cross-linking with proteins and hardening of collagen.
Eucalyptus globulus	Antimicrobial (including *P. acnes*) Anti-seborrheic Penetration enhancer Increases ceramides in stratum corneum	Antimicrobial activities include action against *P. acnes*, possibly due to γ-terpinene and α-pinene (Athikomkulchai, Watthanachaiyingcharoen and Tunvichien 2008). Could control spread of acne by decreasing sebum production via reducing size of sebaceous glands[7] (Bhatt et al. 2011). The penetration-enhancing qualities of 1,8-cineole in the essential oil is mentioned in a review conducted by Guimarães, Quintans and Quintans-Júnior (2013). The leaf extract (ethanolic) increased the level of ceramides (lipids) in keratinocytes in the stratum corneum (Ishikawa et al. 2012).

Plant	Properties	Details
Fennel, sweet (*Foeniculum vulgare* var. *dulce*)	Antifungal (dermatophytes)	Sweet fennel oil has antifungal activity, and could be used in the treatment of fungal nail infections (Patra *et al.* 2002).
Fir, Korean (*Abies koreana*)	Inhibits *P. acnes* and *S. epidermidis* Anti-inflammatory	Yoon *et al.* (2009a) identified that the essential oil was active against both drug-susceptible and drug-resistant *P. acnes* and *S. epidermidis*, and that it was anti-inflammatory; it suppressed secretion of TNF-α, IL-1β, IL-6, NO and prostaglandin E_2. Kanlayavattanakul and Lourith (2011) identified that *A. koreana* could inhibit *P. acnes* and *S. epidermidis*; and that it was anti-inflammatory, therefore a candidate for anti-acne preparations.
Geranium (*Pelargonium* × *asperum*, or *P. roseum* [a hybrid of *P. capitatum* × *P. radens*], *P. capitatum*, *P. radens*, *P. odoratissimum*)	Anti-inflammatory Antibacterial (with tea tree, vs MRSA) Antifungal (*Candida* species)	Edward-Jones *et al.* (2004) investigated the effects of the vapours of patchouli, tea tree, geranium and lavender essential oil, and citricidal (grapefruit seed extract) singly and in combination on *Staphylococcus aureus*, MRSA and epidemic methicillin-resistant *S. aureus* (EMSRA). The oils were tested on dressings of various compositions, over pre-seeded Petri dishes. Citricidal and geranium oil showed the greatest inhibition, and geranium and tea tree was the most active against MRSA. An Algerian-grown, rose-scented geranium essential oil displayed potent anti-inflammatory activity (comparable with diclofenac, the positive control), with a reduction in oedema, and it inhibited inflammatory responses in the skin. It was concluded that rose geranium essential oil has significant potential in the development of novel and safe anti-inflammatory drugs, particularily in the prevention and treatment of acute and chronic inflammatory skin diseases (Boukhatem *et al.* 2013).
Guava leaf (*Psidium guajava*)	Antimicrobial (including *P. acnes*)	The inhibition zones of guava leaf extract were greater than those of tea tree oil for *P. acnes*, and equal for staphylococci, but it was less effective than doxycycline and clindamycin on *P. acnes* (Qadan *et al.* 2005, cited by Azimi *et al.* 2012).
Hemp (*Cannabis sativa*)	Anti-inflammatory	Hadji-Mingalou and Bolcato (2005) investigated its use in a formulation for the replacement of dermacorticoid drugs, and give its components as myrcene (33%), *trans*-β-ocimene (15%), terpinolene, β-caryophyllene and caryophyllene oxide (1.4%). These constituents might also suggest that cannabis essential oil has analgesic potential. It is a 5-LOX inhibitor, and has anti-inflammatory potential (Baylac and Racine 2004).

Immortelle (*Helichrysum angustifolium, H. italicum*)	Anti-haematomal Anti-inflammatory Wound-healing Antimicrobial	Effects often attributed to italidiones (Bowles 2003; Voinchet and Giraud-Robert 2007). Active against the opportunistic micro-organisms *Staphylococcus aureus* and *Candida albicans* (Voinchet and Giraud-Robert 2007).
Inula (*Inula graveolens*)	Anti-inflammatory Wound-healing (potential)	The essential oil contains up to 16% borneol, which is notable for its antimicrobial (against a range of Gram-positive and Gram-negative pathogens and fungi), wound-healing and anti-inflammatory actions; see text above.
Jasmine absolute (*Jasminum grandiflorum, J. sambac*)	Anti-oxidant Inhibitor of HLE Antibacterial (including *P. acnes*) Antiseptic Anti-inflammatory Regenerating Wound-healing	Jasmine has free radical scavenging properties, and may offer protection against UVB-induced skin damage (Baylac and Racine 2003); it inhibits HLE (Baylac and Racine 2004); and has anti-inflammatory, skin protective and regenerative potential. *J. grandiflorum* is active against *P. acnes* (Zu, Yu and Liang 2010). In Ayurvedic medicine, *J. officinale* is used for its ansiseptic, anti-inflammatory and cicatrisant actions (Shukla 2013).
Juniperberry, Phoenician (*Juniperus phoenicia*)	Anti-inflammatory Wound-healing	Tumen *et al.* (2012) conducted an *in vitro* and *in vivo* animal study which investigated the anti-inflammatory and wound-healing actions of the essential oils of several Turkish-grown *Juniperus* and *Cupressus* species[8] in comparison with the reference drug Madecassol[9] and a base ointment. *J. oxycedrus* var. *oxycedrus* and *J. phoenicia* displayed the highest anti-inflammatory activity, and were the only ones that showed a significant wound-healing effect.

Plant	Properties	Evidence
Lavender, true (*Lavandula angustifolia*)	Anti-oxidant Anti-inflammatory Anti-allergic Wound-healing	Yang *et al.* (2010) reported that lavender (from Australia) was significantly more effective against lipid peroxidation than the five other oils studied. In an assay determining free radical scavenging ability (DPPH), lavender exhibited the strongest performance, similar to that of *d*-limonene. Guimarães, Quintans and Quintans-Júnior (2013) noted the anti-inflammatory activity of *l*-linalool, which has a significant presence in the essential oil. The essential oil has anti-allergic activity (Kim and Cho 1999, cited by Tisserand and Young 2014). In a randomised, double-blind, placebo-controlled study exploring the effects of topical lavender oil on recurrent apthous ulceration,[10] it was shown that lavender oil produced a significant reduction in inflammation, ulcer size, overall healing time (2–4 days) and pain relief (mainly from first dose) compared to the baseline and placebo. The oil also showed antibacterial actions against all of the strains tested (Altaei 2012). Lavender essential oil is not recommended in anti-ageing preparations as it displays cytotoxicity in endothelial cells and fibroblasts (Bauman 2007a).
Lemon myrtle (*Backhousia citriodora*)	Antimicrobial (*S. aureus* and *P. acnes*)	The essential oil is active against *S. aureus* and *P. acnes*, as is its constituent citral, and a product containing 1% essential oil showed low toxicity to human skin cells and fibroblasts (Hayes and Markovic 2002, cited by Azimi *et al.* 2012)
Lemongrass (*Cymbopogon citratus*)	Anti-allergic Anti-inflammatory Antifungal	An *in vitro* study demonstrated that lemongrass essential oil had strong anti-allergic and anti-inflammatory activity (Mitoshi *et al.* 2014). Boukhatem *et al.* (2014) evaluated the *in vivo* topical anti-inflammatory effects and the *in vitro* antifungal activity[11] of the essential oil; the results confirmed both actions, and the authors suggested that the oil is a potentially valuable antifungal and anti-inflammatory agent for the prevention and treatment of acute inflammatory skin conditions. They also found that the vapour phase of the oil had good antifungal activity, with advantages over the liquid phase; its greater potency means that lower doses are required. It was suggested that it could be used as an aerial disinfectant.
Marjoram, sweet (*Origanum majorana*)	Anti-inflammatory Wound-healing	Süntar *et al.* (2011) investigated a novel wound-healing ointment based on traditional Turkish knowledge. *Origanum majorana*, in combination with *O. minutiflorum* and *Salvia triloba*, in an ointment containing *Hypericum perforatum* and olive oil and shea butter was shown to have anti-inflammatory and wound-healing effects (much greater than that of *H. perforatum* alone). It did not reduce elastase activity, but inhibited collagenase activity *in vitro*.

Myrrh (*Commiphora myrrha*)	Inhibitor of 5-LOX Inhibitor of HLE Anti-oxidant	Anti-inflammatory (Baylac and Racine 2003). Absolute was anti-inflammatory, with protective and regenerative potential (Baylac and Racine 2004). *C. myrrha* essential oil is a singlet oxygen[12] quencher; it gives excellent protection of squalene[13] peroxidation; squalene peroxidation during solar exposure is due to singlet oxygen more than free radical attack. It was suggested that sun care formulations should use both singlet oxygen quenchers and free radical scavengers (Tonkal and Morsy 2008).
Niaouli (*Melaleuca quinquenervia viridiflora*)	Anti-allergic	The anti-allergic potential of the essential oil was discussed by Schnaubelt (2011).
Orange blossom absolute (*Citrus aurantium* var. *amara*)	Anti-inflammatory	The absolute contains both nerolidol and farnesol – both of which were identified by Baylac and Racine (2003) as inhibitors of 5-LOX – thus indicating anti-inflammatory potential. It also contains phenylethanol, which has anti-inflammatory actions (de Cássia da Silveira e Sá *et al.* 2014) and anti-oxidant actions (Ulusoy, Boşgelmez-Tinaz and Secilmis-Canbey 2009), and can enhance keratinocyte differentiation and thus skin barrier function, texture and moisture levels. Some essential oil components such as nerolidol might increase skin permeability by acting on the lipid bilayer (Cornwall and Barry 1994; Takayama and Nagai 1994).
Orange, Valencia (*Citrus sinensis*; cold pressed)	Antimicrobial Anti-staphyloccocal	Muthaiyan *et al.* (2012b) demonstrated that the vapour of the terpeneless, cold-pressed essential oil, when used on an *in vitro* dressing model with infected keratinocytes, rapidly killed[14] both methicillin-resistant *Staphylococcus aureus* and vancomycin intermediate-resistant *S. aureus*, and showed no cytotoxic effects on keratinocytes.
Patchouli (*Pogostemon cablin*)	Anti-inflammatory Wound-healing	Based on its traditional uses in Chinese, Ayurvedic and Greek medicines, Holmes (1997) noted that the essential oil is indicated for numerous skin disorders and scar tissue. Anti-inflammatory action is suggested by Raharjo and Fatchiyah (2013).
Pine species (*P. pinea* and *P. halepensis*)	Anti-inflammatory Wound-healing	Süntar *et al.* (2012) investigated the wound-healing and anti-inflammatory actions of essential oils from the cones and needles of five Turkish-grown *Pinus* species (*P. brutea*, *P. halepensis*, *P. nigra*, *P. pinea* and *P. sylvestris*). Only *P. pinea* and *P. halepensis* displayed remarkable wound-healing activity, possibly related to their *l*-limonene content. These species also displayed anti-hyaluronidase[15] activity.

Pine, Scots (*Pinus sylvestris*)	Anti-allergic potential	Schnaubelt (2011) suggests that, according to French texts, the oil has cortisone-like qualities.
Pink pepper (*Schinus molle*)	Antimicrobial Anti-dermatophytic Wound-healing	Used in traditional Mexican medicine for coughs, colds, fever, bronchitis and tuberculosis; Pérez-López *et al.* (2011) note its activity against a wide range of bacteria including *Klebsiella pneumoniae*, *Pseudomonas aeruginosa*, *Escherichia coli*, *Listeria monocytogenes*, *Staphylococcus aureus*, *Streptococcus pyogenes*, *Streptococcus pneumoniae*, *Haemophilus influenzae*, *Mycobacterium tuberculosis*, *Bacillus cereus*, and *Salmonella enteritidis*; thus it could be a useful topical antiseptic. It also is active against the dermatophytes *Microsporum gypseum*, *Trichophyton mentagrophytes* and *T. rubrum*. Marongiu *et al.* (2004) note that the essential oil has been shown to have cicatrisant (wound-healing) action. A hydrophilic extract displayed wound-healing activity (C. Schmidt *et al.* 2009).
Plai (*Zingiber cassumunar*)	Antioxidant Anti-inflammatory Anti-dermatophytic Antimicrobial (including *P. acnes*)	Good anti-oxidant capacity (Lertsatitthanakorn *et al.* 2006), which may help reduce potential for scarring. Active against dermatophytes, and a wide range of micro-organisms, including *P. acnes* (Pithayanukul, Tubprasert and Wuthi-Udomler 2007). Shows potential in the management of acne vulgaris, especially in regard to non-inflammatory lesions (Limwattananon *et al.* 2008). Possible wound-healing actions – Chotjumlong (2005) demonstrated than an ethanolic extract of *Z. cassumunar* could reduce tissue hydration and inflammation during the wound-healing process in human oral epithelial cells, but inhibited extracellular matrix hyaluronan and metalloproteinases (the major components of the wound-healing process) in human oral fibroblasts.
Poplar bud absolute (*Populus balsamifera*)	Inhibitor of 5-LOX Anti-inflammatory Regenerative	Used by North American Indians for skin and lung ailments. The resin from the sticky buds was used as a salve – 'Balm of Gilead'. It is an inhibitor of 5-LOX and has anti-inflammatory, protective and regenerative potential (Baylac and Racine 2004).

Rose absolute and oil (*Rosa damascena*)	Anti-inflammatory Anti-oxidant Keratinocyte differentiation-enhancer Inhibitor of *P. acnes*	The absolute is dominated by phenylethanol, which has anti-inflammatory actions (de Cássia da Silveira e Sá *et al.* 2014), anti-oxidant actions (Ulusoy, Boşgelmez-Tinaz and Secilmis-Canbay 2009) and farnesol, which is an inhibitor of 5-LOX (Baylac and Racine 2003); this indicates that the absolute has anti-inflammatory, keratinocyte differention-enhancing, skin texture improving, and skin-regenerating potential. The essential oil contains substantial amounts of citronellol (up to 45%) which has anti-inflammatory (and analgesic) action (Bastos *et al.* 2010). In a review, Kanlayavattanakul and Lourith (2011) identified that *R. damascena* oil could inhibit *P. acnes*; it was anti-inflammatory, and suitable for use in phytocosmeceuticals as a multi-functional ingredient. A topical application of rose oil (from *Rosa* spp.) and *Rubia cordifolia* (common or Indian madder root) extract stimulates keratinocyte differentiation and has skin barrier-reinforcing properties, and so is suitable in phytocosmeceuticals for dry skin (Casetti *et al.* 2011).
Rosemary (*Rosmarinus officinalis*)	Anti-oxidant Anti-inflammatory Inhibitor of HLE Antibacterial (including *P. acnes*)	In a review of botanical extracts and their contribution to skin health, Bauman (2007a) identified rosemary (various extracts) as being of particular interest, by imparting cosmetic benefits and decreasing free radical-induced skin damage. Rosemary absolute has been shown to have strong HLE inhibitory activity (Baylac and Racine 2004). Fu *et al.* (2007) reported that the essential oil was active against *P. acnes*, attributed to 1,8-cineole, α-pinene, camphor and camphene.
Sage, Dalmatian (*Salvia officinalis*)	Anti-inflammatory Antifungal (dermatophytes)	In traditional medicine in Jordan, *S. officinalis* is used to treat skin diseases. Essential oils from Jordan-grown sage belonged to the Group iv category[16] – with 1.8-cineole (40–50%) > camphor (8.0–25%) > α-thujone (1.2–3.7%) > β-thujone (0.1–3.1); this had a low toxicity on macrophages and keratinocytes, indicating that it would be safe for use in topical preparations. This *in vitro* study demonstrated that the essential oil was active against dermatophytes (*Trichophyton rubrum* and *Epidermophyton floccosum*) and the yeast *Cryptococcus neoformans*. It was less active aginst *Candida* and *Aspergillus* species. Moreover, the oil had anti-inflammtory activity; it inhibited NO production (Abu-Darwish *et al.* 2013).
Sage, Greek, Cretan, Turkish (*Salvia triloba*)	Wound-healing	Süntar *et al.* (2011) investigated a novel wound-healing ointment based on traditional Turkish knowledge. *Origanum majorana*, in combination with *O. minutiflorum* and *Salvia triloba*, in an ointment containing *Hypericum perforatum* and olive oil and shea butter, was shown to have anti-inflammatory and wound-healing effects (much greater than the effects of *H. perforatum* alone). It did not reduce elastase activity, but inhibited collagenase[17] activity *in vitro*.

Sage, Sardinian (*Salvia desoleana*)	Antifungal Antidermatophytic	Sokoviç *et al.* (2009) investigated the antifungal activity of the essential oil, given the increasing number of fungal infections in immunocompromised individuals. It was established that the main constituents were linalyl acetate, α-terpinyl acetate, linalool and 1,8-cineole. They observed a correlation between the chemical structure of the essential oil constituents and the antimicrobial activity; it appeared that this affected the potency of each compound. However, what the study revealed was that the complete essential oil of *S. desoleana* was more effective than any of its individual components against all of the fungal pathogens tested; indeed it had strong antifungal activity. This was explained by the synergistic activity of all of the components in the oil.
Sage, wild Somalian (*Salvia somalensis*)	Anti-oxidant Anti-inflammatory	Dominated by bornyl acetate and lacking α- and β-thujone, with a pleasant aromatic and resinous aroma; Villa *et al.* (2009) established that it has a low level of cytotoxicity and would be suitable in cosmetics. Bornyl acetate is noted for its anti-inflammatory actions and has 'extremely high' superoxide dismutase-like activity[18] (Kim *et al.* 2013b).
Sandalwood (*Santalum album*)	Anti-inflammatory Anti-allergic	Inhibitor of 5-LOX (Baylac and Racine 2003). Mitoshi *et al.* (2014) demonstrated that sandalwood essential oil had anti-allergic and anti-inflammatory potential.
Szechuan (Japanese) pepper (*Zanthoxylum piperitum*)	Anti-oxidant	Kim *et al.* (1997) identified that the extract of *X. piperitum* could be a source of anti-oxidants suitable for cosmetic use.
Tea tree (*Melaleuca alternifolia*)	Anti-allergic Anti-inflammatory Antimicrobial	The essential oil and its constituent terpinen-4-ol can suppress histamine release, and cytokine production, which causes allergic symptoms (Brand *et al.* 2002; Koh *et al.* 2002). Excellent potential in the treatment of acne (Enshaieh *et al.* 2007, cited by Sinha *et al.* 2014). 5% tea tree oil reduced the number of inflamed and non-inflamed lesions (comparable with 5% benzoyl peroxide but with fewer adverse effects); terpinen-4-ol, α-terpineol and α-pinene are active against *S. aureus*, *S. epidermidis* and *P. acnes* (Sinha *et al.* 2014).
Thyme, five-ribbed (*Thymus quinquecostatus*)[19]	Anti-oxidant Antibacterial (including *P. acnes*) Anti-elastase Anti-inflammatory	These properties, coupled with a low toxicity in human cell lines, make this species a candidate for acne treatment (Oh, Kim and Yoon 2009, cited by Sinha *et al.* 2014).

Turmeric (*Curcuma longa*)	Antifungal	Active against *Trichophyton longifusus* (Abad, Ansuategui and Bermejo 2007).
Violet leaf absolute (*Viola alba* and *V. odorata*)	Inhibitor of HLE	Violet leaf absolute showed the ability to inhibit HLE (Baylac and Racine 2004), so may have applications on sun-damaged skin, and as an anti-ageing absolute.
Yarrow (*Achillea millefolium*)	Anti-inflammatory Regenerating	Yarrow essential oil has anti-inflammatory effects (Tisserand and Balacs 1995), probably related to its chamazulene and sabinene content. An aqueous extract displayed significant surface-rejuvenating effects (Pain *et al.* 2011).

1. The essential oils were: *Cupressus sempervirens* var. *horizontalis* and *C. sempervirens* var. *pyrimidalis* cones, *Juniperus communis*, *J. excelsa*, *J. foetidissima*, *J. oxycedrus* and *J. phoenicia* berries.

2. Madecassol is an ointment which contains 1% *Centella asiatica* extract.

3. Constituents include kaurene, enemol, γ-eudesmol and sabinene.

4. This study used *in vivo* biological activity models; *J. occidentalis* showed the most significant activity.

5. Superoxide anion radical scavengers.

6. Here, in addition to their activity against *P. acnes*, their anti-oxidant and anti-inflammatory activities were measured, because as well as inhibiting the proliferation of the bacterium, it is also important that pro-inflammatory lipids in sebum and the potential for scar formation is reduced. Pro-inflammatory leukotrienes are derived from the metabolism of arachidonic acid; the enzyme 5-lipoxygenase (5-LOX) is the first enzyme involved in its oxidation. Some essential oils are thought to inhibit this enzyme, and this could go some way towards explaining how they have anti-inflammatory action.

7. Demonstrated in an *in vivo* rat sebaceous gland model (Bhatt *et al.* 2011).

8. The essential oils were: *Cupressus sempervirens* var. *horizontalis* and *C. sempervirens* var. *pyrimidalis* cones, *Juniperus communis*, *J. excelsa*, *J. foetidissima*, *J. oxycedrus* and *J. phoenicia* berries.

9. Madecassol is an ointment which contains 1% *Centella asiatica* extract.

10. Apthous ulceration is the term used to describe benign, usually recurrent mouth ulcers.

11. This study included eight pathogenic *Candida* species and five pathogenic *Aspergillus* species, also one *Penicillium* strain and one *Mucor* strain. It has been suggested that the strong inhibition of *Candida* species might be due to synergism among the constituents, geranial, neral, cymene, terpinene and linalool.

12. Singlet oxygen, also known as dioxygen and dioxidene, is highly reactive, and is often generated with photosensitising agents.

13. Squalene is a lipid produced in human skin; it is an omega 2 oil, also extracted from shark's liver and also vegetable sources (some seeds and olives) for use in cosmeceuticals.

14. The inhibitory actions of the essential oil were due to inhibition of cell wall synthesis (Muthaiyan et al. 2012a).

15. Hyaluronic acid is an important component of the extracellular matrix, and is found throughout connective and epithelial tissues. It contributes significantly to wound healing because it develops from the base of a wound, promotes cell proliferation and encourages the migration of fibroblasts and endothelial cells to the area. Hyaluronidase is an enzyme that breaks down hyaluronic acid, so anti-hyaluronidase activity promotes wound healing (Süntar et al. 2012).

16. Sage oils can be classed in five categories: (i) camphor > α-thujone > 1,8-cineole > β-thujone, (ii) camphor > α-thujone > β-thujone > 1,8-cineole, (iii) β-thujone > camphor > 1,8-cineole > α-thujone, (iv) 1,8-cineole > camphor > α-thujone > β-thujone and (v) α-thujone > camphor > β-thujone > 1,8-cineole (Tucker, Maciarello and Howell 1990, cited by Abu-Darwish et al. 2013). An alternative classification is by dominant constituent: Group I consists of species characterised by α- and β-thujone, such as Dalmatian sage; Group II by linalool and linalyl acetate, such as clary sage; and Group III by 1,8-cineole and camphor, such as Greek, Lebanese and Spanish sage.

17. Collagenase is an enzyme that degrades collagen fibres into fragments, so changes its binding affinities. During re-epithelialisation, it facilitates the movement of keratinocytes over the collagen-rich dermis. Collagenase inhibition may be advantageous in healing chronic rather than acute wounds (Süntar et al. 2011).

18. uperoxide dismutases (SOD) – enzymes that catalyse the dismutation of superoxide (O_2^-) into oxygen and hydrogen peroxide; part of the anti-oxidant defence mechanism. SODs are powerful anti-inflammatory agents – they reduce reactive oxygen species and oxidative stress.

19. Sometimes classed as Thymus serpyllum var. quinquecostatus; also known as 'Desert Thyme'.

Chapter 13

The Psyche

Anxiolytic, Antidepressant and
Cognition-enhancing Actions

It is believed that around 450 million people across the globe have mental or behavioural disorders (World Health Organization 2001, cited by Sayers 2001). In a review of the literature on aromatherapy and its role in the alleviation of psychiatric disorders, Lv *et al.* (2013) noted that, mainly because of recurrent pressures, threats and stresses due to work, illness and life circumstances, many of us suffer from a plethora of disorders, including anxiety, restlessness, depression and insomnia, and also that poor sleep quality is directly related to many mood disorders. They cite the European Brain Council's statistics, which indicate that in the 28 European countries 21 million individuals are affected by depression, costing around 100 billion euros every year.

Symptoms of depression are variable, ranging from low mood, inability to feel pleasure, irritability and erratic thought processes, to loss of concentration, sleep and appetite disturbances and reduced olfactory sensitivity – all of which have an impact on daily life. Suicide can be a consequence of severe depression. Depression can have genetic roots; however, stress, emotional pain, infections, medications[1] and diseases such as cancer can all trigger the occurrence of depression. Anxiety is a common feature of depression, and differential diagnosis can be difficult. De Sousa (2012) notes that anxiety disorders are the most common form of psychopathy, and that the prevalence of anxiety is increasing. Anxiety comprises a group of debilitating disorders, and several explanatory theories have been propsed, but there is no unifying aetiology. Medications developed to treat anxiety[2] have many associated problems, on a spectrum of physical and psychological dependence and side effects, and there is a real need to find new anxiolytic agents (Mesfin, Asres and Shibeshi 2014).

Historically, mankind has used aromatic plants for their calming and mood-enhancing effects, and contemporary research has supported these practices, demonstrating that essential oils offer a broad spectrum of psychoactivity. To explore how essential oils could be used therapeutically in the realm of mental

---

1   Side effects of drugs such as isotretinoin, selective serotonin reuptake inhibitors and α-interferon can trigger depression (Lv *et al.* 2013).

2   These include barbituates (no longer used), benzodiazepines, buspirone, antidepressants and beta-blockers.

health and wellbeing, we first need to look at olfaction and its connections with the central and autonomic nervous systems.

Olfactory connections and the central nervous system

When we examine the effects of essential oils on the psyche, we need to consider their impact on the olfactory system and its neural connections. Odours must be able to evaporate, or exist in vapour form. Once in the atmosphere, odorous molecules are detected by our olfactory organ – thin membranes covered in tiny olfactory hairs, on either side of the bony part of the nasal septum. This extends to the olfactory bulb, the olfactory nerve and the olfactory pathway, which transmits these olfactory signals to the brain. Olfactory neurons project to the limbic system, which is associated with emotions, memories, motivations and pleasure, but where there is no conscious control. The neurons also project to the thalamus, where sensory integration occurs; the hypothalamus, which monitors and maintains bodily functions; the amygdala, the seat of basic emotion; the hippocampus, which is associated with memory; and to the frontal cortex, where recognition of the odour occurs. The frontal cortex is concerned with organising and planning, and the executive, logical and social decisions are made at the prefrontal cortex.

When you consider the olfactory connections with these areas, especially the limbic system (specifically the hippocampus, the hypothalamus and the frontal cortex), it is unsurprising that scents have such a profound influence on us. Berger (1929, cited by Bagetta *et al.* 2010) was the first to correlate electroencephalogram (EEG) patterns with behaviour,[3] and this has been used to identify some of the psychoactive effects elicited by essential oils. For example, the effects of bergamot are specific and reproducible; systemic administration of increasing doses produces a sequence of sedative and stimulatory behavioural effects.

Studies have shown that odours can exert their effects via several mechanisms. Their molecules can act directly and have a pharmacological effect – for example, the sedating, anxiety-relieving effects of lavender. Satou *et al.* (2011a) investigated the potential for anxiolytic effects in mice, via inhalation of the essential oil of *Alpinia zerumbet* (Zingiberaceae).[4] This study considered the time-dependent effects of inhalation, and attempted to elucidate the mechanisms by which this essential oil produced its effects. The olfactory route is mediated through rapid neurotransmission, so any effects due to olfaction would show up fairly quickly. The route through the bloodstream is much slower, because the constituents need to be absorbed and then delivered to the brain, but the potential for sustained

---

3   For example, relaxation is associated with an increase in alpha wave activity, and stimulation with an increase in beta wave activity.

4   The principal chemical constituents were *para*-cymene, 1,8-cineole, limonene, α- and β-pinenes and camphene; an organoleptic evaluation was not given. *A. zerumbet* has been widely used in folk medicine in various subtropical regions, including Okinawa Island, Japan. It has also been used in contemporary herbal medicine specifically for depression, stress and anxiety, including chronic problems associated with female reproductive hormone imbalances.

reaction is increased. Satou *et al.* observed no anxiolytic effect with short (five minutes) duration of exposure, suggesting that the olfactory nerve pathway makes a very small or negligible contribution to the anxiolytic effect. However, longer exposure did produce an anxiolytic effect, which suggests the bloodstream pathway and a pharmacological response. If the exposure continued for 150 minutes, no anxiolytic effect was observed, possibly because the olfactory receptors had become fatigued or habituated, or because receptor desensitisation in the brain was caused by more than tolerable amounts of the constituents. It was concluded that to elicit psychoactivity, an appropriate essential oil inhalation time is required, as well as an optimum dose. Although we will focus on the quasi-pharmacological aspects here, we must bear in mind that other mechanisms are also at work.

Lv *et al.* (2013) reviewed published literature on aromatherapy and the central nervous system, and in the light of their own unpublished studies they proposed some therapeutic mechanisms. In summary, they stressed the importance of the ability of inhaled essential oils to stimulate the production of cerebral neurotransmitters such as serotonin[5] and dopamine,[6] thus regulating mood. Molecular mechanisms were also explored. It has been proposed that our olfactory receptors (ORs) trigger a cascade of reactions in response to odour stimuli, where these odour-coded chemical signals are converted to electrical signals[7] that travel along the nerve-cell's axon to the olfactory bulb, and via its neural connections to the various areas of the cerebrum. The brain responds by releasing neurotransmitters such as serotonin, so we have a 'chemical→electrical→chemical' signalling system. This would imply that, because essential oil molecules can access the brain directly, and can indeed pass through the blood–brain barrier, essential oil vapours have the potential to treat psychiatric disorders.

Olfaction and the autonomic nervous system

Inhalation of aromatic vapours can also affect autonomic functions; for example, heart rate, pulse rate, skin conductance, skin temperature, respiration and breathing rate can all be modulated by fragrance. Haze, Sakai and Gozu (2002) investigated the effects of a range of essential oils specifically on sympathetic activity in normal adults, using the parameters of blood pressure fluctuations and plasma catecholamine levels, demonstrating that fragrance inhalation can modulate sympathetic activity, which in turn affects the adrenal system. It was, however,

---

5   Serotonin, also known as 5-hydroxytrypyamine (5-HT), is derived from *l*-tryptophan, and is found in the brain but also the gut, where it is involved in the regulation of intestinal movements. However, in the brain it modifies mood and contributes to feelings of wellbeing.

6   Dopamine is a neurotransmitter that belongs to the monoamine group; it is associated with reward-motivated behaviour and motor control. Outside of the nervous system, dopamine acts as a vasodilator and a diuretic, and it can reduce gut motility and decrease the activity of lymphocytes (amongst other activities).

7   The signalling pathways cause a cation influx via the opening of cation channels; this produces an action potential, thus converting the chemical signal to an electrical signal.

acknowledged that any effects on sympathetic activity could also be influenced by hedonics, memory, and so on, and also the GABAergic system. This study elucidated some essential oil-specific information that is of direct relevance to aromatherapy practice, identifying oils that either stimulate or inbibit sympathetic activity. Black pepper (*Piper nigrum*), grapefruit (*Citrus × paradisi*), estragon[8] (*Artemisia dracunculus*) and fennel (*Foeniculum vulgare*) all elicited an increase in sympathetic activity by 1.7–2.5-fold; while patchouli (*Pogostemon cablin*) and rose (*Rosa damascena*) produced a decrease of around 40% in comparison with the control. In line with these findings, black pepper inhalation caused a 1.7-fold increase in plasma adrenaline, while rose caused a 30% decrease. Grapefruit inhalation elicited a 1.1-fold increase in adrenaline and a 1.2-fold increase in noradrenalin, but the noradrenalin increase was not statistically significant. All of the findings were consistent with blood pressure fluctuations.[9] The essential oils used in this study were analysed, and it was hypothesised that some of the constituents were implicated in these effects. For example, *d*-limonene, α-pinene and methyl chavivol were present in the stimulating black pepper, grapefruit and estragon oils, and *trans*-anethole dominated the fennel oil. None of these are present in rose or patchouli (which do not have shared constituents); rose is dominated by monoterpene alcohols such as citronellol and geraniol, and patchouli by sesquiterpenes, notably patchouli alcohol. Based on these results, the authors also suggested some therapeutic applications for fragrance inhalation – for example the correction of lifestyle-related disorders such as obesity and hypertension.

Anxiety and depression

Both animal and human studies have led to the conclusion that essential oils can have anxiolytic (anxiety-relieving), calming, tranquillising and sedating, and antidepressant actions. To illustrate this, we can look at two studies on the effects on anxiety of exposure to/inhalation of sweet orange essential oil – one with Wistar rats and one with healthy human volunteers.

Faturi *et al.* (2010) published the results of their study with Wistar rats. Here, male rats were exposed to various doses of sweet orange (*Citrus sinensis*) aroma for a period of five minutes within a Plexiglass chamber, and then subjected to stress in the form of the elevated plus-maze followed by the light/dark paradigm. It was found that the aroma had significant effects on behaviour in both tests – indicated by increased exploration of the open arms of the maze and of the lit chamber of the light/dark paradigm. The study was repeated with tea tree aroma (*Melaleuca alternifolia*), to eliminate the possibility of non-specific aroma effects; tea tree did not have an anxiolytic effect. It was concluded that these results indicated that

---

8   Also known as tarragon; estragon is the name often used in perfumery.
9   Blood pressure fluctuations are generally attributed to the delay in sympathetic vasomotor regulation mediated by the baroreceptor reflex.

sweet orange had an 'acute anxiolytic activity' that gave 'some scientific support to its use as a tranquiliser by aromatherapists' (Faturi *et al.* 2010, p.605).

Goes *et al.* (2012) used healthy volunteers who were exposed to an anxiety-provoking situation (a video-monitored version of the Stroop Color-Word Test or SCWT). In this study the outcome measures included psychological parameters (state-anxiety, subjective tension, tranquilisation and sedation) and physiological parameters (heart rate and gastrocnemius electromyogram). The test group were exposed to the vapour of sweet orange oil (*Citrus sinensis*) at various doses; two control groups were used – the aromatic control was tea tree (*Melaleuca alternifolia*) and the non-aromatic control was water. This study led to the conclusion that sweet orange oil could have an 'acute anxiolytic' effect, but that further studies were needed to establish the clinical relevance. However, it was stated that this gave 'some scientific support to its use as a tranquiliser' (Goes *et al.* 2012, p.798) in aromatherapy.

So here we have two very different studies on sweet orange oil, both leading to the very same conclusions – expressed in the very same words! We can also note that the conclusion is somewhat cautious – is there a reluctance to commit to clinical relevance? Other studies focus on human volunteers who are already stressed and possibly affected by both depression and anxiety. For example:

Itai *et al.* (2000) explored the effects of the aromas of lavender and hiba oils on female chronic hemodialysis patients. In this case the controls were 'natural hospital smells' and an odourless environment. The outcomes were measured by the Hamilton rating scale for depression and the Hamilton rating scale for anxiety. It was found that lavender significantly decreased the score for anxiety, and hiba significantly reduced the scores for both anxiety and depression. (The outcome for the odourless condition was not significantly different from that for the hospital smells.) Although the sample size was small (14 patients), it was concluded that hiba oil was an 'effective, non-invasive means for the treatment of anxiety and depression, and that lavender alleviates anxiety' (Itai *et al.* 2000, p.393).

Preoperative anxiety is another area that has been explored. For example:

Braden, Reichow and Halm (2009) conducted a study to establish whether lavandin essential oil could reduce preoperative anxiety in surgical patients, in comparison with standard care. In this case the sample size was large (150) but the outcomes were measured simply by using a visual analogue scale. It was demonstrated that the lavandin group experienced significantly lower anxiety than either the control (standard care) or the sham (standard care and jojoba) groups, and lavandin was described as a 'simple, low-risk, cost-effective intervention' (Braden *et al.* 2009, p.348).

Akhlaghi *et al.* (2011) explored the potential for neroli (*Citrus aurantium* blossom) to reduce preoperative anxiety. The neroli was delivered orally, with a saline solution administered to the control group; anxiety was measured (prior to and following premedication) using the Spielberger State-Trait Anxiety Inventory and the Amsterdam preoperative anxiety and information scale. The neroli group showed a decrease in anxiety as measured by both scales, while the control showed no significant changes, demonstrating that an oral dose of neroli was effective in reducing preoperative anxiety.

When exploring the literature, it is clear that research designs vary considerably. Yim *et al.* (2009) noted the difficulties in designing aromatherapy/massage research for human subjects, because of the multiple channels of stimulation: olfactory, somatosensory and tactile elements can be present. The studies included in their systematic review on aromatherapy for patients with depressive symptoms highlighted design limitations of the studies; they commented that very few 'well-controlled' randomised clinical trials (RCTs) were available, and that there was a lack of research on patients with primary depression. They concluded that the evidence of the effects of aromatherapy on depressive symptoms was 'insufficient'. Similarly, Perry *et al.* (2012), in their systematic review of RCTs investigating the anxiolytic effects of lavender, were highly critical of the majority of the studies – from the design and methodology to the analyses, discussion and conclusions – again leading to the conclusion that oral administration of lavender 'was promising' but inconclusive, and that lavender administered by aromatherapy, inhalation and massage was 'not currently supported by good evidence of efficacy' (Perry *et al.* 2012, p.834).

Nevertheless, there is a considerable and growing body of research on animal subjects. Tsang and Ho (2010) conducted a systematic review on anxiolytic effects of essential oils on rodents under experimentally induced anxiety models, concluding that 'more standardised experimental procedures and outcome measures are needed in future studies', and that 'translational research to human subjects is recommended'. A similar conclusion was reached by Lee *et al.* (2011) after conducting a systematic review on the anxiolytic effects of aromatherapy on individuals with symptoms of anxiety; they comment that better methodology is needed to identify the clinical effects and clarify the mechanisms. It would appear that many essential oils do have anxiolytic effects without causing adverse events; and although aromatherapists are using essential oils to alleviate anxiety in their clients, there is evidence of further clinical potential. Indeed, Perry and Perry (2006), having reviewed the evidence for aromatherapy in the management of psychiatric disorders, concluded that it provides a 'potentially effective treatment for a range of psychiatric disorders' (Perry and Perry 2006, p.257).

Anxiolytic and sedative effects

It is believed that some essential oil components can bind to various neurotransmitter receptors, including $GABA_A$ (gamma-aminobutyric acid), $5\text{-}HT_{1A}$ (5-hydroxytryptamine) and adenosine A_1. Anxiolytic effects are possibly due to GABAergic modulation, and also serotonergic or adenosinergic modulation.

GABA is the main inhibitory neurotransmitter in the central nervous system, and $GABA_A$ is a receptor subtype. The $GABA_A$ receptor–benzodiazepine complex is a binding site for benzodiazepines. Some essential oils and their constituents potentiate the response of GABA at the receptors, causing anxiolytic, sedative and anticonvulsant effects (Tisserand and Young 2014). Setzer (2009) noted that most of the popular anxiety-relieving essential oils appear to be dominated by the terpenoid alcohols linalool, geraniol and citronellol, and also limonene and citral. Some essential oil constituents have been investigated in relation to their psychoactivity:

Linalool: linalool is implicated in the GABAergic system, which could explain its anticonvulsive and sedative effects, as well as its analgesic activity (Guimarães, Quintans and Quintans-Júnior. 2013). It has been suggested that linalool may inhibit glutamate binding, thus acting as a sedative. *l*-Linalool is certainly considered to contribute to the anxiolytic effects of lavender essential oils, but linalyl acetate, often present in significant amounts, does not appear to have anxiolytic effects when presented independently. However, lavender essential oils that contain both compounds have a greater effect than linalool alone – certainly suggestive of synergism – and indeed both must be present for lavender oil to exhibit anxiolytic action. Takahashi *et al.* (2011) suggested that the synergistic effects of linalyl acetate might be due to the fact that in the limbic system it is hydrolysed by an esterase to linalool. It has also been demonstrated that inhaled lavender essential oils can have anxiolytic-like effects without affecting locomotor functions[10] (Takahashi *et al.* 2011) – highlighting the advantages of aromatherapy over some conventional medications.

Citronellal: citronellal, found in several essential oils such as citronella, lemon-scented eucalyptus, petitgrain combava and lemon balm, has also been investigated with regard to its effects on the psyche. It has a marked depressant action on the central nervous system, coupled with sedative and sleep-inducing properties (Melo *et al.* 2010a; Quintans-Júnior *et al.* 2010).

Carvone: *d*-carvone is a monocyclic monoterpene ketone found in caraway seed, dill seed and white verbena (*Lippia alba*) essential oils. Hatano *et al.* (2012) demonstrated that it was the constituent responsible for the anxiolytic, tranquillising effects of white verbena.[11]

Carvacrol: the isomer of thymol, carvacrol is found in high levels in oregano, savory and numerous *Thymus* species, including *T. zygis* and *T. vulgaris*. These oils are not usually noted for their calming effects; however, Melo *et al.* (2010b)

---

10 Some essential oils, when administered via inhalation, can inhibit locomotor activities. For example, nutemeg oil (*Myristica fragrans*) inhibits locomotor activity in mice and the effect is dose dependent. It was suggested that myristicin, safrole and terpinen-4-ol (which potentiates the $GABA_A$ receptor-mediated response) are involved in the inhibitory effect (Muchtaridi *et al.* 2010).

11 This was an animal study, where rodents were exposed to the essential oil and subjected to the elevated T-maze test.

determined that carvacrol has anxiolytic actions via the $GABA_A$ receptor–benzodiazepine complex.

Limonene: inhalation of *d*-limonene, found in many citrus oils, has anxiolytic actions (Lima *et al.* 2012c, cited by de Sousa 2012), suggesting that it is one of the compounds implicated in the psychoactive effects of sweet orange in animals (Faturi *et al.* 2010) and humans (Goes *et al.* 2012).

Antidepressant effects

Lv *et al.* (2013) note that there are several hypotheses that could elucidate the pathophysiology of depression, but the monoamine deficiency hypothesis (a shortage of noradrenalin and serotonin) is the 'mainstream' model. They suggest that every compound which inhibits noradrenalin and/or serotonin reuptake acts as a clinically successful antidepressant. Additionally, antidepressant drugs such as monoamine oxidase inhibitors and tricyclic drugs, and the new generation of antidepressants that increase monoamines either by inhibiting reuptake by presynaptic neurons, or by acting as antagonists for monoamine receptors,[12] support this hypothesis. Unfortunately, almost a third of patients receiving monoamine-type antidepressants experience undesirable side effects, and the evidence for the benefits of psychological therapies such as cognitive behavioural therapy is limited; we should therefore begin to explore how essential oils might impact on the cerebral neurotransmitters that are implicated in depression, since Lv *et al.* (2103) maintain that aromatherapy should be 'seriously evaluated for the treatment of depression' (p.876).

The 'monoaminergic' systems include the serotoninergic and dopaminergic systems[13] of the brain and CNS – monoamines effectively reduce the availability and indeed uptake of serotonin and noradrenalin. However, it has been suggested that the antidepressant effects of essential oils involve the turnover rate of serotonin in the frontal cortex – in other words, essential oil vapours might be able to regulate serotonin levels – in a way similar to 'the best antidepressants currently available in the therapeutic drug pool' (Lv *et al.* 2013, p.875).

Many essential oils and their components have been described as having significant antidepressant activity. Some, such as bergamot, are thought to stimulate the release of neurotransmitters,[14] while others such as nutmeg and long pepper might inhibit the enzyme monoamine oxidase, which breaks down

---

12 Fluoxetine is a selective serotonin reuptake inhibitor (SSRI).

13 The serotoninergic system influences other neurotransmitters and the dopaminergic and noradrenergic systems.

14 Bergamot can elicit exocytic and carrier-mediated release of amino acids in the hippocampus (Morrone *et al.* 2007, cited by Bagetta *et al.* 2010); lemon essential oil can modulate acetylcholine release in the hippocampus (Ceccarelli *et al.* 2002, cited by Bagetta *et al.* 2010) – both suggestive of activation of olfactory-hippocampal pathways.

neurotransmitters such as serotonin and dopamine. Seol *et al.* (2010) suggested that clary sage exerted antidepressant effects by modulating dopamine activities.

Activating and stress-reducing effects can also be due to the actions of some constituents such as limonene and citral, which can lower the concentrations of serum corticosterone and cerebral monoamines (Fukumoto *et al.* 2007), or via actions on autonomic nerve activity; for example, Shen *et al.* (2005a) demonstrated that the scent of grapefruit had 'activating' effects; the scent of lavender had the opposite effect (Shen *et al.* 2005b). Citral, consisting of the isomers neral and geranial, is found in many essential oils, including lemon myrtle, lemongrass, lemon-scented tea tree, may chang and lemon balm; several studies have demonstrated that citral has motor-relaxing and antidepressant properties (Yim *et al.* 2009).

Cognition

For some time, it has been recognised that essential oil components can impact on cognitive functioning. In 1997 Boddeke, Best and Boeijinga (cited by Bagetta *et al.* 2010) established that activation of glutamate receptors in the hippocampus was implicated in the establishment of coherent beta wave activity, and the potentiation of synaptic transmission – thus influencing both sensory processing and cognitive functioning. Moreover, some essential oil components can bind with both nicotinic and muscarinic cholinergic receptors in brain tissue. Cholinergic systems stimulate the production of acetylcholine (a molecule which is released at the neuromuscular junction and causes contraction), but it has a wider role as a stimulant of the autonomic nervous system, as a vasodilator and cardiac depressant. Kennedy *et al.* (2006) suggested that modulation of the cholinergic system can be beneficial to cognitive functioning.

Impaired cognitive functioning: Alzheimer's disease and dementia

Alzheimer's disease (AD) is a common form of neurodegenerative brain disorder where individuals suffer a progressive and devastating decline in cognitive, behavioural and motor functions. It is thought that the cognitive deterioration is due to a deficit in cholinergic-mediated neurotransmission in the synaptic cleft, and increased levels of acetylcholinesterase and butylcholinesterase have been found in post-mortem brain tissue. Some synthetic and plant-based drugs have been developed to boost cholinergic function by inhibiting acetylcholine degeneration, but so far drugs cannot cure or halt AD, and they can have side effects. However, oxidative stress and inflammation are also factors in the pathology of AD, and indeed it has been observed that the risk of developing AD is reduced in those who use anti-inflammatory medications (Anthony *et al.* 2000, cited by Okonogi and Chaiyana 2012).

Some aromatics, such as narcissus absolute (*Narcissus poeticus*), have been shown to inhibit cholinesterase (Okello *et al.* 2008), as do plai (*Zingiber cassumunar*) essential oil (Okonogi and Chaiyana 2012); terpinen-4-ol, a major constituent of plai (Miyazawa, Watanabe and Kameoka 1997); and lemon (*Citrus limon*) essential oil (Oboh, Olasehinde and Ademosun 2014). The isomers thymol and carvacrol, which dominate some *Thymus* essential oils, are noted for anti-oxidant activity. Azizi *et al.* (2012) investigated their efficacy against induced cognitive defects in rats, providing evidence that they can successfully and safely alleviate cognitive impairments – probably via anticholinesterase, anti-oxidant and anti-inflammatory actions. Therefore anticholinesterase activity coupled with anti-oxidant and anti-inflammatory activities would suggest that some essential oils including narcissus, plai and lemon have therapeutic potential in the management of impaired cognitive function, memory and behaviour.

Lemon balm (*Melissa officinalis*) has also been shown to be of therapeutic value in dementia by calming, reducing agitation and enhancing cognition (Ballard *et al.* 2002); Elliot *et al.* (2007)[15] suggested that this was because it was able to interact with a range of receptors, including 5-HT$_{1A}$, 5-HT$_{2A}$ and GABA$_A$ receptor agonist and channel sites, and histamine H$_3$ receptors. Although the lemon balm and lavender oils used in this study were analysed,[16] it was not determined which of the individual chemical constituents produced the effects. It is likely that the dominant constituents will have effects; indeed we have already established some of the effects of *l*-linalool in lavender oil, and neral, geranial (citral) and citronellal in lemon balm; however, Elliot *et al.* acknowledged the possibility that minor components could also have significant effects, and that synergistic interactions may also be implicated. They suggested that the action of one constituent at a receptor can positively or negatively affect the actions of another constituent via an allosteric[17] effect on the target protein – for example, at the GABA$_A$ receptor. In addition to considering intra essential oil synergy, the effects of lemon balm and lavender combinations were explored – with some interesting results. In terms of binding to receptors, a 1:1 ratio produced additive effects, with one exception – the GABA$_A$–benzodiazepine site. It was concluded that if the effect at this receptor was 'too strong', it might cause over-sedation – an undesirable effect which can lead to falls and social withdrawal in Alzheimer's and dementia patients. These observations offer us an interesting caveat on synergistic blending: we need to be very clear about our objectives when considering combining essential oils, and their doses and ratios.

---

15 This was a laboratory-based study with Wistar rats, to establish the optimum formulation for a clinical trial.

16 The authors noted that there was a variation in essential oils obtained from different suppliers, not only in their chemical composition, but in their efficacy and neurotransmitter modulations.

17 An allosteric effect is where a change in the shape/activity of an enzyme occurs due to binding with a substance at a site other than the active one.

Vigilance and alertness

Inhalation of bornyl acetate, an ester found in several coniferous oils such as hemlock and some spruce and fir species, has effects on cognition, emotion and behaviour. Matsubara *et al.* (2011a) demonstrated that the inhalation of a low dose (279.4µg over a 40-minute period) of *l*-bornyl acetate induced autonomic nerve relaxation and decreased arousal levels in individuals who had undertaken sustained VDT (visual display terminal) work; however, their task performance remained unaffected, because sympathetic nerve activity was not supressed. This would suggest that inhalation of the vapour of bornyl acetate-rich essential oils might be of value for individuals who seek relaxation but need to remain vigilant. However, this study also showed that a higher dose of 716.3µg over the same period induced a decrease in vigilance and performance, possibly because of sedative effects; so it is clear that dosage is an important factor.

Memory enhancement

Before leaving the subject of cognitive functioning, it is worth mentioning a study conducted by Moss *et al.* (2010), where differential effects of the aromas of common sage (*Salvia officinalis*) and Spanish sage[18] (*S. lavandulaefolia*) were examined. It was found that the aroma of common sage produced a 'significant enhancement effect' (Moss *et al.* 2010, p.394) for quality of memory – a cognitive function – compared with the control and the Spanish sage, although both aromas significantly increased alertness (a mood effect) in comparison with the control (no odour). As both aromas were rated as equally pleasant, the hedonic valence mechanism was probably not a factor. It was postulated that the mechanisms involved in the aromatic modulation of mood are distinct from those involved in cognitive effects, and that cognitive effects are probably pharmacological, probably via acetylcholinesterase inhibition. This would seem likely, since Azizi *et al.* (2012) highlighted the cognition-restoring effects of thymol and carvacrol which are found in common sage, while Spanish sage is dominated by 1,8-cineole and camphor.

Essential oil inhalation, mood modulation and wider metabolic influences

An extensive and comprehensive review of the published literature on olfaction and its relationship with the endocrine system and metabolic disorders (Palouzier-Paulignan *et al.* 2012) led to the conclusion that metabolic disorders and body weight modify the physiological response to odours, and that 'the olfactory system is not simply a sensor of external chemical clues, but a parallel detector of internal

---

18   Sometimes called lavender-leaved sage.

chemical clues – the chemistry of metabolism' (p.786). However, to date there have been few published studies on the effects of odour on metabolism.

It is well known that many somatic disorders can be triggered by, or indeed have their roots in, mood disorders such as anxiety and depression. Furthermore, it is probable that oxidative stress is involved in the pathogenesis of psychiatric disorders, including anxiety and depression (Bouayed, Rammal and Soulimani 2009; Ersan *et al.* 2006, cited by Zhang *et al.* 2013; Kuloglu *et al.* 2002; Ng *et al.* 2008). Atsumi and Tonosaki (2007) explored the effects of smelling lavender and rosemary on free radical scavenging activity (FRSA)[19] – a measure of the biological anti-oxidant system. Healthy volunteers sniffed each aroma for five minutes and saliva was collected immediately and analysed for cortisol,[20] secretory immunoglobulin A (sIgA[21]) and α-amylase activity. It was found that the odours of lavender and rosemary significantly increased the FRSA level and decreased cortisol. The total effect of lavender was observed at low concentrations (1000 times dilution) but not at high concentrations (10 times dilution, which was percieived as less pleasant), and that of rosemary at high concentrations but not at low. However, both low and high concentrations decreased cortisol. Lavender stimulates the parasympathetic nervous system, and rosemary the sympathetic, and the authors suggested that both stimulate FRSA, although the former has a weaker effect. Significant effects were not detected for either sIgA or α-amylase activity; it is possible that the short, five-minute exposure was insufficient to elicit any physiological effects. It was concluded that stimulation with a pleasant smell potentiates FRSA and simultaneously decreases cortisol, not always acting via parasympathetic and sympathetic nerves, and thus could protect against oxidative stress.

In 2012 Wu *et al.* demonstrated, for the first time, that the aerial diffusion of essential oils[22] could induce metabolic responses. This was a 'gas chromatography time-of-flight mass spectrometry-metabonomics'[23] study on rats, where behavioural aspects were correlated with metabolic changes. Subtle metabolic changes were recorded, and these included increased carbohydrates and lowered levels of neurotransmitters (tryptophan, serine, glycine, aspartate, tyrosine, cysteine, phenylalanine, hypotaurine, histidine and asparagine), amino acids and

---

19   FRSA decreases in response to exercise fatigue and increases in response to pleasant mental stimulation, including inhalation of a pleasant aroma (Atsumi and Tonosaki 2007).

20   Cortisol is a stress hormone; salivary cortisol is used as a stress marker.

21   Secretory IgA is an antibody important in mucosal immunity; it is the main immunoglobulin found in tears, saliva and sweat. It can survive harsh physiological environments. It is used as a stress marker – it is secreted immediately after a stressful event, and there is also delayed secretion.

22   This was a 'classical formula' (Wildwood 1996): *Lavandula angustifolia*, *Salvia sclarea*, *Santalum album* and *Citrus sinensis*. There were four groups: a control, an anxiety-induced group (the elevated plus maze or EPM), aroma, and aroma plus EPM. The rats in the aroma groups were exposed to the essential oils for 45 minutes every day for ten days.

23   This allowed the researchers to measure endogenous metabolic markers of aroma exposure in the brain and the urine. Essential oil components were not detected, possibly because the concentration was too low to have a detectable level in biofluids and tissues.

fatty acids in the brain, and elevated aspartate, sucrose, maltose, fructose, glucose, nucleosides, lactate and pyruvate in the urine. Brain metabolism is independent of the peripheral circulation, because of the blood–brain barrier; hence the differences in the metabolites in the brain and urine. The significantly increased carbohydrates in brain tissue might be due to the anxiolytic actions of the aroma, as could the decreased levels of brain histamine and its metabolite, phenylalanine. Elevated levels of histamine and phenylalanine are, in humans, associated with 'mind racing', sleep problems and anxiety disorders. It was concluded that inhalation of essential oils could attenuate anxiety-induced metabolic changes; that these changes were concurrent with the behavioural observations; and that this information could lead to a better understanding of the affected pathways in anxiety-related behaviour.

Zhang *et al.* (2013) conducted a study to evaluate the metabolic effects of essential oil inhalation in human volunteers. As in the Wu *et al.* (2012) study, a blend of *Lavandula angustifolia*, *Salvia sclarea*, *Santalum album* and *Citrus sinensis* was investigated; female participants were exposed to the ambient aroma for 45 minutes a day, for ten consecutive days, under controlled conditions. It was found that this daily exposure induced significant metabolic changes in some participants,[24] and all of these were due to endogenous changes rather than inhaled substances. Several metabolic markers[25] in urine were evaluated. It was found, for example, that aroma inhalation elicited a decrease in carbohydrates in urine; this would be consistent with a reduction in anxiety. There was also a reduction in gut microbe-related metabolites, which suggests that the aroma exposure caused an altered gut metabolism, reflecting the relationship between gastrointestinal microbe ecology and gastrointestinal symptoms and anxiety (Haug, Mykletun and Dahl 2002, cited by Zhang *et al.* 2013). It was concluded that the metabolites involved in the TCA (tricarboxylic acid) cycle and gut metabolism were significantly decreased after exposure to essential oil inhalation for ten days, and that this metabolic 'window' could complement the interpretation of behavioural research. We also know that serotonin is found in the gut, and so serotinergic systems are probably involved.

There is no doubt that essential oils have activating, deactivating, harmonising, anxiolytic, antidepressant, sedative and evocative effects. Moreover, the potential to positively influence mood, cognition and behaviour and thus have a beneficial impact on physiology and metabolism is one of aromatherapy's greatest strengths. Table 13.1 provides just some of the evidence that can help inform our choice of aromatics – especially when the I.P. is directed to the psyche, or when refining our selection.

---

24 It was hypothesised that some individuals were more susceptible to the aroma, based on their emotional responses to it.

25 These were carbohydrates, organic acids, amino acids and pyrimidine.

Table 13.1 Effects of essential oils on the psyche

Botanical species	Principal effects	Evidence
Angelica (*Angelica archangelica*)	Anxiolytic	Oral doses of the essential oil had an anxiolytic effect similar to that of diazepam, in mice with experimentally induced anxiety (Chen et al. 2004).
Bay laurel (*Laurus nobilis*)	Mild sedative	In 2003 an animal study conducted by Sayyah et al. (2003) demonstrated that in addition to pain-relieving and anti-inflammatory properties, bay laurel essential oil had mild sedative properties. Inhalation of low levels of volatiles released from bay laurel leaves was rated as pleasant and maintained vigilance performance by facilitating cardiovascular function; higher levels were associated with negative perceptions and did not enhance performance (Matsubara et al. 2011b).
Bergamot (*Citrus aurantium* var. *bergamia* fruct., *C. bergamia*)	Antidepressant Stress reduction	Bergamot essential oil released exocytotic and carrier-mediated discrete amino acids, with neurotransmitter functions, in the hippocampus, and there was evidence of neuroprotection in the case of ischaemia and pain. This supported the use of bergamot in treating the symptoms of cancer pain, mood disorders and stress-induced anxiety (Bagetta et al. 2010). Hand massage with essential oils of bergamot, lavender and frankincense had a helpful effect on pain and depression in hospice patients (Chang 2008). Bergamot, inhaled along with ylang ylang and lavender, reduced psychological stress responses and serum cortisol levels, and reduced the blood pressure of patients with essential hypertension (Hwang 2006).
Black cumin (*Nigella sativa*)	Anxiolytic	Oral administration of the oil can improve cerebral levels of serotonin, and tryptophan in the brain and plasma (Perveen et al. 2009, cited by Lv et al. 2013).
Black pepper (*Piper nigrum*)	Activating	Inhalation of the vapour induced a 1.7-fold increase in plasma adrenaline concentration (Nikolaevskii et al. 1990, cited by Shaaban, El-Ghorab and Shibamoto 2012). Inhalation of the essential oil elicited an increase in sympathetic activity and an increase in plasma adrenaline (Haze, Sakai and Gozu 2002). A randomised controlled trial evaluated inhaled black pepper essential oil[1] and its effects on smoking cessation; it was found that this significantly reduced craving at 3-hour sessions (Kitikannakorn et al. 2013).

Citrus species (peel)	Antidepressant Cognition-enhancing potential	Heuberger *et al.* (2001) showed that both *d*- and *l*-limonene increased systolic blood pressure, but only the *d*-form (in citrus oils) caused subjective alertness and restlessness; the *l*-form had no effects on psychological parameters. Changes in the autonomic nervous system (ANS) and self-evaluation were related to the subjective evaluation of the odours, and both pharmacological and psychological mechanisms contributed to the effects.
		Citrus peel is used in Chinese medicine and African folk medicine in the treatment of degenerative disorders, including neurodegenerative diseases such as dementia. Oboh, Olasehinde and Ademosun (2014) demonstrated that lemon peel oil was an inhibitor of AChE and BChE, inhibited pro-oxidant induced lipid peroxidation, and had anti-oxidant activity – suggesting that it had potential in the management of oxidative-stress-induced neurodegeneration.
Clary sage (*Salvia sclarea*)	Antidepressant	Seol *et al.* (2010) demonstrated that of all the oils tested, clary sage, at a 5% concentration, had the strongest antistressor effect, probably by modulating dopamine activities. They suggest that clary sage could be developed as a therapeutic medication for depression.
Combava peel (*Citrus hystrix*)	Activating Antidepressant	Hongratanaworakit and Buchbauer (2007a) found that massage with *C. hystrix* peel oil caused an increase in blood pressure and decrease in skin temperature compared with the placebo group, and the *C. hystrix* group rated themselves as more alert, cheerful and vigorous than the control; thus the peel oil has activating effects.
		Aris, Taib and Murat (2011) investigated the emotional responses of exposure to the aroma of *C. hystrix* peel oil, which suggested that it has stimulating, activating qualities and may be useful for alleviating mild depression and stress.
Coriander seed (*Coriandrum sativum*)	Anxiolytic Anti-cholinesterase Memory-enhancing effects	Emamghoreishi, Khasaki and Aazam (2005) identified that coriander seed oil has an anxiolytic effect in mice.
		Mahendra and Bisht (2011) explored the potential for coriander seed essential oil and hydroalcoholic extracts as natural anxiolytics to replace benzodiazepines. They proposed that the essential oil components and the flavonoids act via the $GABA_A$ receptor complex, in a similar way to diazepam. They have suggested that because of these anxiolytic effects and also memory-improving effects and anti-cholinesterase activity, coriander seed oil and extracts may have applications in the management of CNS disorders and neurodegenerative diseases.

Plant	Effect	Notes
Fennel, aerial parts (*Foeniculum vulgare*)	Anxiolytic Sedative (higher doses)	Mesfin, Asres and Shibeshi (2014) conducted an animal (mice) study to evaluate the anxiolytic activity of fennel essential oil. They did not analyse the oil, which was hydrodistilled in a laboratory from fresh leaves of an identified species, and cite the composition of bitter fennel seed oil (*trans*-anethole, fenchone[2] and methyl chavicol. It was demonstrated that the essential oil exhibited 'promising' anxiolytic activity; higher doses interfered with locomotor activities and had a sedative effect. The authors suggested that this oil should be studied to establish the optimum dose for use as an anti-anxiety drug. However, their discussion also revolved around the composition and potential active constituents; this is problematical for translation into aromatherapy practice, because the true chemical composition was not established. Moreover, the leaf oil is not commercially available.
Fennel, sweet (*Foeniculum vulgare* var. *dulce*)	Antidepressant Activating	The inhalation of sweet fennel (seed) essential oil can produce a decrease in mental stress, fatigue and depression (Nagai *et al.* 1991). Inhalation of the essential oil elicited an increase in sympathetic activity and an increase in plasma adrenaline (Haze, Sakai and Gozu 2002).
Fir, Korean (*Abies koreana*)	Cognition (memory) enhancing potential	Kim *et al.* (2006) reported the memory-enhancing effects of Korean fir essential oil in mice with scopolamine-induced amnesia; they suggested that terpinen-4-ol was important in this activity.
Fir, Siberian, Japanese (*Abies sibirica*, *A. sachalinensis*)	Anxiolytic	Matsubara *et al.* (2011c) noted that the Siberian fir is used in traditional medicine to maintain health during the severe winters. Their study revealed that inhalation of air containing the essential oil reduced arousal levels after a prolonged visual display terminal (VDT) task. Satou *et al.* (2011b) found that inhalation of *A. sachalinensis* could elicit an anxiolytic-like response (animal study).
Frangipani (*Plumeria* species)	Anxiolytic	In Ayurvedic medicine, frangipani is used to calm fear and anxiety, and also to treat tremors and insomnia (McMahon 2011).
Frankincense (*Boswellia carterii*, *B. socotrana*)	Harmonising Cognition-enhancing potential	Traditional use: Avicenna used frankincense to 'strengthe[neth] the wit and understanding' and the herbalist Culpeper suggested that it helped with depression, poor memory and strengthening the nerves (Lawless 1994). Holmes (1998/1999) theorised that frankincense encompasses four main categories of scent – spicy, sweet, woody and green. The spicy element imparts an uplifting and clarifying effect, while the sweet, woody and green aspects exert a calming, grounding and balancing effect. *Boswellia* species have been used for millennia in traditional medicine for modulation on mood; some species, notably *B. socotrana*, can inhibit acetylcholesterinase[3] (Awadh Ali *et al.* 2014, cited by Hussain *et al.* 2014), and so might have effects on cognition, and perhaps memory.

Plant	Properties	Notes
Geranium (*Pelargonium* × *asperum*, or *P. roseum* [a hybrid of *P. capitatum* × *P. radens*], *P. capitatum*, *P. radens*, *P. odoratissimum*)	Anxiolytic Antidepressant	Inhalation of geranium aroma has been shown to reduce anxiety (Morris, Birtwistle and Toms 1995). Geranium has antidepressant effects (Perry and Perry 2006).
Ginger (*Zingiber officinale*)	Tonic Activating Motivating	Ginger essential oil can restore the humoral immune response in immunosuppressed mice (Schmidt *et al.* 2009). The effects of ginger on the psyche were explored by Holmes (1996), who maintained that the fragrance of ginger combined 'the potential for increased willpower and clarity' (p.19), and so is indicated when there is loss of motivation, apathy, indecision and disengagement.
Grapefruit (*Citrus paradisi*)	Activating	Inhalation of the essential oil elicited an increase in sympathetic activity and an increase in plasma adrenaline (Haze, Sakai and Gozu 2002). Shen *et al.* (2005a) demonstrated that the scent of grapefruit could affect autonomic nerve activity, increasing lipolysis and metabolism, thus reducing weight in rats. This can be interpreted as the fragrance of grapefruit having activating effects. Shen *et al.* (2007) explored the mechanism of changes induced by both grapefruit and lavender scents, where grapefruit stimulated sympathetic nerve activity in white adipose tissue via histamine receptors (H$_1$ receptors).
Hemlock (*Tsuga canadensis*)	Relaxing	Contains 41–43% bornyl acetate (Lagalante and Montgomery 2003), inhalation of which induced autonomic nerve relaxation and decreased arousal levels in individuals who had undertaken sustained VDT work; task performance remained unaffected, because sympathetic nerve activity was not supressed at a low dose. Higher doses had sedative effects (Matsubara *et al.* 2011a).
Hiba wood (*Thujopsis dolobrata*)	Antidepressant Anxiolytic	Itai *et al.* (2000) conducted a clinical trial with chronic haemodialysis patients and the results indicated that aroma of hiba oil was an effective, non-invasive means of treating both depression and anxiety.

Jasmine species (*Jasminum officinale*, *J. sambac*)	Activating Antidepressant	Antidepressant effects (Perry and Perry 2006). Jasmine aroma can regulate mood, enhance alertness and reduce anxiety, and perhaps improve self-confidence and hand–eye coordination (Hirsch *et al.* 2007). Hongratanaworakit (2010) showed that self-administered abdominal massage with *J. sambac* oil not only had a physiologically stimulating effect, but also an increase in subjective behavioural arousal; the jasmine group also felt more attentive, energetic and less tranquillised than the control group. In Ayurvedic medicine *J. officinale* is used as an antidepressant, aphrodisiac and sedative (Shukla 2013).
Juniperberry (*Juniperus communis*)	Activating	Kim *et al.* (2006) demonstrated that the fragrance of juniperberry could suppress weight gain in rats (with no marked difference in 50 minutes of continuous, or short-term, interrupted exposure per day). Rats whose olfactory bulbs were removed did not display suppression of weight gain. It was found that the juniperberry essential oil accelerated sympathetic nerve activity.
Lavandin (*Lavandula × intermedia*)	Anxiolytic	A randomised controlled trial suggested that lavandin could reduce preoperative anxiety, and was a simple, low-risk, cost-effective intervention (Braden, Reichow and Halm 2009).
Lavender, true (*Lavandula angustifolia*)	Stress-reduction Anxiolytic	Itai *et al.* (2000) conducted a clinical trial with chronic haemodialysis patients, and the results indicated that aroma of lavender oil could alleviate anxiety. Shen *et al.* (2005b) demonstrated that the scent of lavender could supress autonomic nerve activity, decreasing lipolysis and metabolism, thus increasing weight in rats. Shen *et al.* (2007) explored the mechanism of changes induced by both grapefruit and lavender scents, where lavender supressed sympathetic nerve activity in white adipose tissue via histamine receptors (H_3-receptors). Lavender, inhaled along with ylang ylang and bergamot, reduced psychological stress responses and serum cortisol levels, and reduced the blood pressure of patients with essential hypertension (Hwang 2006). Exposure to lavender essential oil in the air has an anti-stress effect, with chromogranin A (CgA, a salivary endocrinological stress marker) levels being significantly lowered in the aroma group; no effects on salivary cortisol noted (Toda and Morimoto 2008). Lavender baths for babies can significantly decrease stress in mothers and relax and induce sleep in babies (Field *et al.* 2008). Lavender aroma within an 'optimal soothing environment' prior to gastroscopy minimised patient anxiety (Hoya *et al.* 2008). Inhaled *l*-linalool has an anxiolytic and relaxing effect in mice, with memory affected only by higher doses (Linck *et al.* 2010). Silexan (an oral lavender oil capsule) is as effective as lorazepam (a benzodiazepine) in reducing somatic anxiety and psychic anxiety, but does not have sedative effects and is well tolerated (Woelk and Schläfke 2010).

Lemon (*Citrus limon*)	Activating Antidepressant Cognition-enhancing potential	Lemon oil has antidepressant effects (Perry and Perry 2006). Lemon essential oil, and its components limonene and citral, can decrease both physical and psychological stress by keeping down the concentrations of serum corticosterone and cerebral monoamines (Fukumoto *et al.* 2007). Komori (2009) conducted a study on the effects of the inhalation of lemon and valerian essential oils on the ANS in healthy and depressed male subjects. In the healthy subjects, lemon stimulated sympathetic nerve activity and the parasympathetic nervous system. However, the depressed subjects, who already had enhanced sympathetic activity, showed a decrease relative to the enhanced parasympathetic activity, after inhalation of lemon. Valerian (a sedative) did not stimulate sympathetic activity in any of the test subjects in this study. Lemon can inhibit cholinesterase (Oboh, Olasehinde and Ademosun 2014), and thus has cognition-enhancing potential.
Lemon balm (*Melissa officinalis*)	Anxiolytic Cognition-enhancing	*Melissa officinalis* essential oil reduced agitation in severe dementia, and extended the time spent on constructive activities, while reducing the time of social withdrawal (Ballard *et al.* 2002). Elliot *et al.* (2007) conducted a preliminary investigation to determine the bioactivity of the oil, especially in relation to its ability to bind with the key neurotransmitter receptors that are important in the mediation of agitation. They found that it had a wide receptor binding profile (greater than that of lavender), which could explain its calming and cognition-enhancing actions. They suggested that the topical application or inhalation of *M. officinalis* could be a better way of delivering a treatment for agitation than the usual intramuscular injections or tablets.
Lemongrass (*Cymbopogon citratus*)	Anxiolytic Sedative	A dose of 10mg/kg of lemongrass essential oil had anxiolytic effects in mice, probably via the GABA$_A$ receptor-benzodiazepine complex (Costa *et al.* 2011).[4] Silva *et al.* (2010) found that the essential oil potentiated barbiturate-induced sleeping time in mice.
Lime (*Citrus aurantifolia*)	Anxiolytic	Saiyudthong *et al.* (2009) demonstrated that systolic blood pressure was decreased after a single massage with lime, suggesting the reduction of sympathetic activity and potentiation of the parasympathetic response. It was acknowledged that massage alone could produce these effects, but the lime essential oil potentiated the parasympathetic response.
Long pepper (*Piper longum*)	Antidepressant	Piperine (a pungent constituent of the dried fruit) has 'potent' anti-depressant activity – partially mediated through the inhibition of MAO[5] activity, and is a 'promising candidate' as an antidepressant agent (Zaveri *et al.* 2010).
Marjoram, sweet (*Origanum majorana*)	Anxiolytic Sedating	Mentioned by Perry and Perry (2006) as having comforting, anxiety-relieving and sedating actions.

Plant	Properties	Notes
Nagarmotha (*Cyperus scariosus*)	Antidepressant	In a review of the potential of the herb and essential oil, Bhwang *et al.* (2013) noted that the essential oil has antidepressant action.
Narcissus absolute (*Narcissus poeticus*)	Cognitive effects Sedating	Narcissus absolute was investigated as a potential cholinesterase inhibitor; inhibition was observed at 0.1mg/ml (*in vitro*); it also had behavioural effects in Alzheimer's patients (Okello *et al.* 2008).
Neroli (*Citrus aurantium* var. *amara* flos.)	Anxiolytic	Inhaled neroli was as effective as Xanax (a benzodiazepine) in the treatment of induced anxiety in gerbils (Chen *et al.* 2008). In a randomised double-blind study, it was found that an oral dose of neroli essential oil could reduce preoperative anxiety (Akhlaghi *et al.* 2011).
Orange, sweet (*Citrus sinensis*)	Sedative Anxiolytic	Hongratanaworakit and Buchbauer (2007b) conducted a study that investigated the effects of the transdermal absorption of sweet orange oil, but this time the participants were prevented from smelling the oil. They found that autonomic arousal was decreased, and feelings of cheerfulness and vigour were reported. This type of effect could be due to a quasi-pharmacological mechanism. A study focusing on the use of sweet orange oil in aromatherapy massage concluded that sedative effects were due to olfactory/cognitive influences rather than direct systemic action (Fewell *et al.* 2007). Faturi *et al.* (2010) demonstrated that the aroma of sweet orange oil has acute anxiolytic activity in male Wistar rats. To rule out any non-specific effects of aroma, they also investigated the behavioural responses to the aroma of tea tree – and no anxiolytic effects were observed. Goes *et al.* (2012) evaluated the anxiolytic effect of sweet orange aroma in healthy males submitted to an anxiety-inducing situation (a video-monitored Stroop Color-Word Test, or SCWT), and again the results suggested that it has acute anxiolytic activity.
Osmanthus (*Osmanthus fragrans*)	Antidepressant Activating	Warren and Warrenburg (1993) demonstrated that the scent of osmanthus (synthetic) had stimulating and 'happy' qualities, and could prominently reduce apathy and depression.
Patchouli (*Pogostemon cablin*)	Calming	Inhalation of the essential oil inhibited sympathetic activity and elicited a 40% decrease in plasma adrenaline (Haze, Sakai and Gozu 2002).
Perilla (*Perilla frutescens*)	Antidepressant	Yi *et al.* (2013) demonstrated that oral administration of perilla essential oil could elicit antidepressant effects in mice.
Pink pepper (*Schinus molle*)	Antidepressant	An extract of pink pepper produced an antidepressant-like effect in mice via the monoaminergic systems (Machado *et al.* 2007).

Plai (*Zingiber cassumunar*)	AntiAChE Anti-BChE Cognition-enhancing potential	Okonogi and Chaiyana (2012) investigated the anti-acetylcholinesterase (AChE) and anti-butyrylcholinesterase (BChE) activities of plai essential oil; it was suggested that these actions, coupled with its anti-inflammatory and anti-oxidant activities, would make it a potential candidate for treating Alzheimer's disease. It was suggested that terpinen-4-ol is important in the anti-cholinesterase activity. They also demonstrated that its anti-cholinesterase activities were considerably enhanced when using a microemulsion technique (possibly because of the increased solubility of the oil), and that a topical formulation has advantages in the treatment of Alzheimer's patients.[6]
Roman chamomile (*Anthemis nobilis*)	Calming Sedating	Moss *et al.* (2006) demonstrated that the scent of Roman chamomile had a calming, sedating effect, and reduced subjective alertness. However, as could be expected, these effects were influenced by induced expectancy.
Rose (*Rosa centifolia*, *R. damascena*)	Antidepressant Harmonising Calming Hypnotic	Rose oil has antidepressant effects (Perry and Perry 2006). Hongratanaworakit (2009a) demonstrated that transdermal absorption of rose can produce a state of relaxation, and supported its use in aromatherapy for the alleviation of stress, depression and anxiety, irritability and mood swings. Inhalation of the essential oil elicited a decrease in sympathetic activity and a 40% decrease in plasma adrenaline (Haze, Sakai and Gozu 2002). Maleki, Maleki and Bekhradi (2013) investigated the effects of distilled *R. damascena* essential oil on withdrawal signs in morphine-dependent mice, in comparison with a control group and diazepam group. The essential oil was delivered via intraperitoneal injection, at various concentrations. The results concurred with other studies that suggest that *R. damascena* is an antidepressant that works via the GABA$_A$ system, and that the essential oil can reduce the severity of symptoms of morphine withdrawal. The hypnotic effect of *R. damascena* essential oil is due to its affinity with the GABA$_A$ system (Rakhshandah, Hosseini and Dolati 2004).

Rosemary (*Rosmarinus officinalis*)	Activating Antidepressant	Self-administered abdominal massage with rosemary oil can increase attentiveness, alertness, liveliness, joyfulness, while increasing breathing rate and blood pressure (Hongratanaworakit 2009b). Rosemary promotes alertness, but the effect was short-lived; it can improve speed and accuracy in maths tasks, and rosemary's profile is similar to the effects of oxygen administration and the acute administration of ginseng (Diego et al. 1998; Moss et al. 2003). Moss and Oliver (2012) investigated plasma levels of 1,8-cineole after exposure to rosemary essential oil, finding that the levels correlated with cognitive performance, and concluded that absorbed constituents from rosemary affect cognition and subjective state independently via different neurochemical pathways. Machado et al. (2009) demonstrated that a hydroalcoholic extract of rosemary produced an antidepressant-like effect in mice, and that this was mediated via the monoaminergic system.
Sage, common (*Salvia officinalis*)	Improves quality of memory Cognition-enhancement	The aroma of the essential oil can enhance quality of memory and secondary memory primary outcome factors (Moss et al. 2010). Thymol and carvacrol can restore induced cognition impairment in rats (Azizi et al. 2012).
Sage, Spanish (*Salvia lavandulaefolia*)	Mood and cognition enhancement	A double-blind, placebo-controlled, balanced crossover study revealed that a single oral dose of extract improved both mood and cognitive performance in young, healthy adults (Kennedy et al. 2010).
Sandalwood (*Santalum album*)	Harmonising	Sandalwood fragrance has been used to induce a calm state of mind by all of the Indian spiritual traditions (Morris 1984; Weiss 1997). It is also used to lighten and concentrate the mind (Svoboda 2004) and in Tibetan medicine it is used with other aromatics as a massage oil or incense for insomnia and anxiety (Lawless 1994). Contemporary research has supported the topical use of sandalwood essential oil to elicit both relaxation and behavioural activation simultaneously (Hongratanaworakit, Heuberger and Buchbauer 2004). Heuberger, Hongratanaworakit and Buchbauer (2006) investigated the effects of inhalation of α-santalol, a component of sandalwood oil, and *S. album oil* compared with an odourless placebo. *S. album oil* had an activating effect compared with the α-santalol and the placebo. However, α-santalol produced higher ratings of attentiveness and mood than the essential oil or the placebo. It appears that such effects on arousal and mood are related to perceived odour quality. Both studies support the use of *S. album* as relaxing, antidepressant oil.

Name	Effect	Description
Spikenard (*Nardostachys jatamansi*)	Sedative	The inhalation of agarwood and spikenard oils has sedative effects, and their main constituents also produced such effects, even when administered in lower concentrations than those found in the oils (Takemoto *et al.* 2008). Inhalation of spikenard essential oil was shown to have strong sedative activity, as was its volatile component valerena-4,7(11)-diene. It was suggested that this is a non-harmful method for the treatment of insomnia and ADHD in children (Takemoto, Yagura and Ito 2009).
Tarragon (*Artemisia dracunculus*)	Activating	Inhalation of tarragon essential oil ('estragon') elicited an increase in sympathetic activity and an increase in plasma adrenaline (Haze, Sakai and Gozu 2002).
Turmeric (*Curcuma longa*)	Antidepressant	Curcumin, present in the rhizome, oleoresin and CO_2 extract, has potential antidepressant uses; it compared well with fluoxetine in a randomised controlled trial (Sanmukhani *et al.* 2014). The essential oil does not contain curcumin, but anecdotal reports suggest that the scent has antidepressant, activating qualities.
Verbena, white (*Lippia alba*)	Anxiolytic Tranquillising	In an animal study, *Lippia alba* and its dominant constituent *d*-carvone (present at 40–46%) displayed anxiolytic effects (Hatano *et al.* 2012).
Vetiver (*Vetiveria zizanoides*)	Anxiolytic	In Ayurvedic medicine, the incense and essential oil are used to cool the mind and improve concentration (Svoboda 2004).
Ylang Ylang (*Cananga odorata* var. *genuina*)	Harmonising Stress reduction	Hongratanaworakit and Buchbauer (2004) revealed that ylang ylang has a 'harmonising' effect, where blood pressure and heart rate decreased whilst attentiveness and alertness were increased. Ylang ylang, inhaled along with lavender and bergamot, reduced psychological stress responses and serum cortisol levels, and reduced the blood pressure of patients with essential hypertension (Hwang 2006). Hongratanaworakit and Buchbauer (2006) demonstrated that topical application of ylang ylang significantly decreased blood pressure and increased skin temperature compared with the placebo. The ylang ylang group also reported feeling more calm and relaxed than the control group. Moss, Hewitt and Moss (2008) found that ylang ylang aroma significantly increased calmness, but decreased alertness and reaction times, and impaired memory and processing speed.

1. Inhaled through a hollow plastic tube.

2. The analysis given was from Gulfraz *et al.* (2008); the main constituent was *trans*-anethole at 70.1%, followed by fenchone at 6.9% and methyl chavicol at 4.8%; *d-limonene* was absent. This is not dissimilar to the composition of sweet fennel seed oil; however, sweet fennel oil has limonene at 0.2–21% (Tisserand and Young 2014). It is assumed that Gulfraz *et al.* (2008) analysed bitter fennel (*F. vulgare* var. *amara*); they obtained seeds from a local market in Rawalpindi.

3. The AchE inhibitory effect of this species may be due to the presence of the monoterpenoids (*E*)-2,3-epoxycarene and *para*-menth-1(7)-en-2-one.

4. GABA is the main inhibitory neurotransmitter in the central nervous system, and GABA$_A$ is a receptor subtype. The GABA$_A$ receptor–benzodiazepine complex is a binding site for benzodiazepines. Some essential oils and their constituents potentiate the response of GABA at the receptors, causing sedative and anticonvulsant effects (Tisserand and Young 2014).

5. Monoamine oxidase (MAO) is an enzyme that breaks down serotonin, dopamine, adrenalin and noradrenalin. Some essential oils and their components (such as myristicin and eugenol) are thought to inhibit MAO, hence their antidepressant actions. These should not be administered in conjunction with MAO inhibiting antidepressant drugs or SSRI (selective serotonin reuptake inhibiting) antidepressants (Tisserand and Young 2014).

6. It was suggested that a transdermal delivery would be the ideal approach for treating chronic neurological diseases in the elderly, as it would provide sustained levels of active constituents, is simple to use, and could reduce systemic adverse side effects.

Part III

AROMATICS

In Part III, profiles of a selection of essential oils and absolutes are presented. Here, the aim is to give a summary of their known and likely actions, their directions, traditional uses and notable constituents, with suggestions for expanded practice using related and complementary essential oils and absolutes.

The aromatics are listed by common name and in alphabetical order. If there are several belonging to the same genus – for example, *Thymus* – they will be listed as 'Thyme', with the type following. If, however, the common name refers to oils from different genera or families, as in the case of 'Pepper', each type is listed by its distinguishing characteristic, such as Black pepper, Long pepper, Pink pepper, Szechuan pepper, and so on. If the essential oil that you are considering is not in the main list in Chapter 14, it may be found under 'Expanded Practice Aromatics' in Chapter 15, or in the index.

It is impossible to include every aromatic, so the ones selected here include those that feature prominently in Part II – where we have the makings of an evidence base for practice. Some of these are not currently part of 'mainstream' aromatherapy, but they are commercially available. Oils that are rare and very costly, such as agarwood, have been excluded. Also, some of the more unusual essential oils and absolutes are featured within the profiles under the heading of 'expanded practice', specifically where they might complement and enhance blends from both therapeutic and olfactory perspectives. Some of the oils have associated hazards in specific circumstances, but these oils have been included because it is felt that their therapeutic potential merits this.

In some cases, energetic qualities are mentioned, based on traditional and sacred uses. This may help when a spiritual perspective is being sought, or when 'fine-tuning' blends, or when a number of aromatics are indicated and it is difficult to select the most appropriate ones via more conventional processes.

The main chemical constituents are given, but it should be noted that the percentages are 'typical' and taken from a wide variety of sources (see References); Tisserand and Young (2014) has been used as the main reference text here, especially when there is little consensus among other sources. Variations will certainly be encountered, especially when wild-sourced oils are obtained. It is strongly suggested that if you intend to base your blends on active constituents, you obtain accurate figures from your essential oil supplier. However, bear in mind that the activities of individual constituents may not reflect the actions of the complete essential oil, because of the great potential for synergistic and antagonistic interactions within each and every essential oil.

Essential oil safety is very important, and significant 'cautions' are flagged up. However, safety is not the main focus of this book, so it is suggested that reputable literature is consulted if you are in any doubt as to the hazards presented by any of the oils discussed; Tisserand and Young (2014) is recommended.

Finally, the essential oil combinations mentioned are by no means definitive. They are based on the possibility of compatibility, from the perspective of shared or synergistic constituents, shared actions and directions, and aromas. The blending suggestions are not presented as 'formulae' – that is completely the responsibility of the therapist, who is the only person in a position to create an I.P. Also, these lists are not alphabetical, or presented in order of particular significance, but they do contain 'groups' of compatible oils that you could choose from; for example, herbal, citrus, spice, woods, resins, conifer and floral. It is not the intention to be prescriptive in any way, nor indeed to inhibit creativity – but it is hoped that these suggestions will give you a starting point, and maybe some inspiration.

In Chapter 14 you will find a series of profiles of some of the oils which feature in Part II, consisting of odour descriptions, main constituents, key indications and actions, directions, and blending suggestions for evidence-based practice. Also included, where appropriate, are some suggestions for using alternative and complementary oils, which could expand your scope of aromatherapeutic blending. Chapter 15 consists of abbreviated profiles for the aromatics that feature in these expanded practice suggestions, and more.

Chapter 14

Essential Oils and Absolutes

Evidence-based Practice

Angelica (Umbelliferae)

Angelica archangelica roots; steam-distilled essential oil; contains traces of non-volatiles (including psoralen and bergapten).

Odour: herbaceous, earthy and rich.

Constituents: α-pinene (24%), α- and β-phellandrene (both at 14%–24%), *d*-limonene (up to 13%), δ-3-carene (up to 13%), *para*-cymene, β-myrcene (5–10%) and δ-ocimene (up to 5%); sometimes 1,8-cineole (15%).

Main actions: expectorant, analgesic, anti-nociceptive, antispasmodic, anxiolytic.

Indications: musculoskeletal (fatigue, inflammation, pain), female reproductive (dysmenorrhea), respiratory (congestion), anticarcinogenic potential, psyche (stress and anxiety).

Blending suggestions and expanded practice:

Respiratory: for congestion, consider blending with Atlas cedar, Siberian fir, sandalwood, frankincense, myrtle, spearmint, bergamot.

Musculoskeletal: for aches and pains and toxic accumulations, consider blending with black pepper, nutmeg, coriander seed, clary sage, sweet marjoram, juniperberry.

Female reproductive: for dysmenorrhea, consider blending with plai, thyme, juniperberry, Korean, Siberian or Japanese fir, Douglas fir, palmarosa, rose essential oil.

Psyche: to help reduce stress and anxiety (perhaps due to fear), consider blending with opoponax, pink lotus, patchouli, and vetiver; or to counteract fatigue and anxiety, blend with Siberian fir and bergamot or lemon, or Douglas fir and geranium, palmarosa, rose.

Energetic: evaporate with pink lotus to evoke spiritual support and protection, resilience, peace and transcendence.

Caution: phototoxicity; maximum concentration 0.8%.

Anthopogon (Ericaceae)

Rhododendron anthopogon leaves, twigs and flowers (Nepal); steam-distilled essential oil.

Odour: balsamic, slightly sweet, mild, herbal.

Constituents: constituents include α- and β-pinene (at 37% and 16%) and *d*-limonene (13%), also δ-cadinene (9%) β-ocimene (5%) and other terpenes; these constituents are found in many coniferous essential oils, which share its analgesic and anti-inflammatory properties, and respiratory and musculoskeletal tropisms.

Main actions: antimicrobial (*Bacillus subtilis, Mycobacterium tuberculosis*), antifungal (*Candida* species), analgesic, anti-inflammatory, antiproliferative (tumour cell lines).

Indications: musculoskeletal (sore muscles, rheumatism); respiratory (throat, coughs, congestion, lungs, infections); skin (inflammation, *Candida* infections); energetic (heart and lungs, release of mental and emotional pain, reconnecting with joy, creates a sacred space when diffused).

Blending suggestions and expanded practice:

Musculoskeletal: blend with Scots pine, grand pine, galbanum and blackcurrant bud as a tonic and for musculoskeletal problems, especially when inflammation is involved.

Respiratory: consider bornyl acetate-rich hemlock, black spruce, red spruce, Siberian fir, Japanese fir and silver fir, for diffusion and in treatments directed to the respiratory system.

Skin: for inflammation and acne, blend with white champaca, holy basil, Japanese cedar, combava petitgrain.

Energetic: in Nepal, the Japanese cedar (*Cryptomeria japonica*) is known as *tsugi*, and it is burned as incense. To create a sacred space and peaceful atmosphere, diffuse a blend of anthopogon and Japanese cedar essential oils.

Basil (Lamiaceae)

Ocimum basilicum CT linalool leaves (France); steam-distilled essential oil.

Odour: herbal, slightly anisic, sweet.

Constituents: *l*-linalool (54–58%), eugenol (9–15%), 1,8-cineole (6%), methyl chavicol (up to 2%), traces of methyl eugenol.

Main actions: analgesic, anti-nociceptive, anti-inflammatory, anti-oxidant, immune support, skin penetration enhancement.

Indications: musculoskeletal (pain and inflammation), psyche (stress, fatigue), energetic (promotion of emotional connections with others, final resting places).

Blending suggestions and expanded practice:

Musculoskeletal: for pain and inflammation with stress and anxiety, consider blending with true lavender, clary sage, sweet marjoram and geranium; or with rosemary, bergamot and black pepper if lethargy/burnout is a factor.

Psyche: for anxiety, blend with true lavender and geranium; for fatigue, confusion, or feelings of being overwhelmed you might consider spike lavender, lavandin, rosemary CT cineole, sweet fennel, coriander seed, or the citrus oils bergamot, lemon and lime, or cineole-rich eucalyptus.

Expanded practice: exotic basil, which is also known as Comoran basil, is the estragole (methyl chavicol) chemotype. It contains a substantial amount (73–87%) of this potentially carcinogenic phenolic ether (73–87%) and also methyl eugenol (trace–4%). Methyl chavicol is however credited with antispasmodic properties, and some writers suggest that it is safe to use on the skin in blends for pain; the recommended limit is 0.1%. For the same reasons, tarragon (*Artemisia dracunculus*) could be considered – this contains similar amounts of both constituents. Tarragon also has anticonvulsant and antiplatelet activity.

Basil, holy (Hindu 'Tulsi') (Lamiaceae)

Ocimum sanctum leaves and flowering tops and leaves (India); steam-distilled essential oil.

Odour: aromatic, herbaceous, sweet and clove-like; some varieties have a characteristic cassis (blackcurrant bud) note; there is also a lemon-scented (citral) variety.

Constituents: eugenol – from 40% in Jammu to 71% in Assam, and seasonal variations are noted; also contains methyl eugenol (traces up to approx. 13%), 1,8-cineole (up to approx. 15%), β-bisabolene; traces of β-caryophyllene.

Main actions: antimicrobial (*in vitro*, against *Escherichia coli*, *Bacillus anthracis* and *Pseudomonas aeruginosa*, *Mycobacterium tuberculosis*, *Propionibacterium acnes*), antifungal (*Candida* species) and antiviral, analgesic, anti-inflammatory, anticonvulsive, antispasmodic, vasodilatory, cardioprotective, immunostimulant, anti-allergic, adaptogenic (anti-stress), antioxidant, chemopreventative action, anti-tumoural activity.

Indications: musculoskeletal (sore muscles, tension, spasm, rheumatism, rheumatoid arthritis); circulation (poor peripheral circulation, hypertension); immune (immunosuppression, *Candida* infections, debility, convalescence, allergy); skin (acne, may help prevent scar formation); energetic (purification, inviting divine presence, spiritual protection).

Blending suggestions and expanded practice:

Musculoskeletal: for aches and pains consider blending with black pepper, pink pepper, rosemary, sweet marjoram, lavender; for rheumatoid arthritis consider geranium, coriander seed, ginger, plai and nutmeg.

Circulation: for poor peripheral circulation consider black pepper, pink pepper, Szechuan pepper, and for hypertension/stress consider true lavender, bergamot mint, bergamot, ylang ylang.

Immune: consider lemongrass and ginger for immunostimulation; for *Candida* consider geranium, lemongrass, sweet fennel.

Skin: for acne, consider combava petitgrain, white champaca, ylang ylang, sandalwood.

Expanded practice: may have synergistic effects with antibiotics; African basil (*O. gratissimum*) is also dominated by eugenol at around 54%, with 1,8-cineole (22%); it has similar actions and Indications to holy basil; West Indian bay (*Pimenta racemosa*) contains up to 56% eugenol, and many other constituents which are associated with pain-relieving and anti-inflammatory actions (such as β-myrcene at up to 25%); this could also be considered as an alternative to holy basil for musculoskeletal system applications, but it too merits caution as it also contains small amounts of methyl eugenol.

Caution: the relatively high eugenol content suggests the possibility of interactions with some drugs, including anticoagulants; it may affect blood clotting (oral doses). For dermal use, restrict to 1% and use with caution on clients with sensitive skin or dermatitis.

Bay laurel (Lauraceae)

Laurus nobilis leaves; steam-distilled essential oil and absolute.

Odour:

Essential oil: fresh, sweet, herbal, spicy/clove-like notes and camphoraceous and cineolic notes.

Absolute: herbal, fresh, warm and aromatic with green and spicy notes (preferred in perfumery).

Constituents:

Essential oil: 1,8-cineole (up to 44%) and also α- and β-pinene, α-terpinyl acetate, *l*-linalool (all in general range of 5–15%), eugenol (3%); methyl eugenol is sometimes present, from traces up to 4%; your essential oil supplier can advise.

Absolute: information not available at time of writing.

Main actions: analgesic, anti-nociceptive, anti-inflammatory, expectorant, antiviral (SARS), anti-hypertensive, sedative.

Indications: musculoskeletal (pain and inflammation), respiratory (congestion, infection), psyche (stress, agitation), energetic (divination, vision, prophecy).

Blending suggestions and expanded practice:

Musculoskeletal: for pain and inflammation, rheumatic pain, blend with non-irritant, non-toxic oils such as true lavender, geranium, clary sage, sweet marjoram, juniperberry, rosemary; use in very low concentration (see 'Caution').

Respiratory: for congestion, blend with cineole-rich oils, eucalyptus blue gum, ravintsara, saro, myrtle, hyssop CT 1,8-cineole, or pine and fir species, or bornyl acetate-rich oils such as hemlock; evaporation may be preferable to dermal application.

Psyche: for relaxation and to relieve stress or agitation, blend with ylang ylang, lime, combava peel and labdanum; evaporation may be preferable to dermal application.

Energetic: the smoke was used for its narcotic effects, and the leaves were chewed in preparation for divination; the leaves symbolise academic achievement; evaporate the absolute to enhance meditative practice and promote vision and insight.

Expanded practice: because of the potential hazards, alternatives include nutmeg, basil, holy basil, sweet fennel.

Caution: contains the genotoxic carcinogen methyleugenol (there may be just traces, but it can be present at 4%), so try to obtain a sample that contains only traces, and avoid oils with a higher content. Bay laurel essential oil has been implicated in contact allergic reactions causing redness and severe inflammation. The absolute is used in perfumery, where the levels are voluntarily restricted. The maximum recommended limit for dermal application of the essential oil is 0.5%.

Bergamot (Rutaceae)

C. aurantium subsp. *bergamia* fruit peel; expressed essential oil; available as a furanocoumarin-free (FCF) version.

Odour: citrus, a sharp top note with a sweeter body, with lemony, floral (freesia-like, neroli-like), peppery and herbaceous (lavender-like) notes.

Constituents: variations due to geographical origins; typically linalyl acetate (up to 40%, but as low as 17%), *d*-limonene (27–50%); *l*-linalool (from less than 2% up to 20%); sabinene, γ-terpinene and β-pinene are present from around 5% up to 12%; the non-volatile components include bergapten and occur in traces up to 0.7%.

Main actions: anti-nociceptive, anti-oxidant, anti-atherosclerosis, antidepressant, anxiolytic.

Indications: musculoskeletal (pain), skin (itching, allodynia), psyche (stress, depression, anxiety), energetic (release).

Blending suggestions and expanded practice:

Musculoskeletal: for pain, including pain due to inflammation, blend with true lavender, clary sage, geranium, juniperberry, black pepper, long pepper, pink pepper, coriander seed, or cinnamon leaf or clove bud.

Skin: for itching or pain, blend with true lavender, geranium, immortelle, and consider also citral-rich oils such as may chang (*Litsea cubeba*) or lemon balm (*Melissa officinalis*), or bergamot mint and peppermint or spearmint.

Psyche: for anxiety and depression, perhaps accompanied by pain and stress, consider blending with true lavender, ylang ylang and frankincense; for a refreshing aroma, blend bergamot with lemon, orange, petitgrain bigarade, rosemary and a small amount of neroli – these are classic 'eau de cologne' aromatics.

Energetic: evaporate to diffuse an atmosphere of anger and frustration.

Expanded practice: bergamot mint (*Mentha citrata*) is dominated by *l*-linalool (40%) and linalyl acetate (40%), and has a scent that is reminiscent of petitgrain bigarade, bergamot and lavender; it could be used with bergamot, or in place of it for pain, inflammation, stress relief and anxiety. Yuzu essential oil (*C.* × *junos*, a hybrid of *C. ichangensis*, the Ichang lemon or papeda, and the sour mandarin) is another citrus with floral nuances which could be considered for pain relief, inflammation.

Caution: bergamot essential oil contains traces of phototoxic/photocarcinogenic compounds such as bergapten; limit dermal application to 0.4%, or use rectified oil (bergamot FCF – furanocoumarin free). Its antimicrobial and tissue healing actions may be due to its pro-inflammatory potential – and so the clinical uses of the oil require careful consideration.

Bergamot mint (Lamiaceae)

Mentha citrata leaves: steam-distilled essential oil.

Odour: citrus, lemon-like, light, bright and refreshing, and reminiscent of bergamot, petitgrain bigarade, rosewood, lavender and clary sage.

Constituents: linalyl acetate (40%), *l*-linalool (40%), geranyl acetate (3%), menthol (2%), neryl acetate (2%), also β-myrcene, β-caryophyllene, *d*-limonene, *trans*-β-ocimene, α-terpineol, and others, in traces.

Main actions: anti-nociceptive, anti-inflammatory, anti-oxidant, antimicrobial, antifungal, sedative, anxiolytic (on the basis of the main constituents).

Indications: musculoskeletal (inflammation, pain, tension), skin (prevention of topical infections), psyche (anxiety, stress).

Blending suggestions and expanded practice:

Musculoskeletal: for pain relief, including pain due to inflammation and oedema, consider blending with lavender, clary sage, lemon balm, bergamot, black pepper, pink pepper, coriander seed and juniperberry.

Skin: as an antiseptic for opportunistic bacterial infections, consider blending with *Thymus* species, and tea tree; for fungal infections with carrot seed, holy basil, sweet fennel and tea tree, or with citral-rich oils such as may chang, lemon myrtle, lemon balm.

Psyche: for stress, tension, anxiety, low mood, consider blending with bergamot, combava peel, coriander seed, ylang ylang, geranium, rose, jasmine, golden champaca; for refreshing and activating the senses, consider blending with rosemary CT cineole, basil and peppermint; for calming and aiding sleep, blend with lavender, petitgrain bigarade, neroli.

Expanded practice: bergamot mint has potential as a multi-functional environmental fragrance – it is subtle, mild, fresh and unobtrusive, and has potential as a gentle mood enhancer which could help eliminate unpleasant odours, and might even play a role in discouraging houseflies, thus contributing to a more hygienic environment.

Black cumin (Ranunculaceae)

Nigella sativa seeds; steam-distilled essential oil.

Odour: intense, peppery and spicy, with herbal notes of thyme and oregano.

Constituents: varies according to source; thymoquinone (traces–55%), *para*-cymene (15–60%), *trans*-anethole (up to 38%), α-thujene (2–10%), carvone (trace–4%), *d*-limonene (1–4%), thymol and carvacrol (3%, variable), myristicin (variable), γ-terpinene (13% variable), α- and β-pinene (each 2%), sabinene (trace–2%).

Main actions: anti-oxidant, analgesic, anti-inflammatory, anti-asthmatic (bronchodilatory), chemopreventative, hepatoprotective, anti-atherosclerosis, anticonvulsant.

Indications: musculoskeletal (pain, arthritis, rheumatoid arthritis), respiratory (inflammation, bronchoconstriction, asthma), general wellbeing (LDL cholesterol, liver function, immunity).

Blending suggestions and expanded practice:

Musculoskeletal: for pain, including pain due to inflammation or arthritis, blend with true lavender, geranium, ginger, plai, black pepper, long pepper, pink pepper, coriander seed.

Respiratory: for bronchoconstriction, blend with cardamom, long pepper, pink pepper, ginger, plai, rose absolute, frankincense, thyme, yuzu (inhalation preferred route).

Psyche: for anxiety, consider blending with rose absolute, nagarmotha, patchouli, lemongrass, sweet orange (inhalation preferred route).

Energetic: in Arabic it is known as *Habbah Sadwa* or *Habbat el Baraka*, which translates as 'seeds of blessing'; it is characterised by its ability to impart protection and restore health, and its action on breathing might also suggest a correspondence with the dynamic balance between giving, releasing and receiving.

Caution: thymoquinone is a contact allergen; however, inhalation poses less risk; possibly unsafe in pregnancy; check thymoquinone content with supplier before using.

Black pepper (Piperaceae)

Piper nigrum dried, crushed, almost ripe fruits; steam-distilled essential oil.

Odour: fresh, dry, spicy and woody.

Constituents: vary according to the origin and method of harvesting and drying; terpenoid hydrocarbons (about 70–80%) comprising *d*-limonene (0–40%), β-pinene (5–35%), α-pinene (1–19%), α-phellandrene (1–27%), β-phellandrene (0–19%), sabinene (0–20%), δ-3-carene (trace–15%), myrcene (trace–10%); sesquiterpenes including β-caryophyllene (9–33%), β-bisabolene (trace–5%).

Main actions: analgesic, anti-nociceptive, anti-inflammatory, anti-oxidant, rubefacient, 'warming', activating.

Indications: musculoskeletal (aches and pains, sore muscles, tension, rheumatism), circulation (poor peripheral circulation), wellbeing, energetic (resilience).

Blending suggestions and expanded practice:

Musculoskeletal: for aches and pains consider blending with true lavender, basil CT linalool, clary sage, rosemary, sweet marjoram, peppermint, geranium, juniperberry, coriander seed, nutmeg, galbanum, rose essential oil, citrus (bergamot, lemon, yuzu).

Circulation: for poor peripheral circulation consider lemongrass, West Indian bay, cinnamon leaf, clove bud, ylang ylang.

Expanded practice: there are several alternatives that might be considered: pink pepper (*Schinus molle* of the Anacardiaceae family) contains up to 20% β-myrcene, also α-phellandrene, *para*-cymene, *d*-limonene and β-phellandrene, all of which have analgesic activity and no hazards or known contraindications; it also has anti-inflammatory and antispasmodic actions; Brazilian pepper (*Schinus terebinthifolius raddi* of the Rutaceae family) contains δ-3-carene, α-phellandrene, α-pinene, *d*-limonene and terpinen-4-ol – these are analgesic constituents, with no known hazards or contraindications; Szechuan pepper (*Zanthoxylum piperitum* of the Rutaceae family) is dominated by *d*-limonene (around 40–45%) and has a significant β-myrcene content – again suggesting analgesic activity, with no hazards other than potential sensitisation if an oxidised product is used; it has established anti-oxidant activity, suggesting use in phytocosmeceuticals, and prokinetic actions which would indicate it for gut dysfunction; long pepper (*Piper longum*) contains β-caryophyllene at 18% and piperine, has analgesic (counter-irritant), anti-inflammatory actions (and can reduce oedema associated with inflammation), also anti-asthmatic actions; however, it has anti-fertility actions at 1gm/kg, so should be avoided in pregnancy.

Caution: the oxidised oil can cause skin irritation.

Blackcurrant bud (Grossulariaceae)

Ribes nigrum flower buds, steam-distilled essential oil and solvent-extracted absolute.

Odour: strong, diffusive and penetrating; fruity and green with herbal, cassis (blackcurrant), minty and catty notes.

Constituents:

Essential oil: δ-3-carene (15–35%), β-pinene (trace–24%), β-phellandrene (up to 11%), *d*-limonene (up to 10%), terpinolene (up to 9%), α-pinene (up to 6%); present at less than 5% are γ-terpinene, β-ocimene, *para*-cymene.

Absolute: δ-3-carene (up to 19%), *para*-cymene (up to 15%), sabinene (up to 15%), β-caryophyllene (up to 14%), terpinolene (up to 11%), β-phellandrene (up to 10%), β-ocimene (up to 7%), terpinen-4-ol (up to 6%); present at less than 5% are *d*-limonene, α-caryophyllene (with citronellyl acetate), α-terpinene, β-myrcene, α-terpineol, γ-terpineol, and others.

Main actions: antibacterial (large spectrum of activity, including *Staphylococcus aureus*), anti-pathogenic potential, HLE inhibitor; also analgesic and anti-inflammatory (on basis of major and minor constituents).

Indications: musculoskeletal (pain and inflammation), skin (inflammation, regeneration, sun damage, infection control).

Blending suggestions and expanded practice:

Musculoskeletal: for pain and inflammation, consider blending with Scots pine, grand pine and galbanum, or with juniperberry, rosemary, basil, geranium and bergamot mint.

Skin: for sun-damaged skin, consider blending with helichrysum and violet leaf, or jasmine, cacao; regenerating carriers should be considered; as an antiseptic/infection control, blend with bergamot, coriander seed, pink pepper.

Psyche: in perfumery, the catty element is sometimes described as imparting an animalic, erotic effect, but the oil is not traditionally used as an aphrodisiac.

Expanded practice: the fruity green notes in blackcurrant bud can be used to modify intense green odours, such as that of galbanum and violet leaf.

Caraway seed (Umbelliferae)

Carum carvi dried seeds; steam-distilled essential oil; often rectified to improve odour.

Odour: spicy, intense, warm, sweet (may have a 'weedy' nuance in top note).

Constituents: dominated by *d*-carvone (50–60%) and *d*-limonene (40–50%), with traces of *cis*-dihydrocarvone and β-myrcene.

Main actions: anti-oxidant, hepatoprotective, possibly hypolipidemic, and on the basis of dominant constituents, anxiolytic, anti-inflammatory (inhibitor of 5-LOX); traditional use as digestive and carminative.

Indications: musculoskeletal (pain and inflammation), digestive (support), wellbeing, psyche (anxiety, debility).

Blending suggestions and expanded practice:

Musculoskeletal: consider blending with black pepper, cinnamon, lavender, yuzu.

Digestive: consider blending with Szechuan pepper, pink pepper, sweet fennel, coriander seed, lime, thyme, spearmint or mojito mint.

Psyche: for anxiety, consider blending with jasmine, golden champaca, cassie (Acacia farnesiana) absolute, tobacco absolute or white verbena.

Energetic: caraway seeds are traditionally credited with fortifying and nurturing qualities and are said to confer the gift of 'retention', hence used to restore vigour and protect against loss, theft and infidelity.

Expanded practice: also consider using dill, which contains *d*-limonene and *d*-carvone, with α-phellandrene.

Cardamom (Zingiberaceae)

Elettaria cardamomum sun-dried fruits and seeds; steam-distilled essential oil.

Odour: aromatic, warm and spicy, with a slight camphoraceous/cineolic nuance in the top note.

Constituents: 1,8-cineole (up to 50%, but less is desirable for the olfactory impression), α-terpinyl acetate (24–40%), limonene (6%), also linalyl acetate and linalool, geraniol, α-terpineol and others.

Main actions: expectorant, antitussive, decongestant, anti-oxidant, antimicrobial, anti-nociceptive, analgesic, anti-inflammatory, cognition-enhancement (attributed to 1,8-cineole).

Indications: respiratory (infections, bronchoconstriction, inflammation, congestion, asthma), psyche (mental fatigue, stress, anxiety), energetic (traditional reputation as an aphrodisiac).

Blending suggestions and expanded practice:

Respiratory: for congestion and breathing problems, consider blending with pink pepper, ginger, plai, rose absolute, bay laurel, frankincense, yuzu.

Psyche: for mental fatigue and anxiety, consider blending with jasmine, rose, golden champaca, ylang ylang, bergamot, labdanum, frankincense, sandalwood.

Expanded practice: to replicate the early Arabic formula in the *The Perfumed Garden of Sensual Delight*, combine cardamom with cinnamon, cloves, nutmeg, pepper and a floral oil, such as rose (or carnation absolute if available); or replicate the ceremonial Hindu incense *Abir* by combining with turmeric, cloves and sandalwood.

Carrot seed (Umbelliferae)

Daucus carota subsp. *carota* dried seeds; steam-distilled essential oil.

Odour: spicy, fresh, sweet, intense, persistent, earthy, rooty, woody.

Constituents: vary according to source; carotol (up to 70%), daucol, α-pinene, also geranyl acetate, sabinene, limonene, β-caryophyllene, β-bisabolene, 11-α-(h)-himachal-4-en-1-β-ol.

Main actions: antifungal, antidermatophytic, active against *Candida albicans*.

Indications: skin (dermatophyte infections, *Candida* infections), traditionally used as a digestive tonic (traditional), urinary (traditional).

Blending suggestions and expanded practice:

Skin: a 1:1 ratio of carrot seed to true lavender has synergistic activity against *C. albicans*; for antimycotic actions also consider blending with sabinene-rich plai or yarrow, or with geranium, lemongrass, sweet fennel, pink pepper, sage, black cumin or turmeric.

Digestion: for appetite stimulation and digestive support, consider blending with sweet fennel, coriander seed and lime, also pink pepper, Szechuan pepper, spearmint, ginger.

Expanded practice: the combination of carrot seed and cedarwood essential oils can mimic the scent of orris oil (a 'butter' or concrete), obtained from the dried rhizomes of *Iris pallida*, *I. germanica* and *I. florentina*. Carrot seed also blends well with fenugreek (*Trigonella foenum-graecum*), which contains around 15% camphor – which could increase activity against some dermatophytes.

Cassie (Mimosaceae)

Acacia farnesiana flowers; absolute by solvent extraction.

Odour: a warm, spicy-floral scent with a powdery-floral top note and rich balsamic notes in the dryout.

Constituents: complex and variable in terms of levels of constituents; constituents include benzyl alcohol, methyl salicylate, farnesol, geraniol, linalool, linalyl acetate, geranyl acetate, *para*-anisaldehyde, nerolidol, traces of α- and β-ionones.

Main actions: anti-inflammatory.

Indications: skin (inflammation and oxidative stress), psyche (stress, depression, anxiety).

Blending suggestions and expanded practice:

Skin: for inflammation and damage due to intrinsic and extrinsic ageing, consider blending with violet leaf and blackcurrant bud, or jasmine, rose absolute, poplar bud; regenerating carriers should be considered too.

Psyche: for stress, depression and anxiety consider blending with linden blossom, mimosa, jasmine and perhaps traces of caraway.

Expanded practice: farnesol (a sesquiterpenol) has a delicate floral (lily of the valley-like), green scent and anti-inflammatory potential; consider blending cassie with other farnesol-containing oils, such as linden blossom and mimosa. Cassie contains less than 5% methyl salicylate, which has a sweet fruity/ medicated odour and anti-inflammatory potential, so consider blending with other oils that also contain minor amounts, such as ylang ylang and frangipani absolute, along with small amounts of methyl salicylate-rich sweet birch (*Betula lenta*, 90%); methyl salicylate can inhibit blood clotting, so use with caution.

Cedar, Atlas and Himalayan (Pinaceae)

Cedrus atlantica and *C. deodara* wood; steam-distilled essential oils.

Odour: Atlas (Moroccan) cedar is woody, warm and camphoraceous with soft floral notes; Himalayan cedar is woody, sweet and resinous, but if unrectified has a urinous, slightly 'dirty' quality.

Constituents:

Atlas: α-, β- and γ-himalchenes (70%); other components include α- and γ-atlantone isomers (10–15%), himachalol (2–4%), also δ-cadinene, γ-curcumene.

Himalayan: α- and β-himalchenes (45%), cedrene (16%), α- and γ-atlantone isomers (10%), *cis-* and *trans-*atlantone (up to 7%), *ar-*dihydroturmerone, *d*-himachalol and *d*-allohimachalol.

Main actions: anti-inflammatory, analgesic, antispasmodic, grounding and calming.

Indications: musculoskeletal (pain and inflammation, tension, spasm), psyche (restless mind), traditionally used in the treatment of respiratory, skin and urinary infections.

Blending suggestions and expanded practice:

Musculoskeletal: for tension, pain, consider blending with cypress, juniperberry, Virginian cedarwood, camphor CT nerolidol, frankincense, myrrh, ylang ylang.

Psyche: for agitation, or a restless mind, consider blending with bergamot, mandarin, citron, lavender, frankincense, myrrh, hiba wood, sandalwood, nagarmotha, vetiver, ginger, ylang ylang.

Energetic: The Lebanese cedar symbolised fertility and abundance, and also spiritual strength; the name 'cedar' is derived from the Arabic word *kedron*, which means 'power'; many other cultures valued the ability of cedar to 'preserve'.

Chamomile, German (blue) and Roman (Asteraceae)

Matricaria recutita and *Anthemis nobilis* (*Chamaemelum nobile*) aerial parts and flowers, or dried flowers; steam-distilled essential oils.

Odour:

German: strong, sweet, herbal and fruity, with hay-like notes and a tobacco-like nuance.

Roman: herbal, fruity, sweet, warm, intense, diffusive, with herbaceous, apple-like and tea-like notes.

Constituents:

German: different chemotypes exist, so chemical composition varies widely; active constituents include α-bisabolol (2–60%), α-bisabolol oxide A and B (traces–60%), chamazulene (3–25%), *trans*-β-farnesene (5–30%).

Roman: a very wide variation according to source; isobutyl angelate and butyl angelate (0–35% each), isobutyl butyrate (0–20%) and isoamyl angelate (5–20%), camphene (0–5%), borneol (0–5%) and many others at less than 5%.

Main actions:

German: anti-inflammatory, anti-allergic, antipruritic, antispasmodic, antifungal (yeasts), anti-oxidant, cancer suppression.

Roman: antispasmodic (potential), possibly calming, sedating, reduces subjective alertness.

Indications:

German: musculoskeletal (inflammation, tension, spasm), skin (inflammation, allergy, itching, candidiasis), wellbeing.

Roman: psyche (stress, tension, anxiety, insomnia).

Blending suggestions and expanded practice:

Musculoskeletal: consider blending German chamomile with geranium, lavender, sweet marjoram, clary sage, golden rod, citron, ylang ylang.

Skin: for itching and inflammation, consider blending German chamomile with lavender, bergamot mint, geranium, immortelle, rose essential oil, peppermint, tea tree, niaouli, hops, hemp, guava leaf, vetiver.

Psyche: for tension and headache, consider German chamomile with peppermint; for stress, tension and anxiety, insomnia, consider Roman chamomile with lavender, clary sage, neroli, sweet orange, ylang ylang, hay absolute, labdanum.

Expanded practice: Roman chamomile has a modifying effect on powerful green scents, such as galbanum and violet leaf; an absolute is also available and this has a sweet, warm fruity, herbal aroma which is more robust than the essential oil, sweeter and warmer, and also slightly floral. Blend Roman chamomile with small amounts of tagetes (pungent, warm herbal, sweet, fruity and apple-like, with anti-oxidant and anti-inflammatory properties) to augment its apple-like and fruity notes; emphasise the hay and tobacco notes in German chamomile by blending with hay and tobacco absolutes.

Energetic: Roman chamomile has a long tradition of use for healing and as a companion plant (the 'plants physician'); it was a popular strewing herb that came to represent 'patience in adversity'; its apple-like scent can be hypnotic and evoke feelings of ease.

Champaca, golden and white (Magnoliaceae)

Michaela champaca (golden yellow) and *M. alba* (white, also called magnolia blossom) flowers; absolutes by solvent extraction; *M. alba* essential oil by distillation.

Odour:

Golden: penetrating, warm, smooth and rich indolic floral, with a neroli-like note and spicy, tea-like undertones.

White: powerful, sweet, heady, indolic floral, with notes of lily, hay and orange blossom.

Constituents: complex and variable, over 250 constituents have been identified.

Golden: characterised by 2-phenylethylalcohol (up to 35%), with methyl lineolate, methyl anthranilate, methyl benzoate, benzyl alcohol, α-farnesene, farnesol, *l*-linalool, traces of ionones, and others.

White: characterised by *l*-linalool (up to 75%), 2-phenylethanol (5–10%), and benzyl alcohol, methyl salicylate, farnesol, geraniol, linalyl acetate, geranyl acetate, *para*-anisaldehyde, nerolidol, and traces of α- and β-ionones may be present; white champaca may also contain small amounts (0–2%) methyl eugenol.

Main actions: anti-inflammatory, anti-oxidant (keratinocyte differentiation), antibacterial (*white* is active against *P. acnes*), relaxing.

Indications:

Golden: skin (inflammation, and oxidative stress, dryness, ageing).

White: skin (inflammation, acne), psyche (stress and tension).

Blending suggestions and expanded practice:

Skin:

Golden: for inflammation and damage due to intrinsic and extrinsic ageing, such as impaired barrier function, dryness, wrinkles and thinning skin, consider blending with rose, orange blossom, poplar bud and cacao absolutes, sandalwood, patchouli, vetiver; consider using regenerating carriers such as avocado, blackcurrant seed, *Centella asiatica*, lucuma nut, rosehip seed.

White: for acne, consider blending with jasmine, clary sage, guava leaf, coriander seed and sandalwood, or plai, holy basil, guava leaf, lemon myrtle and eucalyptus blue gum; consider using carriers such as jojoba, blackcurrant seed, raspberry seed, grapeseed.

Psyche: for stress, tension, depression and anxiety consider blending with rose, jasmine, orange flower, frangipani, pink lotus, hay, tobacco (absolutes), ylang ylang, bergamot, coriander seed, caraway seed, nutmeg, sandalwood, nagarmotha, patchouli.

Expanded practice: golden champaca has good phenylethanol content and will be a useful addition to blends when the properties of this constituent are desirable. White champaca has strong activity against *P. acnes*, and could be used in blends for the management of acne where a relaxing floral element is desired, but to minimise any hazard presented by methyl eugenol, use less than 1% in your blend if methyl eugenol is over 2% (check level with your supplier), or use *M. alba* essential oil (often called 'magnolia flower') which is dominated by linalool (70%), with β-caryophyllene and others.

Cinnamon leaf (Lauraceae)

Cinnamomum zeylanicum (*C. verum*) leaves; steam-distilled essential oil.

Odour: harsh, pungent, warm and spicy odour, typical of the spice but also reminiscent of clove, with sweet fruity notes.

Constituents: eugenol (65–90%), with eugenyl acetate, cinnamyl acetate (up to 3%), benzyl benzoate, *cis*-cinnamaldehyde, linalool, may contain traces of safrole.

Main actions: anti-oxidant, analgesic, rubefacient (counter-irritant), anti-inflammatory, antibacterial, antifungal (yeasts).

Indications: musculoskeletal (inflammation, pain), circulatory (poor peripheral circulation), skin (superficial infections), psyche (restorative, aphrodisiac).

Blending suggestions and expanded practice:

Musculoskeletal: for inflammation and pain, and poor circulation, blend cinnamon leaf with non-irritant, anti-inflammatory oils such as geranium, lavender, basil, coriander seed, nutmeg, turmeric, myrrh, frankincense, mandarin, yuzu, orange blossom and rose absolutes, rose essential oil (ratio 1:9).

Skin: a lavender and cinnamon combination with a dominance of lavender may have synergistic activity against *C. albicans*; also additive activity against *S. aureus*, except when cinnamon is dominant (3:7) and synergy might be observed.

Psyche: for stress and feelings of discomfort and vulnerability, combine with ylang ylang or rose, labdanum, vanilla absolute, cacao absolute.

Expanded practice: in ancient cultures, cinnamon was associated with power and wealth; it was considered to be both a panacea and an aphrodisiac. To replicate the early Arabic formula in the *The Perfumed Garden of Sensual Delight*, combine cinnamon with cardamom, cloves, nutmeg, pepper and a floral oil, such as rose (or carnation absolute if available).

Caution: eugenol can interact with medication, inhibit blood clotting, and can also be an irritant; use with care, in low concentration (suggested maximum in the region of 0.5%).

Clary sage (Lamiaceae)

Salvia sclarea flowering tops and leaves; steam-distilled essential oil.

Odour: sweet, warm, herbal with tobacco-like and tea-like notes.

Constituents: linalyl acetate (60–75%), *l*-linalool (10–16%), germacrene D (2%), β-caryophyllene (1–2%), others including sclareol (0%–traces).

Main actions: analgesic, anti-nociceptive, anti-inflammatory, antibacterial (*P. acnes*), antidepressant.

Indications: musuloskeletal (pain, inflammation, tension), female reproductive (dysmenorrhea), skin (acne), psyche (low mood, pessimism, depression).

Blending suggestions and expanded practice:

Musculoskeletal: for inflammation and pain, muscular tension, consider blending with geranium, lavender, basil, bergamot mint, hops, golden rod, juniperberry, coriander seed, cardamom, bergamot, mandarin, yuzu, ylang ylang, black pepper, pink pepper, sandalwood.

Female reproductive: for dysmenorrhea, consider blending with lavender, sweet marjoram, angelica, plai, sweet fennel.

Skin: for acne, consider blending with holy basil, rosemary, also lemon myrtle, combava petitgrain, coriander seed, jasmine, rose, blackcurrant bud.

Psyche: for low mood, depression and anxiety, consider blending with sweet orange, jasmine, golden champaca, rose, ylang ylang, coriander seed, sandalwood, hops, hay, tobacco absolute.

Expanded practice: clary has a long association with the female reproductive system and its disorders, and also as a euphoric agent. There are three broad types of sage, based on their dominant constituents:

> *Group I* consists of species characterised by α- and β-thujone such as Dalmatian sage.

> *Group II* by linalool and linalyl acetate such as clary sage.

> *Group III* by 1,8-cineole and camphor, such as Greek, Lebanese and Spanish sage.

An alternative (for evaporation) is clary sage absolute, which has a sweet, light, warm herbal aroma, with woody and ambra nuances – both subtle and persistent – and can contribute to creating a relaxed and uplifting ambience.

Clove bud (Myrtaceae)

Syzygium aromaticum dried unopened flower buds; water-distilled essential oil.

Odour: directly related to the spice, rich, warm sweet with fruity and woody notes.

Constituents: dominated by eugenol (up to 97%), with β-caryophlyllene (traces to 12%) and others, may be traces of methyl eugenol (check with supplier).

Main actions: anti-inflammatory, analgesic, immunostimulant, antibacterial, antifungal (*Candida* species), anti-oxidant, antiproliferative, anti-atherosclerosis (vasorelaxant).

Indications: musculoskeletal (inflammation, arthritis, pain), immune (compromised immunity, debility, convalescence), wellbeing, skin (topical infections including candidiasis), psyche (relaxing, aphrodisiac).

Blending suggestions and expanded practice:

Musculoskeletal: consider blending with lavender, clary sage, geranium, bergamot, ylang ylang, nutmeg, turmeric, coriander seed, pink pepper, Brazilian pepper, Szechuan pepper or long pepper.

Immune: for prevention of infection, debility, or maintaining wellbeing, consider blending with patchouli, ginger, turmeric, lemongrass, palmarosa.

Skin: for prevention of infection, and topical bacterial and *Candida* infections, consider blending with rosemary, lavender, immortelle, coriander seed, blackcurrant bud.

Psyche: for relaxation and wellbeing, consider blending with rose, jasmine, golden champaca, ylang ylang, pink lotus, coriander seed, turmeric, sandalwood, nagarmotha, patchouli, palo santo.

Expanded practice: create an aromatherapeutic version of the ancient aphrodisiac formula in *The Perfumed Garden of Sensual Delight* by combining clove with cardamom, cinnamon, nutmeg, pepper and a floral oil, such as rose (or carnation absolute if available) to create a sensual, relaxing ambience; or the ceremonial Hindu incense *Abir* by combining with turmeric, cardamom and sandalwood to create a peaceful atmosphere. Or you might like to mimic the 'Mellis accord', which was a traditional perfumery accord that formed the base for spicy oriental perfumes, by blending clove, patchouli and linden blossom. Clove was also found in traditional pain-relieving liniments, often with camphor, wintergreen and origanum. Other eugenol-containing oils that could be used as an alternative are holy basil and West Indian bay.

Caution: Use in small amounts because of the very high eugenol content, in a ratio of 1:9 with other oils that do not contain eugenol.

Combava (makrut lime, kaffir lime) peel (Rutaceae)

Citrus hystrix peel; steam-distilled essential oil.

Odour: vibrant citrus, reminiscent of key lime, fresh and pine-like notes.

Constituents: variable; β-pinene (30–32%), *d*-limonene (5–29%), sabinene (15–21%), citronellal (traces–17%), α-terpineol (6–7%).

Main actions: anti-nociceptive, anti-inflammatory, antimicrobial (including respiratory pathogens), activating, antidepressant.

Indications: musculoskeletal (pain, inflammation), respiratory (infections), psyche (low mood, depression, stress).

Blending suggestions and expanded practice:

Musculoskeletal: for pain, inflammation, tension, consider blending with plai, turmeric, lemongrass, sandalwood, clove bud.

Respiratory: for management and prevention of respiratory tract infections, consider blending with combava petitgrain, eucalyptus blue gum, fragonia, ginger, pink pepper, long pepper, sandalwood.

Psyche: for low mood, depression, stress, consider blending with geranium, ylang ylang, clary sage, rosemary, coriander seed, pink pepper, nagarmotha, patchouli, sandalwood.

Expanded practice: it has been suggested that a combava peel throat spray could be developed as a potential preventative measure or treatment for streptococcal throat infections; this might also help prevent nosocomial-acquired pneumonia in vulnerable patients in hospitals.

Combava petitgrain (makrut lime leaf, kaffir lime leaf) (Rutaceae)

Citrus hystrix leaves; steam-distilled essential oil.

Odour: strong, citronella-like odour, with warm lime-like and floral-rosy nuances.

Constituents: variable; *l*-citronellal (59–82%), citronellol (10–14%), *d*-limonene (up to 6%), citronellyl acetate, *iso*-pulegol, sabinene, linalool (traces to 5%), β-pinene, β-myrcene and γ-terpinene (up to 2%); it is more often the *d*-isomer of citronellal that is found in lemon-scented essential oils such as citronella (*Cymbopogon nardus*) and lemon-scented eucalyptus (Eucalyptus citriodora); it is not clear whether in this instance chirality impacts on the therapeutic actions.

Main actions: anti-nociceptive, anti-inflammatory, anti-oxidant, antibacterial (*P. acnes*), sedative and sleep-inducing properties (based on citronellal content).

Indications: musculoskeletal (pain and inflammation, tension), antimicrobial (respiratory pathogens), skin (acne), psyche (stress, tension, insomnia).

Blending suggestions and expanded practice:

Musculoskeletal: for pain, inflammation and tension, consider blending with combava peel, yuzu, ginger, plai, lemongrass, coriander seed, turmeric, nutmeg, black pepper, pink pepper, vetiver.

Respiratory: for infections and prevention, consider blending with combava peel, eucalyptus blue gum, fragonia, ginger, pink pepper, long pepper, sandalwood.

Skin: for acne, consider blending with holy basil or African basil, guava leaf, petitgrain bigarade, ylang ylang, white champaca, sandalwood, patchouli; a hydrophilic base with aloe and honey might be appropriate for home prescriptions.

Psyche: for tension, and stress, consider blending with combava peel, ginger, lemongrass, palmarosa, ylang ylang, pink pepper, long pepper, coriander seed, turmeric, sandalwood, patchouli, nagarmotha, vetiver.

Energetic: according to folk tradition, combava leaves were used to ward off evil spirits, and in Malaysia combava is important in a bathing ceremony called *mandi berlimau.*

Expanded practice: in traditional medicine, combava leaves are often found in hot herbal compresses for the relief of pain and inflammation, and in bath preparations to improve circulation and reduce muscle tension.

Coriander seed (Umbelliferae)

Coriandrum sativum fully ripe, dried seeds; steam-distilled essential oil.

Odour: fresh, sweet, spicy and woody, with floral and citrus notes.

Constituents: variable; coriandrol, or *d*-linalool (60–88%), α-pinene (trace–10%), γ-terpinene (trace–10%), β-pinene and *para*-cymene (trace–9%), camphor (1.5–7%), geraniol, camphene (trace–5%), also *d*-limonene, geranyl acetate, terpinen-4-ol, α-terpineol.

Main actions: analgesic, anti-inflammatory, antispasmodic, anti-oxidant, antibacterial (*P. acnes, Staphylococcus epidermidis, S. aureus, Streptococcus pyogenes*), anxiolytic, memory-enhancing.

Indications: musculoskeletal (pain, tension, inflammation, osteoarthritis, rheumatic pain), digestive (cramp), wellbeing, skin (acne and oozing dermatitis, traditional), psyche (anxiety, impaired cognition, stress).

Blending suggestions and expanded practice:

Musculoskeletal: consider blending with lavender, clary sage, sweet marjoram, geranium, plai, ginger, lemongrass, turmeric, nutmeg, cardamom, sweet orange, yuzu, black pepper, pink pepper, long pepper.

Digestive: for appetite stimulation, digestive support and relief of cramps, consider blending with sweet fennel, carrot seed, lime, mandarin, Szechuan pepper, spearmint, ginger.

Wellbeing: for health maintenance and enhancement, consider blending with lime, sweet orange, pomelo, bergamot, basil, lemongrass, palmarosa, turmeric, caraway, pink pepper, long pepper.

Skin: consider blending with rose, immortelle, hemp, vetiver; and also with clary sage, combava peel and plai for acne.

Psyche: for anxiety, consider blending with ylang ylang, rose, patchouli and sandalwood, or citrus oils such as sweet orange, mandarin, yuzu, lime, combava peel; for enhancing cognition, consider blending with plai, cardamom and lemon.

Energetic: in ancient times the Chinese maintained that the seeds could confer immortality; the scent of the essential oil can impart a sense of euphoria.

Cypress, Mediterranean (Cupressaceae)

Cupressus sempervirens, C. sempervirens var. *horizontalis* leaves and twiglets, sometimes cones; steam-distilled essential oil.

Odour: woody, resinous and balsamic, with smoky notes.

Constituents: α-pinene (49%), δ-3-carene (22%), limonene (5%), α-terpinolene (5%), myrcene (4%), α-cedrol (3.5%), β-pinene (2.5%), germacrene D (1.5%), sabinene (1%), γ-terpinene (1%), and others.

Main actions: anti-inflammatory, pain-relieving, anti-oxidant, NO scavenger, antiproliferative, antiglycation, antibacterial (antibiofilm), astringent (traditional), wound-healing (potential).

Indications: musculoskeletal, respiratory (traditional), wellbeing, skin.

Blending suggestions and expanded practice:

Musculoskeletal: for inflammation and pain, consider blending with Scots pine, juniperberry, Atlas cedar, clary sage, lavender, sweet marjoram, rosemary, black pepper, nagarmotha.

Respiratory: for prevention of infection, inflammation, consider blending with thyme, Greek sage, rosemary, eucalyptus blue gum, hemlock, long pepper, pink pepper; also rosalina, fragonia, anthopogon.

Skin: for prevention of infection, inflammation and wound healing, consider blending with geranium, rosemary, clary sage, anthopogon, bergamot, sweet orange, lemon, Korean fir, juniperberry, eucalyptus blue gum; could also be included in anti-ageing blends for its antiglycation action, perhaps along with rose, myrrh and yarrow, and regenerating carriers.

Energetic: symbolises grief and mourning, but also transition and transformation.

Eucalyptus 'blue gum' (Tasmanian gum) and eucapharma eucalypts (Myrtaceae)

Eucalyptus globulus var. *globulus* leaves and twigs; steam-distilled essential oil.

Odour: typically powerful, fresh, penetrating, medicinal, cineolic, with camphoraceous and green notes.

Constituents: contain significant amounts of 1,8-cineole; 'blue gum' 1,8-cineole (56–85%) with α-pinene (up to 15%), *d*-limonene (up to 10%), and others including *para*-cymene (up to 4%).

Main actions: 1,8-cineole is significant; it is a skin penetration enhancer, a decongestant and an antitussive, a licenced product for the treatment of bronchitis, sinusitis, respiratory tract infections and rheumatic conditions; it has anti nociceptive activity which does not involve the opioid system; high doses can have adverse effects on locomotion and low doses elicit nociception at spinal and supraspinal levels; it is a potent anti-inflammatory agent with an excellent peripheral analgesic effect; it has anaesthetic qualities (acting directly on sensory nerves and blocking excitability); 'cooling' sensations may be due to its activation of specific ion channels; it is expectorant, a bronchodilator and antitussive agent, with action against respiratory pathogens; antifungal (including yeasts), and mentally stimulating; *E. globulus* has skin-penetration-enhancing actions, and is astringent and anti-seborrheic (acting by decreasing sebum production by reducing the size of sebaceous glands); the eucapharma oils will probably share these properties.

Indications: musculoskeletal (pain, inflammation), respiratory (congestion, infection), skin (acne), psyche (mental fatigue).

Blending suggestions and expanded practice:

Musculoskeletal: for pain and inflammation, consider blending with lavender, lavandin, spike lavender, rosemary CT cineole, rosemary CT myrcene, sweet marjoram, *Thymus vulgaris*, clove bud, black pepper, pink pepper, plai, ginger, lemon.

Respiratory: for congestion, infections, consider blending with myrtle, Atlas cedar, bay laurel, cajeput, niaouli, ravintsara, saro, rosalina (type 2), sweet fennel, thyme, peppermint, Greek sage, fir (Siberian, Japanese, balsam or silver), fragonia, ginger, plai, long pepper, hemlock, lemon, yuzu.

Skin: for acne-prone and oily skin, consider blending with basil, holy basil, Korean fir, rosemary, camphor CT nerolidol, lemon myrtle, combava petitgrain, lemon, yuzu, sandalwood.

Psyche: to enhance alertness, consider blending with rosemary CT cineole, peppermint, juniperberry, common sage, Spanish sage, grapefruit, lemon, black pepper.

Expanded practice: as an alternative to blue gum, consider using one of the other eucapharma oils – blue-leaved mallee (*E. polybractea*), green mallee (*E. viridis*), gully-gum or Smith's gum (*E. smithii*), or *E. camadulensis*; the 'industrial eucalypts', namely the broad-leaved peppermint (*E. radiata*) and narrow-leaved peppermint (*E. dives*), could also be considered, especially for their expectorant and antimicrobial actions. Other alternatives might include cajuput, niaouli, ravintsara (asthma) and myrtle. Some, such as niaouli, ravintsara and the broad-leaved peppermint are also said to embody the 'cold and flu' synergy, because of their relative proportions of monoterpenes, monoterpene alcohols and 1,8-cineole.

Caution: 1,8-cineole-rich oils present a hazard to small children and babies – they can cause breathing difficulties and affect the CNS; cineole-rich oils should not be applied near their faces. In cases of dermatitis, the maximum recommended dermal limit is 1%.

Fennel, Sweet (Umbelliferae)

Foeniculum vulgare var. *dulce* dried seeds; steam-distilled essential oil.

Odour: fresh, sweet, spicy, anisic and earthy.

Constituents: *trans*-anethole (50–90%), *d*-limonene (up to 20%), fenchone (trace –8%), methyl chavicol (1–4.5%), with α-pinene, α-phellandrene and *cis*-anethole.

Main actions: analgesic, anti-inflammatory, vasorelaxant, antithrombotic, chemopreventative, hepatoprotective, anti-oxidant, antibacterial, antifungal (dermatophytes and yeasts), antispasmodic, activating, antidepressant.

Indications: musculoskeletal, respiratory, digestive, female reproductive, skin, wellbeing, psyche.

Blending suggestions and expanded practice:

Musculoskeletal: for pain, inflammation, spasm, tension, consider blending with basil, lavender, sweet marjoram, geranium, ginger, plai, black pepper, pink pepper.

Respiratory: for bronchial spasm and coughs, consider blending with thyme, rosemary CT 1,8-cineole, peppermint, or rosalina, yuzu and rose, long pepper, ginger, galangal.

Digestive: for colic, cramp, spasm, consider blending with thyme, spearmint, peppermint, mojito mint, ginger, coriander seed, lime.

Female reproductive: for dysmenorrhea, consider blending with plai, angelica, pink pepper.

Skin: for dermatophytic and superficial infections (not mucous membranes), consider blending with plai, carrot seed, sage CT 1,8-cineole, geranium, lemongrass.

Psyche: to enhance alertness, and combat mental fatigue, consider blending with rosemary, black pepper, lemon, lime; for wellbeing and depression, blend with coriander seed, cardamom and rose.

Energetic: in ancient times, fennel was associated with longevity, strength and courage, for helping the sight, and to avert the evil eye.

Expanded practice: you might also consider the other 'anisic' oils – anise (*Pimpinella anisum* seeds) and star anise (*Illicium verum* dried fruits) – but these and sweet fennel should be used with care due to their high anethole content and the presence of methyl chavicol (estragole).

Caution: sweet fennel, anise and star anise essential oils can interfere with medication (anti-diabetic, diuretic and anticoagulant) – and should be avoided in pregnancy, breastfeeding, endometriosis, oestrogen-dependent cancers, bleeding disorders, children and babies.

Check with your supplier regarding the methyl chavicol content; if it is in the region of 5%, limit dermal applications to 1.5–2.0%.

Fir (balsam, grand, Korean, Japanese, Siberian and silver) (Pinaceae)

Abies balsamea, *A. grandis*, *A. koreana*, *A. siberica*, *A. sachalinensis* and *A. alba* young shoots and needles, sometimes cones; steam-distilled essential oils.

Odour: generally, fir essential oils have fresh, typically coniferous, pine-like scents, sometimes with a lemony aspect, and lacking the resinous base notes of the pines and junipers; there are subtle differnces – for example, Siberian fir has a fresh, sweet, coniferous and pine-like odour, with balsamic and citrus nuances; grand fir has an orange note; the balsam fir is sweet, balsamic and forest-like, with a fruity note; and the silver fir is sweet and rich, with balsamic notes.

Constituents: varies according to species; typical constituents are α- and β-pinene, bornyl acetate, camphene, *d*-limonene, β-myrcene, δ-3-carene and β-phellandrene.

Siberian fir: bornyl acetate (31%), camphene (24%).

Japanese fir: bornyl acetate (30%), camphene (18–19%).

Balsam fir: β-pinene (up to 56%), bornyl acetate (5–16%).

Silver fir: bornyl acetate (30%), camphene (20%), δ-3-carene (14%), tricyclene (13%), *d*-limonene (7.5%), and α-pinene, β-caryophyllene, β-phellandrene and α-terpinene as minor constituents, present at 1.0–5.0%.

Main actions: analgesic, anti-inflammatory, anti-oxidant, antimicrobial (some species), anxiolytic.

Indications: musculoskeletal, respiratory, skin, wellbeing, psyche.

Blending suggestions and expanded practice:

Musculoskeletal: for inflammation and pain, rheumatism, consider blending with bornyl acetate-rich hemlock, black, red and white spruce; Scots pine, rosemary, spike lavender, lavandin, also galbanum, blackcurrant bud, bergamot, lemon.

Respiratory: for inflammation, cough, prevention of infection, blend with bornyl acetate-rich oils such as hemlock, black, red and white spruce, labdanum, cistus, rosemary, thyme, Greek sage, blue gum, cypress, long pepper, also rosalina (type 2), fragonia, anthopogon.

Skin: for acne, inflammation, consider blending Korean fir with Japanese cedar, Lebanese cedar, rosemary, poplar bud.

Psyche: for anxiety, prevention of mental fatigue, relaxation, consider blending with hemlock, Douglas fir, hiba wood, juniperberry, frankincense, rosemary, lemon, black pepper.

Energetic: hemlock, spruce and fir oils have been used in traditional spiritual and health-sustaining practices. Folk wisdom indicated that these conifers and their oils conferred strength and resilience, clarity and purpose, and happiness; and that they acted specifically on the lungs, joints and muscles, often being used to alleviate respiratory problems, rheumatism and arthritis.

Frankincense (olibanum) (Burseraceae)

Boswellia carterii (or *B. sacra*), *B. serrata*, *B. papyrifera* gum resin; steam-distilled essential oil.

Odour: terpenic, lemony, woody, spicy, borderline balsamic.

Constituents: variable, *B. carterii* and *B. sacra* typically α-pinene (20–50%), α-phellandrene traces–40%), *d*-limonene (5–22%), β-myrcene (traces–20%), β-pinene (traces–10%), *para*-cymene (traces–15%), β-caryophyllene (2–10%), and many more including terpinen-4-ol, sabinene, linalool, bornyl acetate, δ-3-carene, δ-cadinene, camphene, α-caryophyllene and others.

Main actions: anti-inflammatory, anti-arthritic, anti-oxidant, antiproliferative, apoptosis-inducing, antibacterial, antifungal, harmonising, cognition-enhancing potential.

Indications: musculoskeletal, respiratory (traditional), skin (traditional), wellbeing, psyche.

Blending suggestions and expanded practice:

Musculoskeletal: for inflammation, joint pain, consider blending with balsam fir, Korean fir, Scots pine, cypress, juniperberry, sweet marjoram, lavender, coriander seed, cinnamon leaf, clove bud, ginger, bergamot, lemon, mandarin, myrrh, black pepper, pink pepper, jasmine, cassie absolute.

Respiratory: to aid breathing, and support the system, consider blending with rose and cardamom, or consider ginger, fragonia, rosalina type 2 and long pepper.

Skin: for inflammation and protection, consider blending with bergamot, jasmine, rose, myrrh, pink pepper, or with violet leaf, galbanum and blackcurrant bud.

Wellbeing: for health maintenance and enhancement, immune support, consider blending with mastic, opoponax and myrrh; also clove bud, patchouli, lemongrass, jasmine, cassie absolute.

Psyche: for mood elevation and cognition enhancement, consider blending with bergamot, lime, grapefruit, combava peel, coriander seed, juniperberry, Spanish sage, Siberian fir, hiba wood, narcissus, frangipani, rose, ylang ylang, sandalwood.

Energetic: frankincense is the archetypal incense, it has psychoactive properties; the ancient Greek philosopher, Pythagoras, used frankincense to enable him to prophesy. The cross-cultural observations of the effects of incense on the psyche, such as heightened senses and awareness, have since been explained in terms of neurophysiology. Avicenna used frankincense to 'strengtheneth the wit and understanding', and the herbalist Culpeper suggested that it helped with depression, poor memory and strengthening the nerves. In terms of Fragrance Energetics, frankincense encompasses four main categories of scent – spicy, sweet, woody and green; the spicy element imparts an uplifting and clarifying effect, while the sweet, woody and green aspects exert a calming, grounding and balancing effect. Therefore the scent of frankincense creates a dynamic balance, but the net balancing effect is provided by the sweet and green notes.

Geranium (Geraniaceae)

Pelargonium × *asperum, P. roseum* (a hybrid of *P. capitatum* × *P. radens*), *P. capitatum, P. radens, P. odoratissimum* leaves; steam-distilled essential oil.

Odour: depends on the botanical and geographical source:

The *Bourbon, Réunion* essential oil (rose geranium) is fresh, rosy with herbaceous, green, vegetable and minty nuances.

Moroccan oil has a sweet, rosy and herbaceous aroma.

Egyptian oil has a similar aroma to that from Morocco.

Oil from *China* is more variable in quality because of the differences in distillation methods and also the number of variants under cultivation; generally, Chinese oil has a harsher odour than Réunion, and is more lemony and rosy, sweet and herbaceous.

Constituents: a typical rose geranium from Réunion has citronellol (20–48%), geraniol (up to 30%), *l*-linalool (up to 15%), *iso*-menthone (up to 10%), γ-eudesmol (up to 8%), and numerous others, including geranyl esters, menthone, β-myrcene, β-caryophyllene and *cis*-rose oxide.

Main actions: analgesic, anti-inflammatory, hypotensive, vasorelaxant, antifungal (including yeasts), antibacterial, anxiolytic, antidepressant.

Indications: musculoskeletal (inflammation, pain, oedema), skin (inflammation, pain, infections), psyche (stress, tension, anxiety, depression).

Blending suggestions and expanded practice:

Musculoskeletal: for inflammation with oedema, blend with bergamot mint, lavender, clary sage, thyme, peppermint, immortelle, lemon balm, lemongrass, yuzu, long pepper, pink pepper.

Skin: for inflammation, pain, soft tissue damage, bruising, blend with lavender, immortelle, basil, bergamot, Lebanese cedar, Virginian cedar, juniperberry, rose, patchouli; for prevention of bacterial infections blend with tea tree, consider blackcurrant bud, rosemary, clary sage, coriander seed, Korean fir, combava petitgrain, lemon myrtle; for dermatophytes consider Sardinian sage, carrot seed, sweet fennel, lemongrass, plai, pink pepper.

Psyche: for stress, anxiety and depression consider blending with Douglas fir, balsam fir, grand fir, sweet orange, yuzu, bergamot, bergamot mint, clary sage, jasmine, ylang ylang, rose, sandalwood, patchouli.

Energetic: often associated with balance, and creativity.

Expanded practice: despite the variations in scent, geranium oils will have very similar actions and Indications. It is possible, therefore, to align the scent of the oil with those that you intend to blend with. For example, you might use the Chinese oil with citral or citronellal-rich oils, the Egyptian or Moroccan with herbal oils, and the Réunion oil with floral, herbal, green or minty-scented oils.

Ginger (Zingiberaceae)

Zingiber officinale unpeeled, dried and powdered rhizomes; steam-distilled essential oil.

Odour: a lemony, spicy top note, a warm, spicy and woody body, with a spicy, balsamic dryout.

Constituents: zingiberene (38–40%), *ar*-curcumene (17%), β-sesquiphellandrene (7%), camphene (5%), β-phellandrene, borneol, 1,8-cineole, α-pinene, β-elemene and others; sometimes farnesene.

Main actions: analgesic, anti-inflammatory, anti-emetic, antispasmodic, anti-oxidant, anti-tumoural, immunostimulant, decongestant, bronchodilator, activating, motivating.

Indications: musculoskeletal (pain and inflammation, osteoarthritis), digestive (nausea, cramp), wellbeing, immune, respiratory (congestion, bronchoconstriction), psyche (fatigue, lethargy, apathy).

Blending suggestions and expanded practice:

Musculoskeletal: for pain and inflammation, consider blending with lavender, rosemary, geranium, lemongrass, may chang, yuzu, bergamot, Atlas cedarwood, turmeric, galangal, black pepper, long pepper, pink pepper; for osteoarthritis also consider plai.

Digestive: inhale ginger for nausea; for digestive cramps, consider blending with sweet fennel, sweet marjoram, spearmint, peppermint, mojito mint, coriander seed, galangal, lime.

Respiratory: for congestion, inflammation, bronchoconstriction, consider blending with plai, galangal, cardamom, sweet fennel, black cumin, anthopogon, sweet marjoram, rosemary, long pepper, yuzu, kewda, rose absolute.

Immune: for immune support, consider blending with turmeric, clove bud, frankincense, lemongrass, patchouli.

Wellbeing: consider blending with angelica root, black cumin, frankincense, bergamot, grapefruit, pomelo, palmarosa, galangal, turmeric, poplar bud, nagarmotha, patchouli, ylang ylang, ginger lily.

Psyche: for fatigue, lethargy, feeling undermined, lack of clarity and direction, consider blending with frankincense, coriander seed, lime, grapefruit, sweet orange; rose, jasmine, golden champaca, ginger lily absolutes.

Energetic: the scent of ginger essential oil can support the will and impart clarity; it can be helpful for loss of motivation, apathy, indecision and feelings of disengagement.

Expanded practice: create an aromatherapeutic version of *Trikatu* (an Ayurvedic formula for increasing digestive fire, treating cold and fevers, and relieving respiratory congestion) by blending with black pepper and long pepper; evaporate ginger with ginger lily rhizome (*Hedychium spicatum*) and white ginger lily flower (*H. coronarium*) to create a relaxing ambience. Galangal (*Alpinia galanga*) could also be considered – either blended with ginger, or as an alternative for the musculoskeletal and respiratory systems.

Grapefruit (Rutaceae)

Citrus × paradisi peel; cold-expressed essential oil.

Odour: sharp citrus top notes, a sweet, fresh citrus, orange-like body, but distinctively 'grapefruit' – due to traces of a sulphur-containing compound called nootkatone.

Constituents: *d*-limonene (up to 95%), with β-myrcene, α-pinene, sabinene, *d*-linalool, geraniol and nootkatone (trace–1%).

Main actions: anti-nociceptive, anti-inflammatory (inhibitor of 5-LOX), anti-oxidant, hepatoprotective (potential), cancer suppression (all based on high *d*-limonene content), activating, anxiolytic.

Indications: musculoskeletal (pain and inflammation), wellbeing, psyche (lethargy, anxiety and depression).

Blending suggestions and expanded practice:

Musculoskeletal: for tension, stress, pain, inflammation, consider blending with bergamot, basil, lavandin, rosemary, sweet fennel, cardamom, black pepper, long pepper, pink pepper, plai, ginger.

Wellbeing: consider blending with pomelo, palmarosa, black pepper, ginger, turmeric, patchouli.

Psyche: for lethargy, low mood, anxiety, consider blending with lemon, bergamot, pomelo, citron, geranium, rosemary, juniperberry, ginger, pink pepper, black pepper.

Expanded practice: the grapefruit 'note' is difficult to work with; although the major constituent of the peel oil is *d*-limonene, the grapefruit-scented nootkatone (which is an isomeric form of a ketone based on a terpenylcyclohexanol structure) and traces of a sulphur-containing compound give the oil its distinctive aroma. It has been suggested that the yellow type is preferable to the pink or red variants, because this contains slightly more nootkatone; however, this is a matter of personal preference.

Hemlock (Pinaceae)

Tsuga canadensis needles and twigs; steam-distilled essential oil.

Odour: sweet, clean and coniferous, with pine-like and green-earthy nuances, completely lacking in any harsh, disinfectant-like characteristics.

Constituents: bornyl acetate (41–43%), α-pinene (13%), camphene (8%), with β-pinene, β-myrcene, α- and β-phellandrene, *ortho*-cymene, *d*-limonene, *cis*-ocimene, borneol, piperitone, β-caryophyllene, α-humulene, γ- and δ-cadinene (all at less than 5%), and others.

Main actions: analgesic, anti-nociceptive, anti-inflammatory, antitussive, expectorant, relaxing.

Indications: musculoskeletal (inflammation and pain), respiratory (congestion, coughs), psyche (stress, tension, focus), energetic (strength, resilience, clarity, will).

Blending suggestions and expanded practice:

Musculoskeletal: for pain, inflammation, tension, fatigue, consider blending with bornyl acetate-rich fir, spruce; also Douglas fir, Scots pine, rosemary

CT bornyl acetate or CT myrcene, spike lavender, golden rod, galbanum, blackcurrant bud, bergamot, lemon.

Respiratory: for coughs, congestion, consider blending with bornyl acetate-rich fir, spruce, inula, golden rod, valerian; cypress, rosemary CT bornyl acetate or CT 1,8-cineole, thyme, labdanum, cistus, long pepper, anthopogon.

Psyche: for fatigue, lack of focus and concentration, tension, consider blending with rosemary CT 1,8-cineole, lime, grapefruit, lemon, Douglas fir, balsam fir, pink pepper; for relaxation consider lavender and valerian.

Energetic: hemlock, spruce and fir oils have been used in traditional spiritual and health-sustaining practices; folk wisdom indicated that these conifers and their oils conferred strength and resilience, clarity and purpose, and happiness, and that they acted specifically on the lungs, joints and muscles, often being used to alleviate respiratory problems, rheumatism and arthritis.

Expanded practice: evaporate hemlock essential oil when undertaking work (perhaps at a VDT or computer screen) that requires sustained focus; perhaps with Douglas fir to evoke clarity of thought.

Immortelle (Asteraceae)

Helichrysum angustifolium, or *H. italicum* subsp. *italicum* flowering tops; steam-distilled essential oil.

Odour: powerful, rich, sweet, honey-like, fruity and tea-like, with a warm and herbaceous dryout.

Constituents: neryl acetate (35–40%), γ-curcumene (6–13%), with variable amounts of α-pinene (traces to 20%), *d*-limonene (3–10%), *ar*-curcumene (traces–12%), italidiones (up to 8%), and *d*-linalool, nerol, and others.

Main actions: analgesic, anti-inflammatory, antibacterial (*Staphylococcus* and *Streptococcus* species), wound-healing, anti-haematomal.

Indications: musculoskeletal (pain and inflammation), skin and soft tissues (inflammation, pain, soft tissue damage, bruising).

Blending suggestions and expanded practice:

Musculoskeletal: for pain and inflammation, including arthritis, consider blending with lavender, geranium, golden rod, hops, ginger, plai, pink pepper, nutmeg, clove bud.

Skin: for inflammation, pain, soft tissue damage, bruising, blend with lavender, sweet marjoram, bergamot, Lebanese cedar, Virginian cedar, inula, rose, orange blossom absolute, patchouli, pink pepper; for prevention of infection consider anthopogon and blackcurrant bud; consider regenerating carriers including rosehip seed; for allergic responses consider tea tree and German chamomile.

Expanded practice: neryl acetate is not often found as a major constituent, but it is believed that it contributes to the pain-relieving and anti-inflammatory actions of immortelle; to augment neryl acetate, consider blending with fenugreek (which contains 15% neryl acetate), also lemon balm (up to 4%), orange flower absolute (up to 4%), and petitgrain bigarade (2–3%), where appropriate.

Jasmine (Oleaceae)

Jasminum grandiflorum, J. sambac, J. auriculatum (and others), flowers; absolutes via solvent extraction, CO_2 extracts available.

Odour:

J. grandiflorum from France: heady, intense, diffusive, rich and heavy, warm floral (jasmine), indolic, with fruity, animalic, waxy, spicy, tea-like and green notes.

J. sambac from India: sweet, delicate, fresh, light top notes, but body is a heady, intense, diffusive, rich indolic floral (jasmine), with lily-like, tea-like, fruity and green notes.

Constituents:

J. grandiflorum: benzyl acetate (15–25%), benzyl benzoate (8–20%), with others including *d*-linalool, indole (up to 4%), *cis*-jasmone (up to 4%).

J. sambac: α-farnesene, indole (up to 14%), *d*-linalool (up to 15%), methyl anthranilate (5%), benzyl acetate (4–5%), phenylethanol (2–3%), and others.

Main actions: activating, antidepressant, relaxing, euphoric, aphrodisiac, antioxidant, inhibitor of HLE, antibacterial (including *P. acnes*), antiseptic, antiinflammatory, regenerating, wound-healing, antispasmodic.

Indications: skin (acne, intrinsic and extrinsic ageing, inflammation, damage), psyche (depression, low mood).

Blending suggestions and expanded practice:

Musculoskeletal: for stress-related tension, spasm, consider blending with clary sage, Roman chamomile, yuzu, ginger, black pepper, long pepper, pink pepper, Szechuan pepper, sandalwood.

Female reproductive: for premenstrual syndrome, dysmenorrhea, consider blending with sweet fennel, plai, angelica, rose, palamarosa, pink pepper.

Skin: for acne, consider including white champaca, coriander seed, clary sage, plai and yuzu in the blend; for skin damage and regeneration, consider blending with blackcurrant bud absolute, rose absolute, cypress, myrrh, patchouli, sandalwood, and include regenerating carriers.

Psyche: for low mood, depression, poor self-esteem, lack of confidence, anxiety, consider blending with clary sage, Roman chamomile, nagarmotha, patchouli, sandalwood, coriander seed, black pepper, long pepper, pink pepper, sweet orange, grapefruit, lime, combava peel, frankincense, ginger, turmeric, ylang ylang, kewda, pink lotus, frangipani and golden chamapca absolutes.

Energetic: since ancient times, fragrant jasmine flowers were used in garlands, as hair decorations, in worship and ritual, strewn at feasts, and used to scent bathwater; according to a South Indian folktale there was once a king whose laugh would spontaneously spread the fragrance of jasmine for miles around; jasmine was considered to be an aphrodisiac, but was also a muscle relaxant and used to facilitate childbirth; jasmine could be considered as one of the most significant scents associated with 'feeling good'.

Expanded practice: jasmine has been well-researched, and the actions cited above are based on evidence as well as tradition. You will find that *sambac* is more heady and indolic than *grandiflorum*, and perhaps better suited to blends where you would like to emphasise its relaxing, euphoric and indeed sensual aspects, while *grandiflorum* might be well suited in skin care blends. There are many other varieties of jasmine to explore. To give an indolic facet to blends, you might also consider using red or golden champaca, orange flower absolute, tuberose, white ginger lily, or honeysuckle (if available, very scarce) absolutes. In India jasmine was used to scent ointments, body oils, hair dressings and perfumes; the *gandhika* (perfume dealer) had an important role in society. You might enjoy recreating a perfumed body oil by blending sesame oil with *sambac*, coriander seed, cardamom, holy basil, kewda, turmeric, red or golden champaca and clove bud; or you could create an aromatherapeutic blend inspired by *Iasmelaion*, a perfume of ancient Rome, by blending sesame oil, *grandiflorum*, cardamom, cinnamon, turmeric and myrrh.

Juniperberry (Cupressaceae)

Juniperus communis berries; steam-distilled essential oil.

Odour: terpenic, coniferous (pine-like), resinous, woody, balsamic, fresh.

Constituents: α-pinene (25–55%), sabinene (up to 30%), β-myrcene (up to 25%), terpinen-4-ol (up to 18%), *l*-limonene (up to 10%), and others such as γ-terpinene, δ-3-carene, *para*-cymene, β-caryophyllene, α-terpineol.

Main actions: analgesic, anti-nociceptive, anti-inflammatory, histamine suppression, antispasmodic (potential), antimicrobial, antifungal (including dermatophytes, due to presence of sabinene with α-pinene), anti-oxidant, activating.

Indications: musculoskeletal (inflammation, pain), respiratory (histamine-induced bronchoconstriction and spasm), skin (inflammation, dermatophytes), urinary (traditional), psyche (stress).

Blending suggestions and expanded practice:

Musculoskeletal: for pain, inflammation, stress-related tension and spasm, arthritis and rheumatic pain, consider blending with basil, clary sage, lavender, geranium, rosemary, thyme, sweet marjoram, coriander seed, sweet fennel, frankincense, ginger, plai, nutmeg, lemongrass, palmarosa, cypress, Himalayan cedar, hemlock, camphor CT nerolidol, bergamot, black pepper, pink pepper, long pepper.

Respiratory: for bronchoconstriction, consider blending with plai, ginger, tea tree, sweet marjoram, kewda, black cumin, yuzu, German chamomile, yarrow.

Skin: for inflammation, dermatophyte infection, consider blending with Sardinian sage, carrot seed, sweet fennel, lemongrass, palmarosa, plai, pink pepper.

Energetic: in folk tradition juniper has been used to drive away evil, to assist prayer, in ritual and ceremony, to evoke protection from natural elements; herbalists believed that the berries could restore the brain and nerves, and indeed restore youth.

Expanded practice: juniperberry essential oil is activating, and was able to supress weight gain in rats. Unwanted weight gain is a complex problem; however, evaporation of a combination of juniperberry and grapefruit (and perhaps rosemary) essential oils might be supportive for those who wish to lose weight. Phoenician juniperberry oil is anti-inflammatory and has wound-healing actions; this also could be considered in blends directed to the skin.

Kewda (Kewra) (Pandanaceae)

Pandanus odoratissimus, P. fascicularis 'flowers' (male spadix, enclosed in a long, fragrant bract); hydrodistilled essential oil (known as *rooh kewra*).

Odour: powerful, sweet, lilac, green and honey-like.

Constituents: variable; the main constituent responsible for the aroma is phenylethyl methyl ether (65–75%), terpinen-4-ol (up to 20%), *para*-cymene, α-terpineol, γ-terpinene; may also contain phenylethanol, benzyl alcohol (and its esters benzyl acetate, benzyl benzoate and benzyl salicylate), linalool and geraniol, linalyl acetate, santalol, guaicol and ω-bromstyrene.

Main actions: anti-nociceptive, anti-inflammatory, histamine suppression, antispasmodic, bronchodilatory (potential, based on main constituents).

Indications: musculoskeletal (pain, inflammation), respiratory (histamine-induced inflammation and bronchoconstriction, asthma), skin (inflammation and allergy).

Blending suggestions and expanded practice:

Musculoskeletal: for pain and inflammation, rheumatism, tension, consider blending with holy basil, sweet marjoram, geranium, juniperberry, sweet fennel, Himalayan cedar, clove bud, nutmeg, turmeric, frankincense, galbanum, nagarmotha, sandalwood, patchouli, blackcurrant bud, lime, rose absolute, jasmine, black pepper, long pepper, pink pepper.

Respiratory: for allergy, bronchoconstriction, asthma, consider blending with rose absolute, plai and sandalwood.

Skin: for inflammation, consider blending with geranium, palmarosa, rose absolute, jasmine, frankincense, patchouli, sandalwood.

Energetic: the flowers are used to make oils, perfumes and lotions; they are used in garlands and hair ornaments, but they are not offered in worship, because they are said to have been cursed by the Lord Shiva; *rooh kewra* is costly and valued as a perfume, but is also used in medicine as an antispasmodic and stimulant; it is used to treat headache and rheumatism.

Expanded practice: recreate an aromatherapeutic version of *Attar kewra*, by combining with true sandalwood oil; or create natural therapeutic perfumes by combining with tropical flowers such as frangipani, ylang ylang, jasmine, and golden champaca with pink lotus, labdanum, frankincense and vanilla; or with perilla, geranium, clove bud, pink pepper, nagarmotha and patchouli.

Lavender, true (Lamiaceae)

Lavandula angustifolia, *L. officinalis* or *L. vera* (subspecies include '*delphinensis*' and '*fragrans*', flowering tops); steam-distilled essential oil; an absolute is also available.

Odour: sweet, fresh, light, herbal (lavender), with floral, woody and fruity notes.

Constituents: *l*-linalool (20–45% depending on origin; French oils usually range from 30–45%), linalyl acetate (typically 40–42%, although some oils contain less, and some high-altitude French oils may have as much as 50–52%, giving rise to a fruity, 'pear drops', bergamot-like note), lavandulyl acetate, β-caryoplyllene, terpinen-4-ol, β-ocimene and others (check with supplier; the absolute contains linalyl acetate (45%) and linalool (30%) and others.

Main actions: analgesic, anti-nociceptive, anti-inflammatory, anti-oxidant, antimicrobial, anxiolytic.

Indications: musculoskeletal (pain and inflammation), female reproductive (dysmenorrhoea), circulatory (atherosclerosis), immune (support), skin (inflammation, allergy, infection), psyche (anxiety and its somatic manifestations, insomnia).

Blending suggestions and expanded practice:

Musculoskeletal: for pain and inflammation, including joints, consider blending with bergamot, bergamot mint, geranium, clary sage, basil CT linalool, rosemary, thyme, sweet marjoram, golden rod, juniperberry, frankincense, coriander seed, sweet fennel, nutmeg, ginger, plai, lemongrass, palmarosa, cypress, Himalayan cedar, hemlock, camphor CT nerolidol, clove bud, holy basil, cinnamon leaf, black pepper, long pepper, pink pepper.

Female reproductive: for dysmenorrhoea, consider lavender with clary sage and marjoram (2:1:1 ratio, 3%, abdominal massage); you might also consider sweet fennel and plai.

Circulatory: for atherosclerosis, consider lavender with monarda or bergamot, mandarin and lemon, mastic, clove bud, thyme, *Pinus mugo* (skin irritant – therefore evaporation would be the preferred route), and tea tree.

Immune support: consider lavender with sweet marjoram and cypress (3:2:1); or clove bud, holy basil, ginger, lemongrass, palmarosa.

Skin: consider blending with essential oils such as anthopogon, bergamot, geranium, guava leaf, patchouli; for inflammation/infection, trauma, with immortelle and a macerated oil of *Rosa rubiginosa*; for inflammation/allergy with German chamomile or niaouli; for infections with tea tree and/or *Thymus zygis* cultivars (including fungal infections, but perhaps not for MRSA); for topical infections consider lavender and cypress or lavender and may chang (1:1) for *Candida albicans*; for *C. albicans* and *Staphylococcus aureus*, consider lavender in 1:1 combinations with carrot seed, Virginian cedar, cinnamon or sweet orange.

Psyche: for anxiety, insomnia, consider blending with bergamot, clary sage, frankincense and ylang ylang, also rose and geranium, or fir and vetiver.

Energetic: directed to the thorax and heart, soothing, cooling, purifying, instils tranquillity and acceptance, dispels melancholy.

Expanded practice: lavender absolute is also dominated by linalyl acetate (45%) and *l*-linalool (28%) with coumarin (4–5%) and others; its scent is perhaps closer to that of the flowering herb than the essential oil, and it could be used for its psychotherapeutic effects via inhalation. You might also consider using lavandin, which also has anti-nociceptive and anxiolytic actions; there are three varieties: 'Abrialis', 'Grosso' and 'Super'; exercise caution with anticoagulant medication and bleeding disorders. Spike lavender lacks linalyl acetate, which is synergistic with linalool as far as anxiolytic action is concerned, therefore it should not be substituted with this intention; French lavender (*L. stoechas*) is dominated by camphor, *d*-fenchone and 1,8-cineole, with only small amounts of *l*-linalool (2%), and often linalyl acetate is absent; therefore it should not be considered as an alternative for true lavender.

Lemon (Rutaceae)

Citrus × limon, *C. limonum* peel, cold-expressed essential oil.

Odour: fresh, sharp citrus top with a sweet, fresh lemony body, little tenacity or depth.

Constituents: *d*-limonene (up to 76%), β-pinene (15%), γ-terpinene (12–13%), α-terpineol (8%), with geranial, α-pinene, *para*-cymene, sabinene, β-myrcene, and others; traces of non-volatile phototoxic constituents such as oxypeucedanin, bergamottin and bergapten.

Main actions: anti-inflammatory (inhibitor of TFN-α), anti-oxidant, LDL anti-oxidant (γ-terpinene), anticholinesterase, activating, antidepressant.

Indications: musculoskeletal (inflammation), psyche (cognition, depression).

Blending suggestions and expanded practice:

Musculoskeletal: for inflammation, consider blending with lavender, geranium, yuzu, plai, ginger, frankincense, black pepper, Szechuan pepper, pink pepper, patchouli.

Psyche: for impaired cognitive processes, blend with plai, narcissus, terpinen-4-ol-rich oils (sweet marjoram, kewda, juniperberry); also consider thyme, rosemary, Spanish sage, coriander seed, sweet fennel; for low mood or depression, consider blending with citron, combava peel, bergamot, grapefruit, clary sage, geranium, frankincense, coriander seed, ginger, turmeric, Korean fir, black pepper, pink pepper, jasmine, golden champaca, osmanthus, ylang ylang, patchouli, sandalwood.

Expanded practice: lemon itself has little tenacity; if you are creating a therapeutic perfume, use with citron or yuzu to augment the citrus element, or with may chang and Szechuan pepper to carry the lemon note into the heart of the scent; bear in mind that lemon is phototoxic.

Lemon balm (Lamiaceae)

Melissa officinalis leaves; steam-distilled essential oil.

Odour: citrus, herbal top notes and a herbal body.

Constituents: variable, dominated by citral (up to 64%), geranial (up to 38%) and neral (up to 26%), with β-caryophyllene (up to 20%), citronellal (up to 14%), and many others including geraniol, β-ocimene, neryl acetate (up to 4%).

Main actions: anti-inflammatory, analgesic, antispasmodic, antiviral, anti-cancer, sedative, sleep-inducing.

Indications: musculoskeletal (pain, inflammation, tension), skin (allergy, itching, inflammation), wellbeing, psyche (stress, tension, agitation, anxiety, insomnia).

Blending suggestions and expanded practice:

Musculoskeletal: for tension, pain, inflammation, consider blending with lavender, clary sage, bergamot mint, golden rod, hops, geranium, immortelle, Szechuan pepper, pink pepper.

Skin: for allergy, itching and inflammation, consider blending with lavender, lemongrass, palmarosa, immortelle, German chamomile, jabara, sandalwood.

Wellbeing: consider blending with palmarosa, lemongrass, ginger, plai, patchouli.

Psyche: for agitation, stress, anxiety, insomnia, consider blending with lavender, spikenard, patchouli, frankincense, narcissus, rose, neroli, white verbena, sweet orange.

Energetic: lemon balm was known to the ancient Greeks and Romans; Pliny and Dioscorides suggested that it could close wounds and supress inflammation. The early herbalists knew it as 'balm' and it was highly regarded for disorders of the nervous system; the herbalist John Evelyn maintained that 'balm is sovereign for the brain, strengthening the memory and powerfully chasing away melancholy' and that balm steeped in wine 'comforts the heart and driveth away melancholy and sadness' (Grieve 1992, p.76); hence, it has a reputation for aiding cognitive functions and uplifting the spirits.

Lemongrass (Poaceae)

Cymbopogon citratus (West Indian), *C. flexuosus* (East Indian) grass-like leaves; steam-distilled essential oil.

Odour: a tenacious, strong, lemony herbal aroma, with an herbal, oily dryout.

Constituents: vary according to type:

C. citrates: geranial (45–55%), neral (30–36%), geranyl acetate (up to 4%), geraniol (up to 4%), limonene (up to 4%) with caryophyllene oxide, 6-methyl-5-hepten-2-one and *l*-linalool.

C. flexuosus: geranial (37–60%), neral (25–35%), β-myrcene (5–20%), geraniol (up to 7%), limonene oxide (up to 7%), 1,8-cineole (up to 3%), with 6-methyl-5-hepten-2-one, geranyl acetate and *l*-linalool.

Main actions: analgesic, anti-nociceptive, anti-cancer (apoptosis-inducing, antiproliferative, chemopreventative), immunostimulant (preventative), anti-allergic, anti-inflammatory, antifungal, anxiolytic, sedative.

Indications: musculoskeletal (pain, inflammation, stress-induced tension), wellbeing, skin (inflammation, allergy, acne, dermatophyte infection), psyche (anxiety, stress, insomnia).

Blending suggestions and expanded practice:

Musculoskeletal: for pain and inflammation, stress, tension, consider blending with palmarosa, ginger, plai, turmeric, galangal, nutmeg, clove bud, coriander seed, Szechuan pepper, pink pepper, long pepper, black pepper, basil, lavender, geranium, frankincense, juniperberry, combava petitgrain and peel, nagarmotha, patchouli, sandalwood.

Wellbeing: consider blending with lime, pomelo, yuzu, mandarin petitgrain, palmarosa, ginger, plai, turmeric, galangal, nutmeg, clove bud, Szechuan pepper, pink pepper, basil, lavender, perilla, mastic, frankincense, juniperberry, patchouli, sandalwood.

Skin: for allergy and inflammation, consider blackcurrant bud, basil, lavender, geranium, rose, immortelle, Virginian cedarwood, sandalwood, hemp, patchouli, vetiver; for dermatophytes, consider plai, carrot seed, sweet fennel, pink pepper, Sardinian sage; for acne, consider clary sage, combava petitgrain, guava leaf, plai, coriander seed, jasmine, white champaca.

Psyche: for anxiety, insomnia, stress, consider blending with lime, lavender, rose, ylang ylang, frangipani, frankincense, patchouli, sandalwood, angelica, spikenard, vetiver.

Lime (Rutaceae)

Citrus aurantifolia or *C. medica* var. *acida* peel, steam-distilled essential oil (expressed oil occasionally available).

Odour: fresh, sharp, terpenic top with a sweet, fruity citrus, distinctive lime character.

Constituents: variable, *d*-limonene (up to 50%) and occuring with 1,8-cineole, α-terpineol, γ-terpinene, terpinolene (all up to around 10%), with *para*-cymene, terpinen-4-ol, α-terpinene, α- and β-pinene, borneol and others.

Main actions: antispasmodic, vasorelaxant (potential), antiproliferative, anxiolytic.

Indications: musculoskeletal (tension), digestion (cramp, spasm), circulation (hypertension), wellbeing (LDL anti-oxidant, anti-atherosclerosis), psyche (anxiety and stress).

Blending suggestions and expanded practice:

Musculoskeletal: for tension, spasm, consider blending with basil, holy basil, coriander seed, ginger, plai, jasmine, nagarmotha, vetiver, pink pepper.

Digestion: for cramp and spasm, consider blending with lemon balm, spearmint, thyme, coriander seed, sweet fennel, ginger, pink pepper.

Circulation: for hyptertension, consider blending with bergamot, sweet marjoram, geranium, rose, clove bud.

Wellbeing: consider blending with yuzu, ginger, turmeric, lemongrass, lemon balm, frankincense, mastic, patchouli.

Psyche: for stress, tension and anxiety, consider blending with frangipani, ylang ylang, coriander seed, black pepper, ginger, white verbena, linden blossom, yuzu, sweet orange, grapefruit, black pepper, frankincense, labdanum, vetiver, patchouli, sandalwood.

Energetic: in Ayurvedic medicine the lime is a panacea; it is sour, bitter, astringent and cooling, and it is claimed that there is no disease that this fruit does not have the potential to treat.

Expanded practice: you might also consider using some other species that are known as 'lime', such as sweet lime (*C. limetta*), which has a lemon-like scent. The Australian finger lime (*C. australasica*) is dominated by *d*-limonene, with *iso*-menthone, and citronellal – a composition unique in the citrus family. *C. medica* var. *sarcodactylis*, is called 'Buddha's hand' or the 'fingered citron'; the fruit is highly fragrant, and is used in China and Japan to scent rooms and clothing; the closed hand form, which resembles the prayer position, is offered in Buddhist temples.

Mandarin (Rutaceae)

Citrus reticulata peel; cold-expressed essential oil.

Odour: intense, sweet, soft citrus, with fruity, orange-like, very occasionally amine (fishy) notes; an amine note is due to nitrogen-containing compounds such as trimethylamine.

Constituents: *d*-limonene (up to 75%), γ-terpinene (up to 23%), with α- and β-pinene, β-myrcene, *para*-cymene, and others including short chain fatty aldehydes C_8, C_{10} and C_{12}, and methyl-*N*-methyl anthranilate.

Main actions: anti-inflammatory (inhibitor of 5-LOX), LDL anti-oxidant (γ-terpinene), antidepressant, calming.

Indications: musculoskeletal (pain and inflammation), circulatory (anti-atherosclerosis), psyche (stress, tension, low mood, insomnia).

Blending suggestions and expanded practice:

Musculoskeletal: for stress and tension, inflammation, consider blending with lavender, nutmeg, coriander seed, clove bud, black pepper, pink pepper, Szechuan pepper.

Circulatory: consider blending with other oils that are rich in γ-terpinene, such as cumin seed, mandarin petitgrain, narcissus absolute, lemon, yuzu.

Psyche: for low mood, consider blending with jasmine, orange blossom or neroli, also coriander seed, pink pepper, Szechuan pepper, clary sage, Roman chamomile.

Expanded practice: the unripe green fruits yield the oil that is preferred in perfumery; when creating therapeutic perfumes, consider including green mandarin in top note citrus accords – it can add sharpness to floral blends. You could also consider using *Citrus tachibana* essential oil; this is related to mandarin and has a sweet, green citrus aroma.

Marjoram, sweet (Lamiaceae)

Origanum majorana, O. hortensis dried flowering herb; steam-distilled essential oil.

Odour: warm, typically herbal, slightly camphoraceous odour with woody and spicy notes.

Constituents: variable, depending on source; dominated by terpinen-4-ol (15–32%), *trans*-sabinene hydrate, linalyl acetate (up to 10%), with others including α-terpineol, γ-terpinene, sabinene, *l*-linalool, *para*-cymene.

Main actions: analgesic, anti-inflammatory, antispasmodic, smooth muscle relaxation, vasodilator, histamine suppression, bronchodilatory, wound-healing, anxiolytic, sedative.

Indications: musculoskeletal (pain, inflammation, tension, spasm); female reproductive (dysmenorrhea), circulatory (hypertension), respiratory (allergy, bronchoconstriction, asthma), skin (inflammation, allergy and wound healing), psyche (stress, tension, anxiety, insomnia).

Blending suggestions and expanded practice:

Musculoskeletal: for muscular and joint pain and inflammation, stress-related tension and spasm, consider blending with rosemary, lavender, spike lavender, lavandin, basil, lemon balm, clary sage, thyme, peppermint, camphor CT nerolidol, cypress, juniperberry, ginger, plai, nutmeg, black pepper, pink pepper.

Female reproductive: for dysmenorrhea, consider Roman chamomile, sweet fennel, angelica, nutmeg, plai, pink pepper.

Circulatory: for hypertension, consider blending with bergamot, geranium, mojito mint.

Respiratory: for bronchoconstriction, allergy, consider blending with rose absolute, plai, ginger, long pepper, or spearmint, peppermint, thyme, rosemary, myrtle, rosalina type 2, hemlock, fir, spruce, juniperberry, tea tree.

Skin: for inflammation and wound healing, consider blending with cypress, Lebanese cedar, Virginian cedar, camphor CT nerolidol, juniperberry, pink pepper, or poplar bud, immortelle, inula, rose, patchouli, sandalwood.

Psyche: for stress, tension, anxiety, insomnia, consider blending with lavender, lemon balm, white verbena, sweet orange, rose, ylang ylang, spikenard, patchouli, sandalwood.

Energetic: folk history suggests that, since ancient times, sweet marjoram has been associated with encouraging sleep and contentment.

Expanded practice: you could consider using wild Spanish marjoram – *Thymus mastichina* – as a mucolytic and expectorant. You could also recreate an aromatherapeutic version of a traditional Turkish wound-healing ointment by combining sweet marjoram, *O. minutiflorum* (if available) and Greek sage with hypericum-infused oil, and olive oil.

Myrrh (Burseraceae)

Commiphora myrrha, *C. molmol* and others, oleo-gum resin; steam-distilled essential oil (liquid when fresh, but becomes sticky and resin-like upon exposure to air).

Odour: sweet, spicy, slightly medicinal, borderline balsamic; with age, becomes mellower and loses the sharp medicinal quality of fresh oil.

Constituents: variable, and dependent on variety; furanodienes (50%), lindestrene, β- and δ-elemene, germacrenes, curzerene, β-caryophyllene, γ-cadinene and others.

Main actions: analgesic, anti-inflammatory (inhibitor of 5-LOX and HLE), anti-cancer (apoptosis-inducing); hypolipidemic (potential), anti-oxidant (singlet oxygen quencher).

Indications: musculoskeletal (pain and inflammation, arthritis), skin (inflammation, ageing, sun exposure, infections – traditional), wellbeing.

Blending suggestions and expanded practice:

Musculoskeletal: for pain and inflammation, arthritis, consider blending with frankincense, galbanum, juniperberry, cypress, geranium, lavender, sweet marjoram, lemon, turmeric, clove bud, cinnamon leaf, rose, cassie, black pepper, pink pepper.

Skin: for inflammation, regeneration, intrinsic and extrinsic ageing and damage, possibly wound healing, consider blending with Japanese cedar, cypress, geranium, jasmine, rose, poplar bud, pink pepper, sandalwood, patchouli.

Wellbeing: consider blending with frankincense, mastic, galangal, labdanum, cistus, Japanese cedar, rose, pink lotus.

Energetic: myrrh is often associated with frankincense, because of their common habitat and botanical similarities; this led to their similar cultural uses, but myrrh was not as valuable as frankincense, and was symbolic of suffering and death. Myrrh was an important incense ingredient; it was present in the ancient Egyptian *kyphi* and the Hebrew holy incense. Many cultures included it in their perfumes, such as *stakte* (the simple, uncompounded perfume of ancient Egypt), and several compounded therapeutic perfumes of ancient Rome such as *Mendesium*, which was also used to ease aching muscles; a myrrh perfume called *Murra* was valued as a skin cleanser and hair tonic. Myrrh has a long association with purification, and the fragrance was also used to purify (deodorise) the atmosphere.

Expanded practice: for relaxation and meditation, consider evaporating opoponax, the myrrh of ancient times, with frankincense; or, to create an aromatherapeutic interpretation of *Mendesium*, combine opoponax, cardamom and galbanum.

Narcissus (Amaryllidaceae)

Narcissus poeticus flowers; absolute via solvent extraction.

Odour: sweet, heavy, narcotic floral, with earthy, herbaceous and hay-like notes (best appreciated in high dilution).

Constituents: complex and highly variable; constituents include γ-terpinene (up to 28%), *trans*-methyl cinnamate (trace–16%), *l*-linalool (trace–12 %), benzyl acetate (9–10%), benzyl benzoate (trace to 9%), *para*-cymene (trace–9%), δ-3-carene (6–9%), α-terpineol (trace–7%), with others including benzyl alcohol, γ-methyl ionone, anisaldehyde, phenylethanol, and traces of indole.

Main actions: anti-atherosclerosis (γ-terpinene is an LDL anti-oxidant), cognition enhancement (inhibits cholinesterase), sedative (traditional), narcotic (in excess).

Indications: psyche (cognitive impairment, impaired memory, agitated behaviour), wellbeing.

Blending suggestions and expanded practice:

Psyche: use on its own, in very low concentration for topical application or evaporation; for agitation, stress, anxiety, insomnia, you might also consider blending it with lavender (also absolute), clary sage (also absolute), spikenard, nagarmotha, patchouli, sandalwood, galbanum, opoponax, hay, genet, tuberose, rose, neroli, orange blossom, white verbena, bitter orange, petitgrain bigarade; for emotional shock it could be combined with cistus.

Energetic: it is named, not after the Narcissus of myth, who gave us the concept of narcissism, but from the Greek *narkao*, because the plant has narcotic properties; Socrates called it the 'chaplet of the infernal gods' because of its effects; an extract of the bulbs, if applied to open wounds, caused staggering, numbness of the nervous system and paralysis of the heart. Perhaps from a more positive energetic perspective we might prefer to use the words 'comfortably numb', indicating its potential to calm disturbing or painful emotions.

Expanded practice: you could create natural therapeutic perfumes by blending narcissus with galbanum, blackcurrant bud, vanilla and sandalwood; and with tuberose or jasmine, orange blossom, hay, genet, mimosa, tobacco, labdanum and cedar. If available, you could also consider jonquil absolute, which has a fresh top note, a heavy, narcotic, sweet, honey, green floral heart – similar to narcissus, and obtained from the 'rush daffodil', *Narcissus jonquilla*.

Neroli bigarade and orange blossom (Rutaceae)

Citrus aurantium var. *amara* flowers; essential oil by stream distillation and absolute via solvent extraction.

Odour:

Neroli bigarade essential oil has a strong, light, floral citrus top note, a floral green, bitter body and no perceptible dryout.

Orange blossom absolute has a fresh top, a heady, intense, rich and heavy indolic floral (orange flower) body and a floral dryout (it is best appreciated in dilution).

Constituents:

Neroli essential oil: *l*-linalool (45–55%), *d*-limonene (6–10%), linalyl acetate (5–10%), with β-ocimene, α-terpineol, β-pinene and geranyl acetate (all around 5%), and others including *trans*-nerolidol, geraniol, *trans-trans*-farnesol, neryl acetate and others.

Orange blossom absolute: phenylethanol (5–35%), *l*-linalool (30%), linalyl acetate (up to 17%), methyl anthranilate (up to 15%), *trans-trans*-farnesol (up to 8%), nerolidol (up to 8%), with *d*-limonene, β-ocimene, α-terpineol, geraniol, nerol, neryl acetate and indole (up to 1%).

Main actions: analgesic, anticonvulsant, anti-inflammatory, anti-nociceptive, reduces cardiovascular responses to stress, regenerating (enhances keratinocyte differentiation), may enhance skin penetration (potential, based on actions of main constituents), anxiolytic, antidepressant (traditional), vasomotor actions (reduces menopausal hot flushes).

Indications: hypertension (including stress-induced), menopause (hot flushes, low libido), infection (control of skin infections), musculoskeletal (pain and inflammation), skin (inflammation, stress, ageing), psyche (anxiety, stress and depression).

Blending suggestions and expanded practice:

Menopause: for hot flushes, anxiety and low libido, neroli can be used on its own, or blended with ylang ylang and used in massage and skin care applications.

Musculoskeletal: for pain and inflammation, tension and stress, consider blending neroli or orange blossom with lavender, bergamot mint, petitgrain bigarade, bergamot, yuzu, lemon, coriander seed, frankincense, myrrh, opoponax, pink pepper.

Skin: for inflammation, damage, impaired texture and barrier function, consider blending orange blossom absolute with jasmine (*J. grandiflorum*), rose, poplar bud, blackcurrant bud, or golden champaca absolutes, sweet orange, cypress, myrrh, violet leaf, and regenerating carriers.

Stress and hypertension: neroli can be used on its own, or perhaps blended with lavender, ylang ylang and marjoram for massage.

Psyche: for anxiety, blend neroli with lavender, bergamot mint, Roman chamomile, cistus, petitgrain bigarade, bergamot, bitter orange, mandarin; and for stress, depression, consider blending orange blossom with jasmine (*J. sambac*), clary sage, sweet orange, labdanum, coriander seed, pink pepper.

Energetic: the scent of orange blossom has been used as an aphrodisiac, yet paradoxically is also associated with virginity, purity and chastity; this possibly reflects the contrast between the pure white, delicate blossoms and the sensual, indolic facet to their aroma.

Expanded practice: in perfumery, neroli is an important ingredient in classic eaux de Cologne; it is often combined with bergamot, orange and ylang ylang.

Orange blossom absolute is more indolic, and could be combined with other white flower oils to create a sensual, heady and more robust therapeutic perfume.

Studies have demonstrated that inhalation of neroli can be effective for reducing anxiety and the somatic manifestations of stress (such as elevated blood pressure and pulse rate), and for alleviating some menopausal symptoms. You might like to use an essential oil 'pendant' or 'necklace' for continuous, longer-term delivery of neroli in these circumstances.

Nutmeg (Myristicaceae)

Myristica fragrans fruit kernels; steam-distilled essential oil.

Odour: fresh, warm and spicy, with sweet, pine-like, ethereal notes.

Constituents: there are two types of nutmeg essential oil which are commercially available; in perfumery, the 'East Indian' oil from Indonesia and Sri Lanka is preferred over the 'West Indian' oil from Grenada; both are dominated by sabinene with α- and β-pinene – the myristicin content differs, being higher in the East Indian (at up to 14%) than the West Indian (at 0.5–1.0 %), and sabinene can be present at higher levels in the West Indian type. East Indian essential oil contains sabinene (15–45%), α-pinene (18–27%), β-pinene (9–18%), myristicin (4–14%), terpinen-4-ol (up to 10%), γ-terpinene (up to 8%) and many others including *l*-linalool, *d*-limonene, α-terpinene, elemicin, β-myrcene, α-thujene, *para*-cymene, β-phellandrene, δ-3-carene, terpinolene, α-terpineol; there are two potentially hazardous constituents – safrole (trace–3.5%) and methyleugenol (trace–1.2%), check with supplier.

Main actions: anti-inflammatory, anticonvulsant, chemopreventative, antiproliferative, psychotropic, aphrodisiac (traditional).

Indications: musculoskeletal (pain and inflammation), wellbeing, psyche (stress, insomnia).

Blending suggestions and expanded practice:

Musculoskeletal: for inflammation, aches and pains, joint inflammation, consider blending with juniperberry, cypress, plai, ginger, frankincense, lavender, lavandin, clary sage, geranium, bergamot mint, camphor CT nerolidol, petitgrain bigarade, coriander seed, clove bud, kewda, sweet orange, lime, yuzu, black pepper, pink pepper.

Wellbeing: for enhanced wellbeing and immune support, consider blending with saro, holy basil, clove bud, frankincense, mastic, ginger, lime, lemongrass, palmarosa, patchouli.

Psyche: for stress, tension, depression, insomnia, consider blending wtith rose absolute, tuberose, ylang ylang extra, bay laurel, pink pepper, frankincense, mastic, nagarmotha, patchouli, sandalwood.

Energetic: the Hindus used nutmeg as an intoxicant – its Ayurvedic name is *made shaunda*, meaning 'narcotic fruit'; however, despite its reputation, nutmeg's narcotic effects have not been widely exploited or abused; it is possible that myristicin and elemicin are responsible; *in vitro*, these are converted into trimethoxyamphetamine (TMA) and 3-methoxy-4, 5-methoxyamphetamine (MMDA), and this is possibly what happens in the body; however, used in small amounts, the effects are very mild indeed, and have really only been exploited as a soporific in bedtime drinks.

Expanded practice: you might also consider using mace essential oil; this is very similar to nutmeg, but less pine-like in the top notes; it is obtained from the 'aril', the red husk that surrounds the nutmeg; it too may be psychtropic.

Caution: safrole and methyleugenol are carcinogenic; this has not been found with the essential oil; however, caution is suggested and low doses are recommended.

Orange, sweet (Rutaceae)

Citrus × *sinensis* (a hybrid, probably a cross between *C. maxima* (pomelo) and *C. reticulata* (mandarin)); peel oil obtained by cold expression; various cultivars are available, such as 'blood orange' (*C. sinensis* cv. '*Sanguinelli*' and cv. '*Moro*').

Odour: fresh, fruity and very similar to the peel when scarified; the top note is sweet, light, fresh and citrus, the middle is citrus and aldehydic, the dryout is faint and pithy.

Constituents: variable, according to source and cultivar; typically *d*-limonene (90–95%), β-myrcene (1–5%), octanal and decanal have a significant impact on the odour, linalool, octyl and neryl acetate are also present.

Main actions: anti-inflammatory, anti-oxidant (hepatoprotective), antibacterial (anti-staphylococcal), sedative, anxiolytic.

Indications: skin (antiseptic, anti-inflammatory), wellbeing, psyche (stress, anxiety).

Blending suggestions and expanded practice:

Skin: as an antiseptic and for superficial infections and/or inflammation, consider blending with lavender (1:1) or perhaps with clove (1:9), or in skin care with jabara, geranium, immortelle, palmarosa, clary sage, neroli, patchouli, sandalwood.

Wellbeing: consider blending with black, pink or long pepper, ginger, coriander seed, nutmeg, sweet fennel, lemon balm, palmarosa, poplar bud.

Psyche: consider blending with jasmine, orange blossom or neroli, also coriander seed, pink pepper, clary sage, Roman chamomile.

Expanded practice: although some research has specifically supported the use of sweet orange as an anti-inflammatory (it is a 5-LOX inhibitor) and anxiolytic, it is likely that other species will share these properties. Bitter orange (90% *d*-limonene) has a fresh, delicate aroma, with sweet floral and green notes; it is more subtle, fresh and tenacious than sweet orange. For good tenacity, citron (cédrat) could also be considered – perhaps in a therapeutic perfume where you would like to emphasise the citrus element. You might also consider pomelo with its good anti-oxidant activity, or the mild, sweet, gentle clementine, or the sweet, green *C. tachibara* essential oil. Also, for anti-inflammatory action in conjunction with soothing and anti-allergic actions, *C. jabara* could be used along with sweet orange.

Palmarosa (Poaceae)

Cymbopogon martinii var. *martinii* grass-like leaves; steam-distilled essential oil.

Odour: fresh, sweet, delicate, floral (rosy), with woody, violet and oily notes.

Constituents: variable, typically geraniol (75–80%), geranyl acetate (up to 10%), *trans-cis*-farnesol (up to 6%), *l*-linalool (up to 5%), with β-ocimene, β-caryophyllene, β-myrcene, geranial and others.

Main actions: anti-nociceptive, anti-inflammatory, antifungal (yeasts), anti-cancer (potential), modifier of bacterial resistance.

Indications: musculoskeletal (pain and inflammation), skin (inflammation), wellbeing.

Blending suggestions and expanded practice:

Musculoskeletal: for pain and inflammation, consider blending with geranium, lavender, lemon balm, lemongrass, combava leaf, ginger, plai, Virginian cedarwood, pink pepper, patchouli, nagarmotha, sandalwood.

Skin: for inflammation, and also superficial yeast infections, consider blending with geranium, immortelle, rose, patchouli, nagarmotha, plai, lemongrass, carrot seed; for pain and itching combine with may chang and lavender.

Wellbeing: consider blending with clove bud, coriander seed, lime, ginger, rose, patchouli.

Expanded practice: the main constituents are noted for their rosy scents; geraniol is rosy and geranyl acetate is sweet, rosy and fruity; for this reason palmarosa blends very well with other botanicals with a rose aspect to their aromas; these include rose otto and absolute (phenylethanol is soft, petal-like and rosy, and citronellol is warm, vibrant and rosy, geranium (citronellol, geraniol and geranyl esters), immortelle (nerol is a harsher, fresh rosy, and neryl acetate is fruity and rosy); and also the rosy-scented woods such as guiaicwood and rosewood. To create a relaxing, therapeutic perfume, blend with rose absolute, guaiacwood, sandalwood, patchouli, nagarmotha and tobacco leaf absolute.

Patchouli (Lamiaceae)

Pogostemon cablin semi-dried and lightly fermented leaves; steam-distilled essential oil.

Odour: unique, distinctive and complex, patchouli has a rich, intense, rounded, smooth, persistent, slightly sweet scent, with earthy, balsamic, woody, spicy, rooty, herbaceous, green, bitter chocolate, peppery and wine-like notes.

Constituents: patchouli alcohol (up to 33%), α-bulnesene (up to 21%), α-guaiene (up to 15%), seychellene (up to 10%), with α- and β-patchoulene, aromadendrene and others.

Main actions: anti-inflammatory, antiplatelet, antiproliferative (apoptosis-inducing), wound healing, calming.

Indications: musculoskeletal (inflammation, stress, tension), skin (inflammation, wounds, damage), wellbeing, psyche (stress, tension, agitation, depression, anxiety).

Blending suggestions and expanded practice:

Musculoskeletal: for stress-related inflammatiom and tension, consider blending with lavender, geranium, clary sage, lemongrass, ginger, nutmeg, clove bud, black pepper, nagarmotha, sandalwood.

Skin: for inflammation, wounds, damage and ageing, consider blending with rose, jasmine, blackcurrant bud, plai, hemp, vetiver, sandalwood, myrrh, cypress, Lebanese cedar.

Wellbeing: consider blending with palmarosa, lemongrass, lime, ginger, nutmeg, frankincense, mastic.

Psyche: for relaxation, stress reduction, depression, anxiety, consider blending with rose, frangipani, ylang ylang, combava peel, sweet orange, lime, lavender, hay, pink lotus, spikenard, nagarmotha, sandalwood.

Energetic: patchouli has been used for its scent for thousands of years, beginning in Asia and the Far East; the herb was used in India and China by Buddhist monks to make a purifying bath, and it was also used as an ingredient in the water used to bathe images of the Buddha; in China, patchouli was used to make a perfumed ink for writing on scrolls; the leaves were dried, pulverised and used as incense, and its oil was used as perfume. Its scent was exotic, mysterious and sensual, and in the West became loved by many – from the

Empress Josephine to the painters and poets of the Romantic period. The herb is used in Chinese medicine and in Ayurvedic and Greek traditions, for gastrointestinal deficiency, pain, insomnia, anxiety, varicose veins and haemorrhoids, scar tissue and numerous skin disorders.

Expanded practice: create relaxing therapeutic perfumes by combining patchouli with florals such as rose, jasmine, golden champaca, frangipani or ylang ylang; with rich, smooth absolutes of vanilla, cacao, tobacco; patchouli also combines well with hay, hops, pink lotus, opoponax, labdanum, tobacco absolute.

Peppermint (Lamiaceae)

Mentha × *piperita* leaves and twigs (a cross between spearmint (*M. spicatum*) and watermint (*M. aquatica*), steam-distilled essential oil.

Odour: strong, fresh, penetrating, medicinal and mentholic odour, with green and herbaceous notes.

Constituents: *l*-menthol (20–55%), menthone (10–30%), and many others including *l*-menthyl acetate, 1,8-cineole, *iso*-menthone, menthyl *iso*-valerate, terpinen-4-ol, *l*-limonene.

Main actions: antispasmodic, anti-oxidant, antiviral, decongestant, mucolytic.

Indications: digestive (spasm, colic), respiratory (bronchial and sinus congestion).

Blending suggestions and expanded practice:

Digestion: for spasm, colic, irritable bowel, consider blending with spearmint, sweet fennel, coriander seed, lime, lemon, ginger, Szechuan pepper.

Respiratory: for bronchial and sinus congestion, consider blending with other mucolytic oils such as inula, Greek sage, *Thymus mastichina*, hyssop; also can blend successfully with 1,8-cineole-rich eucalypts, rosemary, sweet marjoram, spike lavender.

Expanded practice: because of its 'cooling' effects, peppermint essential oil is best suited to local applications and inhalation rather than for body massage. If you would like a gentle minty note in therapeutic perfumes or in massage blends, consider using mint absolute (*M.* × *piperita*), which has a fresh, soft, minty, green aroma without sharpness or harshness. For respiratory congestion you could also consider blending peppermint essential oil with broad-leaved peppermint (*Eucalyptus dives*) essential oil – the piperitone-rich varieties have a fresh, camphoraceous, minty odour – and narrow-leaved or black peppermint (*E. radiata*) essential oil – the phellandrene-rich varieties have a penetrating, peppery-camphoraceous, minty odour.

Pine, Scots (Pinaceae)

Pinus sylvestris needles, twigs and cones; steam-distilled essential oil.

Odour: fresh, somewhat harsh, strong, coniferous (pine), with woody, resinous, balsamic, terpenic notes.

Constituents: α-pinene (20–45%), β-pinene (2–35%), δ-3-carene (0.5–30%), β-phellandrene camphene and δ-cadinene (each traces–10%), and many others including *l*-limonene, bornyl acetate, β-myrcene, β-caryophyllene, α-terpinene, ocimene, 1,8-cineole.

Main actions: analgesic, anti-inflammatory, anti-allergic (potential), wound-healing (potential).

Indications: musculoskeletal (pain, inflammation), respiratory (bronchial and sinus congestion, traditional), skin (inflammation, damage).

Blending suggestions and expanded practice:

Musculoskeletal: for pain and inflammation, consider blending with Atlas cedarwood, Virginian cedarwood, rosemary CT myrcene, sweet marjoram, juniperberry, cypress, lemon, black pepper.

Respiratory: for bronchial and sinus congestion, use on its own or blend with rosemary CT 1,8-cineole or CT bornyl acetate, spike lavender, juniperberry, cajuput, niaouli, myrtle, rosalina type 2, fir, hemlock and spruce species.

Skin: for wound healing, consider blending with rosalina type 1, poplar bud, Greek sage, sweet marjoram, juniperberry, cypress, Korean fir, Virginian cedarwood, Japanese cedar, Lebanese and Himalayan cedarwood, lavender.

Expanded practice: dwarf pine essential oil from *Pinus mugo* var. *pumilo* and *P. montana* is dominated by terpinolene; it is sweet, woody and balsamic, and more tenacious than other pine oils; sometimes described as 'unique' and much preferred in perfumery, but not aromatherapy because it has a reputation as an irritant and sensitizer. It could, however, be used via inhalation.

Plai (Zingiberaceae)

Zingiber cassumunar fresh rhizomes, steam-distilled essential oil.

Odour: initially a slightly pungent, diffusive, spicy odour, reminiscent of black pepper and ginger but with distinctive tea tree-like and green/fresh notes; after 24 hours the tea tree/fresh/green notes are absent, replaced by a spicy green/ginger, cinnamon and clove dryout.

Constituents: sabinene (25–45%), terpinen-4-ol (25–45%), γ-terpinene (5–10%), α-terpinene (2–5%), trans-1-(3,4- dimethoxyphenyl) butadiene (DMPBD)

(1–16%), with α- and β-pinene, β-myrcene, *para*-cymene, β-phellandrene, β-terpinyl acetate, α-terpineol.

Main actions: anti-inflammatory (inhibitor of NO, inhibitor of COX-2 and PGE2), analgesic, reduces oedema, antispasmodic, anti-oxidant, anti-cancer, antihistaminic, anti-asthmatic, antimicrobial (yeasts and dermatophytes), wound-healing, anticholinesterase.

Indications: musculoskeletal (pain, inflammation, osteoarthritis, rheumatoid arthritis), digestive and female reproductive (spasm, irritable bowel, pain, dysmenorrhea), wellbeing, respiratory (allergy and asthma), skin (dermatophytes, inflammation, wounds), psyche (impaired cognition, dementia), energetic (support, balance, purification).

Blending suggestions and expanded practice:

Musculoskeletal: for chronic inflammatory joint diseases and soft tissue injury, plai can be incorporated into creams or gels at relatively high concentrations (15%), or combined with ginger at 4%; or consider blending with sabinene-rich nutmeg, yarrow, black pepper, juniperberry; also consider blending with lemon, sweet orange, Himalayan cedar, camphor CT nerolidol.

Digestive and female reproductive: for spasm, cramp, irritable bowel, consider blending with coriander seed, lime, lemon balm, peppermint, spearmint, clary sage; for dysmenorrhea, consider blending with black cumin, combava peel, ginger, Szechuan pepper, black pepper; also angelica, sweet fennel, sweet marjoram, clary sage, linden blossom, lime, sweet orange.

Respiratory: for reduction of inflammation, antihistaminic action, and asthma consider blending with terpinen-4-ol rich tea tree, sweet marjoram, juniperberry, kewda; or black cumin, cardamom, ginger, long pepper, niaouli CT 1,8-cineole or CT viridiflorol, ravintsara, rosemary CT 1,8-cineole or CT bornyl acetate, thyme, rose absolute.

Skin: for acne, consider blending with combava petitgrain, lemon myrtle, holy basil, clary sage, Japanese cedar, Lebanese cedar, Korean fir, white champaca, blackcurrant bud; for dermatophyte infections, consider blending with carrot seed, lemongrass, sage (*Salvia officinalis* Group IV, 1,8-cineole > camphor > α-thujone > β-thujone).

Wellbeing: for health maintenance and stress reduction, consider blending with combava peel, lime, lemongrass, palmarosa, coriander seed, ginger, long pepper, pink pepper, Szechuan pepper, sandalwood, vetiver, patchouli, nagarmotha, mastic.

Psyche: for impaired cognition or dementia, use on its own or consider blending with narcissus absolute, lemon, lemon balm, thyme, and terpinen-4-ol-rich sweet marjoram, juniperberry, kewda.

Expanded practice: in traditional Thai bodywork, to treat joint and muscle pain, plai is often used in combination with Thai herbs; we could emulate this in aromatherapy practice by blending with turmeric, lemongrass, combava peel, ginger, black pepper and sandalwood.

Rose (Rosaceae)

Rosa × centifolia (France, 'Rose de Mai') and *R. × damascena* (Bulgaria, Turkey) flowers; absolute via solvent extraction and steam-distilled essential oil ('otto').

Odour:

Absolute: rich, sweet, smooth rose, with waxy, honey and spicy notes.

Essential oil: deep, sweet, warm, rich, rosy, waxy; less spicy than the absolute, and the Moroccan oil is in turn less spicy than oils from Bulgaria or Turkey.

Constituents:

Absolute: phenylethanol (65–75%), *l*-citronellol (10–12%), geraniol (5–7%), nerol (up to 3%), eugenol (up to 3%), *trans-trans*-farnesol (up to 2%), may contain traces of methyleugenol (<1%).

Essential oil: *l*-citronellol (up to 45%), geraniol (up to 25%), nerol (up to 9%), with others including *l*-linalool (up to 3%), citronellyl acetate (up to 2%), geranyl acetate (up to 2%), *trans-trans*-farnesol (up to 1.5%), eugenol (up to 1.5%) and others; methyleugenol variable, depending on source (up to 3.5%).

Main actions: analgesic, anti-inflammatory, vasorelaxant, hypotensive, anti-asthmatic, bronchodilator, antitussive, anti-oxidant, enhances keratinocyte differentiation, inhibits *P. acnes*, antidepressant, harmonsising, calming, hypnotic.

Indications: musculoskeletal (inflammation, pain), wellbeing (stress, hypertension), respiratory (asthma, bronchoconstriction, inflammation, coughs), skin (texture, barrier function, acne), psyche (depression, anxiety, stress, insomnia).

Blending suggestions and expanded practice:

Musculoskeletal: for pain and inflammation, consider blending with clove bud, cinnamon leaf, long pepper, black pepper, pink pepper, ginger, turmeric, coriander seed, sweet fennel, star anise, Himalayan cedar, sandalwood, patchouli, kewda, immortelle, basil CT linalool, thyme, clary sage, lavender, bergamot, sweet orange, mandarin, yuzu.

Wellbeing: for stress, tension and high blood pressure, consider blending with bergamot, bergamot mint, geranium, palmarosa, sweet marjoram, sweet fennel, clove bud, guiaicwood.

Respiratory: for coughs, bronchoconstriction, inflammation and asthma, consider blending with anthopogon, black cumin, cardamom, ginger, plai, long pepper, fragonia, cistus, kewda, inula, juniperberry, sweet marjoram, yuzu.

Skin: for inflammation, allergy, consider blending with German chamomile, yarrow, hemp, geranium, immortelle, inula, sandalwood, lavender; for acne consider clary sage, eucalyptus blue gum, combava petitgrain, lemongrass, white champaca; for wound healing consider basil, Greek sage, bergamot, patchouli, pink pepper; for regeneration/damage/anti-ageing consider jasmine, blackcurrant bud, violet leaf, poplar bud, cacao, myrrh, cypress, with regenerating carriers.

Psyche: for relaxation, anxiety, insomnia, consider blending with lavender, sweet orange, Roman chamomile, cistus, genet, mimosa, linden blossom, patchouli, bay laurel, frangipani, tuberose, spikenard, valerian, labdanum; for harmonising mood, consider blending with ylang ylang, coriander seed, frankincense, sandalwood, labdanum, opoponax, vanilla; for depression and low mood consider bergamot, grapefruit, clary sage, rosemary, geranium, sweet fennel, perilla, black pepper, pink pepper.

Energetic: the rose is imbued with powerful symbolism – love, beauty, purity and passion, secrecy and clandestine activities ('*sub rosa*').

Expanded practice: for a simple therapeutic perfume, recreate a traditional attar by combining rose and sandalwood. There are many different types of rose essential oils and absolutes; their fragrances and energetic signatures are subtly different, influenced by their biology and geographical origins. You might also like to try the very beautiful white rose (*Rosa alba*) or the Japanese rose (*Rosa rugosa*).

Rosemary (Lamiaceae)

Rosmarinus officinalis fresh flowering tops; steam-distilled essential oil.

Odour: typically, a strong, fresh, herbal, resinous top note, and a herbal, woody, balsamic middle note with a dry herbal dryout (dependent on chemotype).

Constituents: there are several chemotypes; the most commonly available appears to be the cineole CT, which contains 1,8-cineole (40–58%), with camphor (up to 15%), α- and β-pinene (combined 20%), and α- and β-caryophyllene, borneol, camphene, α-terpineol, *para*-cymene, *d*-limonene, *l*-linalool, and others; camphor CT (up to 28% camphor), bornyl acetate CT (up to 15% bornyl acetate but dominated by α-pinene at up to 30%, with up to 14% 1,8 cineole); borneol CT (up to 16% borneol but dominated by 1,8-cineole at up to 20%, with 15% camphor); myrcene CT (up to 55% β-myrcene with α-pinene and *d*-limonene and up to 5% camphor); verbenone CT (up to 13% verbenone but dominated by camphor at up to 15%).

Main actions: analgesic, anti-nociceptive, anti-inflammatory, antispasmodic, anti-hypertensive, expectorant, anti-oxidant, inhibitor of HLE, antibacterial (*P. acnes*), activating, antidepressant.

Indications: musculoskeletal (pain, inflammation, arthritis), circulatory (hypotension), wellbeing, respiratory (congestion), skin (ageing, loss of elasticity, acne), psyche (loss of motivation, low mood, depression).

Blending suggestions and expanded practice:

Musculoskeletal: for pain, inflammation, arthritis, consider blending the myrcene, bornyl acetate or cineole chemotypes with lavender, lavandin, sweet marjoram, basil, thyme, juniperberry, pine, spruce, fir, hemlock, bergamot mint, golden rod, hops, hemp, frankincense, lemon, grapefruit, combava peel, Szechuan pepper, pink pepper, black pepper.

Wellbeing: for stress, tension, lethargy, consider blending with peppermint, spearmint, spike lavender, bergamot mint, juniperberry, Korean or Siberian fir, sweet fennel, combava peel, lemon, grapefruit, black pepper.

Respiratory: for congestion, consider blending the cineol CT with cineole-rich eucalypts, cajuput, fragonia, niaouli, rosalina type 2, myrtle, spike lavender, Greek sage; or the bornyl acetate CT with hemlock, spruce, fir, pine, juniperberry, cypress, sweet marjoram, Spanish marjoram, thyme, anthopogon, long pepper.

Skin: for inflammation, sun damage, ageing, and also acne, you might consider the borneol CT and blend with cypress, Japanese cedar, Virginian cedar, Korean fir, eucalyptus blue gum, juniperberry, cade, camphor CT nerolidol, jabara, bergamot, lemon, geranium, clary sage, basil, five-ribbed thyme, Somalian sage, inula, yarrow, guava leaf, Szechuan pepper, violet leaf, blackcurrant bud.

Psyche: for loss of motivation, poor concentration and focus, depression, consider blending with Korean or Siberian fir, thyme, bergamot mint, combava peel, lime, lemon, grapefruit, black pepper.

Energetic: since ancient times rosemary has been associated with improving the memory; rosemary also came to symbolise fidelity and remembrance; the virtues of rosemary were perfectly summed up by the herbalist William Langham in his 1579 work, *The Garden of Health*: 'Seethe much Rosemary, and bathe therein to make thee lusty, lively, joyfull, likeing, and youngly.'

Expanded practice: in addition to the suggestions given above, it is worth giving consideration to matching the chemotypes with oils that can augment their desirable components, especially β-myrcene, bornyl acetate and borneol. Exercise approptiate cautions in relation to the presence of camphor, and when 1,8-cineole dominates.

Sage, Dalmatian (Lamiaceae)

Salvia officinalis leaves; steam-distilled essential oil.

Odour: often said to be a typical representative of the herbaceous family, sage oil is warm, herbal, camphoraceous; sometimes slight urinous nuances are perceived.

Constituents: there are three broad types of sage, based on their dominant constituents:

Group I consists of species characterised by α- and β-thujone such as Dalmatian sage.

Group II by linalool and linalyl acetate such as clary sage.

Group III by 1,8-cineole and camphor, such as Greek, Lebanese and Spanish sage.

Dalmatian sage: camphor (10–50%), α-thujone (15–50%), borneol (trace–25%), 1,8-cineole (trace–20%), β-thujone (5–20%); with β-caryophyllene, camphene, bornyl acetate, α- and β-pinene.

Main actions: analgesic, anti-inflammatory, antiproliferative and apoptosis-inducing (Lebanese), antimicrobial, antidermatophytic, wound-healing (Greek), expectorant, mucolytic, cognition and memory enhancement.

Indications: musculoskeletal (pain and inflammation), wellbeing, respiratory (congestion), skin (wound healing, inflammation, dermatophyte infection), psyche (impaired cognition, impaired memory).

Blending suggestions and expanded practice:

Musculoskeletal: consider blending with lavender, geranium, bergamot mint, clary sage, sweet marjoram, rosemary, juniperberry, cypress, bergamot, grapefruit, jabara, lemon, black pepper.

Respiratory: consider using Greek sage and blending with lemon, rosemary, sweet marjoram, thyme, inula, myrtle, rosalina type 2, black spruce, fir, hemlock, juniperberry, bay laurel, long pepper.

Skin: for wound healing consider using Greek sage, with marjoram and hypericum fixed oil; for dermatophytes, consider blending Sardinian sage with carrot seed, sweet fennel, juniperberry, pink pepper; to counteract oxidative stress, consider using Somalian sage with immortelle.

Psyche: for enhancing memory and cognition, consider blending with lemon, rosemary.

Energetic: long considered to be a sacred herb; in the *Tabula Salerni*, there is a proverb: *Cur moritur cui Salvia crescit in horto?* This translates as 'Why should he die who has sage in his garden?' reflecting the belief that sage conferred immortality. *Salvia* is from the Latin *salvere* which means 'to be saved', and in past times it was referred to as 'Sage the Saviour', alluding to its healing properties; in the ancient Salerno School of Medicine, it was said that *Salvia salvatrix, natura concilatrix* – '*Salvia* is a cure with a calming effect.'

Expanded practice: numerous studies have elucidated *Salvia* species' therapeutic and medicinal potentials as antimicrobial agents, as spasmolytics and hypotensives, anti-oxidants and anti-inflammatories, for prolonging sleep, and for treating Alzheimer's disease. Sage essential oils that are commercially available for aromatherapeutic use include Dalmatian sage, Greek sage (*S. triloba*), Lebanese sage (*S. libanotica*) and Spanish sage (*S. lavandulaefolia*). Despite their therapeutic potential, some of their dominant constituents are neurotoxic (see below). However, it would appear that Somalian sage (*S. somalensis*) is without hazard, and has anti-inflammatory and anti-oxidant actions; it could be used to combat oxidative stress in the skin, and therefore may be useful in anti-ageing formulae; it also appears that Sardinian sage (*S. desoleana*) presents no hazards and has considerable potential as an antidermatophytic agent.

Caution: Groups I (Dalmatian sage) and III (Greek, Lebanese and Spanish sage) are characterised by the neurotoxic constituents α- and β-thujone and camphor, therefore must be used with care and caution. Tisserand and Young (2014) suggest:

Dalmation sage: neurotoxic; contraindicated in pregnancy and breastfeeding; maximum dermal limit of 0.4%.

Greek sage: the presence of α- and β-pinenes (combined around 14%) may mitigate the neurotoxic effects of β-thujone (1.6%); contraindicated for young children; a maximum dermal limit was not suggested (Lebanese sage will be similar).

Spanish sage: neurotoxic; camphor can be present at 11–36%, with 1,8-cineole at 10–30% and traces of thujones; however, it also contains *cis*-sabinyl acetate, which has abortifacient actions; contraindicated in pregnancy and breastfeeding; suggested maximum dermal limit is high, at 12.5%, based on camphor content.

Sandalwood, white, East Indian (Santalaceae)

Santalum album heartwood and roots; water or steam-distilled essential oil.

Odour: white sandalwood lacks a top note; persistent, soft, sweet and woody, with balsamic, fatty, animalic, milky, musky and urinous notes (some individuals may experience partial anosmia with sandalwood).

Constituents: *cis*-α-santalol and *cis*-β-santalol (combined 66–90%), *cis*-nuciferol, *cis*-α-*trans*-bergamotol, α- and β-santalal, and others.

Main actions: anti-inflammatory, antiproliferative, apoptosis-inducing, anti-allergic, harmonising, calming.

Indications: musculoskeletal (stress, tension, inflammation), wellbeing, skin (inflammation, allergic responses), psyche (stress, tension, anxiety, depression, inhibitions).

Blending suggestions and expanded practice:

Musculoskeletal: for inflammation and somatic manifestations of stress, consider blending with ginger, plai, nutmeg, coriander seed, black pepper, pink pepper, lemongrass, geranium, bergamot, juniperberry, Virginian cedarwood, kewda.

Wellbeing: consider blending with turmeric, ginger, plai, clove bud, nutmeg, black pepper, pink pepper, caraway, black cumin, lemongrass, palmarosa, frankincense, mastic, patchouli, vetiver, cypress, juniperberry, lime, sweet orange, poplar bud.

Skin: for inflammation and healing, consider blending with rose, poplar bud, myrrh, immortelle, geranium, patchouli, vetiver, hemp, Lebanese cedar, Virginian cedar; for allergy consider lavender, German chamomile, lemongrass.

Psyche: for harmonising mood, consider blending with rose, ylang ylang, geranium, frangipani, sweet orange, mandarin, lime, labdanum; for calming include spikenard, vanilla, patchouli, tuberose; for elevating consider jasmine, golden champaca, nagarmotha, kewda.

Energetic: sandalwood and its oil have been used for over 2500 years, and before that it certainly would have had ritual and ceremonial uses; the fragrance has been used by all of the Indian spiritual traditions to induce a calm state of mind; the wood, incense and perfume are a feature of Brahmin, Buddhist and Hindu religious rituals, and Hindu erotic arts; the yogis maintain that sandalwood is the scent of the 'subtle body', and in Tantric practice it is used by males to awaken *kundalini* energy and transform this into an enlightened mind; in Ayurvedic medicine sandalwood is classed as bitter, sweet, astringent and cool, and is used to control the doshas, but has more physical effects on *Pitta*; in Tibetan medicine it is used with other aromatics as a massage oil or incense for insomnia and anxiety; in Islam sandalwood is used in aromatic incense that is placed in a censer at the feet of the dead, to carry the soul to heaven.

Expanded practice: in recent times availability of true sandalwood has been limited because of over-exploitation; at time of writing availability is increasing. If *S. album* oil is unavailable, substitutes include Western Australian *S. spicatum* (soft, woody, extremely tenacious, balsamic and sweet, with a dry, spicy, resinous top note) and New Caledonian *S. austrocaledonicum* (woody, sandalwood-like, amber nuances, less resinous than *S. spicatum*). The New Caledonian is closest to white sandalwood in composition; the Western Australian oil is sometimes extracted with solvents. Sandalwood oil was, and still is, used in traditional perfumery; when combined with rose otto it made a purification fragrance known as *aytar*, which was used at the end of the Hindu year to symbolically remove past influences and prepare for a fresh start. It is also the base of the attars, where it is co-distilled with other aromatics to make traditional perfumes. You could create therapeutic perfumes based on the attars by blending sandalwood with rose or the floral absolutes – especially jasmine, golden champaca, frangipani, tuberose or kewda and pink lotus.

Caution: can very occasionally cause adverse skin reactions; suggested maximum dermal limit of 2%.

Spruce, black (Pinaceae)

Picea mariana needles and twigs; steam-distilled essential oil.

Odour: characteristically coniferous, fresh and very penetrating, with green and 'forest floor' notes.

Constituents: *l*-bornyl acetate (35–40%), β-pinene and α-pinene (each 14–15%), with camphene (8%), *d*-limonene (5%), camphor (5%), δ-3-carene (3–4%), β-myrcene (3%), β-phellandrene (2%) and borneol (1–2%).

Main actions: analgesic, anti-nociceptive, anti-inflammatory, decongestant, expectorant, antitussive, relaxing (based on known actions of constituents), endocrine stimulant (traditional).

Indications: musculoskeletal (inflammation and pain), respiratory (congestion, coughs), psyche (stress, tension, focus), energetic (strength, resilience, clarity, will).

Blending suggestions and expanded practice:

Musculoskeletal: for pain, inflammation, tension, fatigue, consider blending with bornyl acetate-rich hemlock, fir; also Douglas fir, Scots pine, rosemary CT bornyl acetate or CT myrcene, spike lavender, golden rod, galbanum, blackcurrant bud, bergamot, lemon.

Respiratory: for coughs, congestion, consider blending with bornyl acetate-rich hemlock, fir, inula, golden rod, valerian; cypress, rosemary CT bornyl acetate or CT 1,8-cineole, thyme, labdanum, cistus, long pepper, anthopogon.

Wellbeing: for severe and prolonged stress and adrenal 'burnout', consider blending with Scots pine, galbanum and blackcurrant bud.

Psyche: for fatigue, lack of focus and concentration, tension, lack of stamina, consider blending with rosemary CT bornyl acetate, lavender, lime, grapefruit, lemon, Douglas fir, silver fir, balsam fir, pink pepper.

Energetic: hemlock, spruce and fir oils have been used in traditional spiritual and health-sustaining practices; folk wisdom indicated that these conifers and their oils conferred strength and resilience, clarity and purpose, and happiness, and that they acted specifically on the lungs, joints and muscles, often being used to alleviate respiratory problems, rheumatism and arthritis; black spruce has been recommended for its 'opening and elevating, through grounding, quality' (Lavabre 1990, p.64).

Expanded practice: you could also consider using red spruce (*P. rubens*), which contains 16–17% bornyl acetate – it has a lighter, fresher aroma with underlying citrus notes; or white spruce (*P. alba* or *P. glauca*), which is dominated by α- and β-pinenes (together at around 40%) with bornyl acetate and limonene – its scent has a liberating effect on the senses.

Thyme, common (Lamiaceae)

Thymus vulgaris, flowering tops and leaves; steam-distilled essential oil; the first distillate from *T. vulgaris* is red in colour and cloudy in appearance, and this is called 'red thyme oil'; it is then filtered and redistilled to produce 'white thyme oil', which has a sweeter top note; there are several chemotypes, including thymol, carvacrol, carvacrol/thymol, linalool and geraniol.

Odour: the thymol and carvacrol types have sharp, warm and penetrating herbal (thyme type) odours, with woody, spicy and tobacco-like notes; thymol itself has a powerful, medicated and herbaceous odour; carvacrol itself has a tar-like odour; the linalool CT is herbal (thyme), with a softer, sweeter, woodier odour; the geraniol CT is herbal (thyme) with a sweeter odour and rosy notes.

Constituents:

Thymol CT: thymol (50–63%), carvacrol (up to 20%), *para*-cymene (up to 20%), with γ-terpinene, β-caryophyllene, *l*-linalool, α-terpinene, α-pinene.

Carvacrol CT: carvacrol (up to 42%), thymol (10%), with *para*-cymene (27–28%), γ-terpinene (10–11%), *l*-linalool, α-pinene, β-myrcene, α-terpinene and others.

Linalool CT: *l*-linalool (70–80%), with linalyl acetate, α-terpineol, borneol, thymol and carvacrol (5%), *para*-cymene, camphene and others.

Geraniol CT: geranyl acetate (36–37%), geraniol (25%), β-caryophyllene (6%), with *l*-linalool, terpinen-4-ol, myrtenyl acetate, geranyl propionate, geranyl butyrate, γ-terpinene and *cis*-sabinene hydrate (note absence of thymol and carvacrol).

Main actions:

Thymol, carvacrol and linalool chemotypes: analgesic, anti-nociceptive, anti-inflammatory (inhibits prostaglandin synthesis, COX-1 inhibitor), antispasmodic, anti-oxidant, antibacterial, antifungal (yeasts), antiviral, broncholytic, expectorant, wound-healing (all based on actions of essential oils and thymol).

Geraniol CT: analgesic, anti-nociceptive, anti-inflammatory, antifungal (yeasts and dermatophytes), anxiolytic (all based on known actions of major constituents).

Indications:

Thymol, carvacrol and linalool chemotypes: musculoskeletal (inflammation and pain), digestive (spasm and cramps), wellbeing, prevention of infection, respiratory (congestion, coughs, infections).

Geraniol CT: musculoskeletal, skin, psyche.

Blending suggestions and expanded practice:

Musculoskeletal: for pain, inflammation, arthritis, consider blending thymol, carvacrol and linalool chemotypes with lavender, geranium, bergamot mint, lemon balm, sweet marjoram, rosemary CT myrcene, bergamot, lemon; consider blending the geraniol CT with palmarosa, coriander seed, or use in conjunction with the thymol-containing types.

Digestive: for pain, spasm, irritable bowel syndrome, consider blending with peppermint, spearmint, lavender, sweet marjoram, clary sage, sweet orange, lime, Szechuan pepper.

Wellbeing: for prevention of infection, consider blending thymol-rich types with terpinen-4-ol-containing tea tree, plai, sweet marjoram, kewda, juniperberry, nutmeg, and linalool-rich rosewood, thyme linalool CT, wild marjoram, basil CT linalool, bergamot mint, rosalina type 1, lavender; for stress and immune support, consider blending the geraniol CT with palmarosa, neroli, coriander seed.

Respiratory: for congestion, coughs, consider blending the thymol-containing types with rosemary, sweet marjoram, wild marjoram, spearmint, inula, plai, myrtle, rosalina type 2, fragonia, juniperberry, fir, spruce, hemlock, cypress.

Skin: for dermatophyte infection, consider blending the geraniol CT with carrot seed, Sardinian sage, juniperberry, pink pepper.

Psyche: for anxiety and stress, consider blending the geraniol CT with palmarosa, geranium, rose, neroli.

Energetic: early civilisations used thyme not so much as a culinary herb but for its scent and smoke – the genus name is derived from the Greek word *thymon* or *thuein*, which meant 'to make a burnt offering'; thyme was thought to invigorate and inspire courage; it was a sacred herb of the Druids, who used it to lift the spirits and dispel negativity; in folklore the thyme plant was the fairies' playground, and often a patch of thyme would be left undisturbed for their use.

Expanded practice: in addition to the chemotypes of *T. vulgaris*, there are other *Thymus* species and their chemotypes that you could consider using: these include Moroccan thyme (*T. saturoides* borneol CT), wild thyme (*T. serpyllum*), Spanish thyme (*T. zygis*) and Spanish marjoram (*T. mastichina*); also Spanish oreganum (*T. capitatus*), but this may contain high levels of carvacrol (70–85%). If a thyme fragrance element is desirable in a therapeutic perfume, you might also consider *T. vulgaris* absolute, which is sweet, light, warm and subtle, herbal and persistent, with woody and ambra nuances, and only small amounts will be required.

Caution: the isomers thymol and carvacrol interfere with blood clotting, and the oral use of thymol/carvacrol-rich thyme oils is contraindicated if anticoagulants are being taken or if bleeding disorders are present; they are also skin and mucous membrane irritants; the maximum dermal limit should be in the region of 1%, and the phenol rule applies.

Turmeric (Zingiberaceae)

Curcuma longa rhizomes; steam-distilled essential oil.

Odour: the essential oil has a fresh, spicy aroma, with woody notes; it is reminiscent of the ground spice, and has a distinctive yellow colour.

Constituents: turmerone (up to 28%), *ar*-turmerone (up to 28%), zingiberene (up to 17%), α-phellandrene (up to 13%), also β-curcumene, 1,8-cineole, α- and β-caryophyllene, terpinolene, sabinene and others (traces to around 5%).

Main actions: analgesic, anti-nociceptive, anti-inflammatory, anti-arthritic, anti-oxidant, anti-cancer, antifungal, antidepressant.

Indications: musculoskeletal (inflammation, pain, arthritis), wellbeing, psyche (depression, nervousness).

Blending suggestions and expanded practice:

Musculoskeletal: for inflammation, pain, arthritis, consider blending with ginger, plai, galangal, *Alpinia calcarata* (if available), clove bud, cinnamon leaf, nutmeg, black pepper, pink pepper, Szechuan pepper, black cumin, frankincense, patchouli, kewda, cassie, mimosa, linden blossom, rose, lime, yuzu.

Wellbeing: consider blending with palmarosa, lemongrass, plai, ginger, galangal, nagarmotha, sandalwood, patchouli, vetiver, frankincense, labdanum, mastic, clove bud, cardamom, nutmeg, kewda, ylang ylang, rose, lime.

Psyche: for depression, apprehension, nervousness, consider blending with sandalwood, labdanum, spikenard, nagarmotha, patchouli, frankincense, mastic, rose, jasmine, ylang ylang, frangipani, pink lotus.

Energetic: in Ayurvedic medicine turmeric is classified as bitter, astringent, pungent and hot, and is used to purify and protect, and as an antiseptic; it is used for body painting in the Pacific Islands, and in India followers of Vishnu use turmeric to make a perpendicular mark on their foreheads.

Expanded practice: create an aromatherapeutic version of the pungent, aromatic Ayurvedic *Trikatu* by combining turmeric, ginger, black pepper and long pepper; or the Hindi *Abir* by combining turmeric with sandalwood, cloves and cardamom. The anticarcinogenic compound curcumin (a curcuminoid) is not present in the essential oil, but it does occur in the oleoresin and the CO_2 extract; this has potential aromatherapeutic use for general wellbeing, and health recovery and maintenance.

Caution: *ar*-turmerone and turmeric essential oil inhibit glucosidase enzymes better than some anti-diabetic drugs; possible interaction with anti-diabetic medication (Tisserand and Young 2014, p.458).

Vetiver (Poaceae)

Vetiveria zizanoides roots and rhizome; steam-distilled essential oil.

Odour: there is considerable variety, depending on the geographical origins; in perfumery, oils from Réunion (and India) are favoured over the more readily available Java oil; typically, vetiver has a smooth, strong, sweet, rich, woody and earthy aroma, with rooty, musty nuances reminiscent of sliced raw potato; it shares some of these qualities with patchouli.

Constituents: extremely complex composition; only one constituent is present at over 10%, and that is khusimol (3–15%), with isonootkatol (up to 8%); numerous other sesquiterpenoids are present; the odour is influenced by α- and β- vetivone and khusimone.

Main actions: analgesic, anti-inflammatory, immunostimulant, wound-healing, antidepressant, sedative –all traditional aromatherapeutic uses.

Indications: musculoskeletal (arthritis, pain, inflammation, rheumatism), wellbeing (health recovery and maintenance), skin (inflammation, acne and dermatitis, eczema), psyche (depression, anxiety, insomnia) – all traditional aromatherapeutic uses.

Blending suggestions and expanded practice:

Musculoskeletal and wellbeing: for pain, inflammation, arthritis, rheumatism, and general wellbeing, consider blending with ginger, plai, turmeric, lemongrass, palmarosa, patchouli, hemp, nagarmotha, coriander seed, black pepper, pink pepper, bergamot, lime, sweet orange, combava peel, combava petitgrain.

Skin: for acne, consider blending with combava petitgrain, petitgrain bigarade, ylang ylang, white champaca, sandalwood, patchouli; for dermatitis, consider blending with Himalayan or Lebanese cedar, cypress, geranium, immortelle, cassie, lemongrass, rose, sandalwood, patchouli, hemp.

Psyche: for anxiety, depression, insomnia, consider blending with lavender, spikenard, nagarmotha, patchouli, opoponax, labdanum, cistus, rose, ylang ylang, pink lotus, frangipani.

Energetic: in Ayurvedic medicine, vetiver is classed as a bitter, sweet and very cooling remedy. In the hot season bundles of the roots are soaked in water and placed in front of electric fans to both cool and scent rooms. The roots can also be soaked in drinking water to make a cooling drink, which prevents *Pitta* (one of the doshas) 'flare-up'; in India and Sri Lanka vetiver is known as 'the oil of tranquillity'.

Ylang ylang 'extra' (Anonaceae)

Cananga odorata var. *genuina* flowers; steam-distilled essential oil; the first fraction is termed 'extra', followed by a 'first', then 'second' and 'third' fractions; 'complete' is a combination of all four fractions; sometimes sold as cananga oil; an absolute via solvent extraction is also available.

Odour: varies according to geographical source (Comoro and Madagascar); typically a diffusive, strong, sweet, heady, smooth and rich tropical-floral scent, with underlying fruity, medicated and spicy notes; extra is believed to have the finest odour, but the third fraction is also used in perfumery; cananga oil is sweet and floral, with medicated, woody and oily notes; the absolute has very similar odour profile to the essential oil, but is rounder and softer.

Constituents: complex composition; germacrene D (17%), benzyl acetate (12–13%), *para*-cresyl methyl ether (8–9%), *l*-linalool (8–9%), α-farnesene (8%), β-caryophyllene (5%), with geranyl acetate, methyl benzoate, cinnamyl acetate, benzyl salicylate and others in lesser quantities.

Main actions: the constituent profile suggests pain-relieving and anti-inflammatory actions; mood enhancement.

Indications: skin care (traditional), general wellbeing, tension and stress reduction, psyche (harmonising, depression, anxiety, inhibitions).

Blending suggestions and expanded practice:

Wellbeing: for muscular tension, inhibitions, frustration, out of touch with physical needs, ylang ylang can be used on its own; also consider blending ylang ylang with rose, palmarosa, sandalwood, labdanum, opoponax, frankincense, patchouli.

Psyche: for depression and anxiety, consider blending with clary sage, violet leaf, petitgrain bigarade, rose, jasmine, frangipani, patchouli, sandalwood, labdanum, opoponax, frankincense, tobacco, lime.

Energetic: The flowers have an intense, floral, narcotic fragrance, and they are used for personal decoration and to scent fabrics, homes and clothing; in Indonesia it is a folk custom to perfume the bed linen of newly married couples with ylang ylang flowers; it has long been considered an aphrodisiac.

Expanded practice: its unique scent is very relaxing, yet highly euphoric – and so it can help to connect the emotions and feelings with the senses and the physical realm. Ylang ylang has a 'harmonising' effect, where blood pressure and heart rate decrease while attentiveness increases. However, it can also decrease alertness and reaction times; this profile of actions makes ylang ylang one of the most useful oils for aromatherapy massage, and for creating a relaxing ambience. If it is felt that the fragrance is too sweet and intense, combine with violet leaf, which can 'tone it down'; alternatively the sweet-floral facet can be augmented by blending with vanilla.

Caution: ylang ylang presents a risk of skin sensitisation, and must be used with caution on sensitive skin, or where the barrier function is impaired; avoid using it on children.

Yuzu (Rutaceae)

Citrus × junos peel (a hybrid of the Ichang lemon or papeda (*C. ichangensis*) and the sour mandarin); expressed essential oil.

Odour: a strong, aromatic citrus with floral notes, in the manner of bergamot, but more intense.

Constituents: *d*-limonene (60–65%), γ-terpinene (12–13%), β-phellandrene (5–6%), with β-myrcene, *l*-linalool, α- and β-pinene, *trans*-β-farnesene, bicyclogermacrene; two constituents have recently been identified as important in its unique odour: undecatriene-3-one, and 1,3,5,7-undecatetriene, which contributes to the green aspects; phototoxic constituents are absent.

Main actions: analgesic, anti-inflammatory, anti-atherosclerosis (γ-terpinene is an LDL anti-oxidant), broncholytic, anti-stress/antidepressant (likely).

Indications: musculoskeletal (pain and inflammation, tension), wellbeing, respiratory (anti-inflammatory, asthma), psyche (depression, anxiety, stress).

Blending suggestions and expanded practice:

Musculoskeletal: for pain, inflammation, stress-related tension, consider blending with galbanum and blackcurrant bud, also clove bud, cinnamon leaf, nutmeg, coriander seed, star anise, black pepper, pink pepper, Szechuan pepper, plai, ginger, frankincense, geranium, palmarosa, lemongrass.

Wellbeing: consider blending with lime, bitter orange, grapefruit, pomelo, mandarin petitgrain, bergamot mint, clove bud, nutmeg, caraway, turmeric, plai, ginger, mastic, frankincense, Szechuan pepper, pink pepper, narcissus, perilla, patchouli, sandalwood.

Respiratory: for inflammation, asthma, consider blending with plai, ginger, sweet fennel, long pepper, rose, jasmine, kewda, sandalwood.

Psyche: for depression, anxiety and stress, consider blending with narcissus, jasmine, ylang ylang, frangipani, orange blossom, neroli, bitter orange, Szechuan pepper, sandalwood, patchouli.

Energetic: in Japan, on *Tōji*, the winter solstice, it is customary to bathe with yuzu oil or the cut fruit in the bathwater; the yuzu bath is called *yuzuyu* or *yuzuburo*, and is a cleansing and fortifying ritual.

Expanded practice: create a 'single note' bath preparation for use on the winter solstice; blend a citrus 'fantasy' therapeutic perfume by blending yuzu with grapefruit, sweet orange, bitter orange, orange blossom, mandarin petitgrain and Szechuan pepper.

Chapter 15

Expanded Practice Aromatics

Abbreviated Profiles for Synergistic Blending

African basil (*Ocimum gratissimum* leaves, Lamiaceae family): dominated by eugenol at around 54%, with 1,8-cineole (22%); it has similar actions and directions to holy basil; for acne-prone skin use a hydrophilic base, and with honey or aloe vera.

African bluegrass (*Cymbopogon validus*, Poaceae family): anti-inflammatory and analgesic potential due to dominance of β-myrcene (15–20%); also contains up to 10% borneol, which is notable for its antimicrobial (against a range of Gram-positive and Gram-negative pathogens and fungi), wound-healing and anti-inflammatory actions; caution – traces of methyl eugenol may be present; check with supplier.

Anise (*Pimpinella anisum* seeds, Umbelliferae family): the essential oil has a warm, spicy, sweet anisic odour; *trans*-anethole (75–90%), *d*-limonene (up to 5%), methyl chavicol 0.5–5%) and others; similar to sweet fennel in actions; cautions apply.

Bitter orange (*Citrus × aurantium* peel, Rutaceae family): this is the Seville orange; the peel oil has a subtle, fresh, delicate but tenacious aroma, with sweet floral and green notes; dominated by *d*-limonene (90–95%) with linalool and β-myrcene; it has anticonvulsant activity.

Blue-leaved mallee (*E. polybractea* leaves and twigs, Myrtaceae family): sweet, fresh and cineolic with camphoraceous nuances; 1,8-cineole (90%), *para*-cymene (2–3%), terpinen-4-ol, α- and β-pinene, *d*-limonene and sabinene; constituents suggest properties similar to eucalyptus blue gum.

Brazilian pepper (*Schinus terebinthifolius raddi* dried fruits, Rutaceae family): contains δ-3-carene, α-phellandrene, α-pinene, *d*-limonene and terpinen-4-ol – these are analgesic constituents; no known hazards or contraindications.

Broad-leaved peppermint (*Eucalyptus dives* leaves and twigs, Myrtaceae family): an 'industrial eucalypt'; one variety is rich in piperitone (54%), with α-phellandrene, *para*-cymene, terpinen-4-ol and others; piperitone is isolated and used as a raw material for the production of synthetic menthol and thymol.

Cacao (*Theobroma cacao* seeds, Malvaceae family): cacao absolute is balsamic, rich and warm, with chocolate nuances, but vanilla element is absent; although cacao is one of the most important botanicals from the perspective of human wellbeing, it is not so well known as an aromatic and fragrance; it has fixative properties, it imparts 'edible' or 'gourmand' effects in blends and is used in base accords; use to impart feelings of comfort and wellbeing; blends very well with patchouli, vanilla, tobacco, rose and sweet orange.

Cajuput (*Melaleuca cajuputi* leaves and twigs, Myrtaceae family): strong, sweet and camphoraceous; dominated by 1,8-cineole (40–70%), with α-terpineol, *para*-cymene, terpinolene, γ-terpinene, *l*-limonene and others; pain-relieving, anti-inflammatory, antimicrobial and expectorant actions.

Camphor (Hon-sho, *Cinnamomum camphora* wood and twigs, several chemotypes including *1,8-cineole, linalool, safrole, nerolidol*, Lauraceae family): the odour is distinctive and camphoraceous, penetrating and pungent, clean, fresh and sharp.

CT 1,8-cineole: 1,8-cineole (76%), α-pinene (20%) with α-terpinene.

CT linalool: known as ho oil, dominated by linalool (80%), with 10% monoterpenes.

CT safrole: safrole (80%) and 10% monoterpenols (not for therapeutic use).

CT nerolidol: nerolidol (40–60%), with monoterpenoids (20%) and sesquiterpenoids (20%); the nerolidol type is possibly anti-inflammatory and nerolidol is an inhibitor of 5-LOX.

Chinese cedarwood (*Cupressus funebris* wood, Cupressaceae family): also known as the Chinese weeping cypress; the essential oil contains *iso-* and thujopsene, with cedrenol, longifolene, α-cedrene and others; these constituents are not yet associated with any particular actions; however, they are not hazardous and they are also found in other members of the *Cupressaceae* family. Chinese cedar essential oil may have an affinity with the respiratory system and the skin.

Cistus or **Rock rose** (*Cistus ladaniferus, C. creticus*, Cistaceae family): distilled from the aerial parts of the flowering plant; warm, sweet and woody; composition is variable but the oil can be dominated by α-pinene (up to 55%), camphene, bornyl acetate, aromadendrene (viridiflorol), sabinene, *para*-cymene and many others; consituents suggest an affinity with the respiratory system and probable pain-relieving qualities (in alignment with traditional medicine uses); the flower remedy is used for trauma and numb feelings.

Citron or cédrat (*Citrus medica* peel, Rutaceae family): one of the 'ancestral' citrus species; the essential oil has a sharp, characteristic citrus odour with intensity and depth, and better tenacity than other citrus species; dominated by *d*-limonene. It is mentioned in Islamic texts; in ancient Greece it was macerated in wine to counteract poisoning; it does not have a history of aromatherapeutic use. Use in therapeutic perfumes for its tenacity and depth.

Citronella (*Cymbopogon nardus* (Sri Lanka), or *C. winterianus* (Java) leaves, Poaceae family): the Sri Lankan essential oil has a sweet, fresh, lemony odour; the Java type has a lemony, floral, grassy and woody odour; citronella is an 'industrial oil' used in insect repellents, household and industrial cleaning products, and the isolation of aromachemicals. Dominated by citronellal (up to 46%), with geraniol, *l*-citronellol, *l*-limonene, camphene, citronellyl acetate, borneol and others; from this we can expect anti-nociceptive, anti-inflammatory, antimicrobial, vasorelaxant, possibly hypotensive and sedative actions.

Clementine (*Citrus reticulata* var. *clementina* peel, Rutaceae family): a sweet, mild, gentle citrus aroma; dominated by *d*-limonene (around 95%); we might expect actions similar to those of sweet orange essential oil.

Dill (*Anethum graveolens* seed, Umbelliferae family): a light, fresh, spicy, slightly minty, caraway-like odour; contains *d*-limonene (35–65%), *d*-carvone (30–50%) and α-phellandrene; *d*-carvone has anxiolytic action. During the Middle Ages dill was hung at doors and windows to protect against witchcraft, but it was also used in spells, including love potions. The modern name comes from the Old Norse word *dilla*, which means 'to lull' – alluding to its widespread reputation for soothing colicky babies.

Douglas fir (*Pseudotsuga menziensi* (British Columbia), *P. taxifolia* (the Oregon Douglas fir, Oregon balsam), Pinaceae family): the essential oil from the needles and twigs has a very fragrant, fresh coniferous/lemon aroma, with a note that is reminiscent of pineapple; constituents are variable and unusual for a coniferous oil: geraniol (31–32%), and also α- and β-pinene (24%), camphene (15%), bornyl acetate (10%), with sabinene, terpinen-4-ol, *d*-limonene, γ-terpinene, citronellol, and citronellyl acetate, and others – suggesting anti-oxidant, anti-inflammatory, anti-nociceptive and analgesic actions, an affinity with the respiratory system, and anxiolytic and cognition-enhancing potential.

Eucalyptus camadulensis (leaves and twigs, Myrtaceae family): very similar to *E. globulus*; contains 1,8-cineole (50–85%), with α- and β-pinene, *d*-limonene, α-terpineol and others; could be considered as an alternative to eucalyptus blue gum.

Exotic (or Comoran) basil (*Ocimum basilicum* CT estragol, leaves, Lamiaceae family): the estragole (methyl chavicol) chemotype contains a substantial amount (73–87%) of this potentially carcinogenic phenolic ether, and also methyl eugenol (trace–4%). Methyl chavicol is, however, credited with antispasmodic properties, and some writers suggest that it is safe to use on the skin in blends for pain; the recommended limit is 0.1%.

Fenugreek (*Trigonella foenum-graecum* seeds, Fabeaceae family): the essential oil and absolute both have an intense, woody odour, initially reminiscent of curry but quickly becoming warm, rich and walnut-like; the essential oil is characterised by virtually equal parts (15%) of neryl acetate, camphor, β-pinene and β-caryophyllene; it probably has pain-relieving actions (neryl acetate and β-caryophyllene, which are also anti-inflammatory), and the presence of camphor could increase the antifungal activity of other essential oil constituents; an α-amylase and maltase inhibitor.

Fragonia (*Agonis fragrans* fresh leaves and twigs, Myrtaceae family): this trademarked essential oil has a cineolic, herbaceous/balsamic odour, with cinnamon-like notes; it contains 1,8-cineole (26–33%), α-pinene (22–27%) and monoterpene alcohols such as α-terpineol (5–8%), linalool, geraniol and terpinen-4-ol; this is considered to be the ideal ratio of these compounds for the treatment of respiratory infections. It also contains γ-terpinene, *para*-cymene, *d*-limonene and β-myrcene; based on this profile of constituents, it could be expected that fragonia will have pain-relieving and anti-inflammatory actions; it has a pleasant odour and does not necessarily need to be blended with other oils.

Frangipani (*Plumeria* species, *P. rubra* (red) and *P. acuminata* (white) flowers, Apocynaceae family): the absolute has a diffusive, strong, heady, sweet, rich, tropical floral scent, with honey, fruity, spicy, green and citrus notes; the composition is complex and variable, including benzyl salicylate, neryl phenylacetate, phenyl ethyl benzoate and phenyl ethyl cinnamate, also pehenylethanol, *trans*-nerolidol, linalool and geranial; anxiolytic – in Ayurvedic medicine it is used to bring comfort, impart inner peace and release tension, calm fear and anxiety, and to treat tremors and insomnia. *Plumeria* is among the traditional plants that have been found to possess anti-tumoural and antimicrobial properties; it might also be effective against parasitic infestations. In Thailand, an infusion of the flowers is applied to the skin after bathing, as a cosmetic; in India, incense sometimes contains *Plumeria* species, indicated by the word *champa*; perhaps 'Nag Champa' is best known in the West; this combines frangipani with sandalwood and the water-absorbing resin of *Ailanthus malabarica*.

French lavender (*Lavandula stoechas* subsp. *stoechas*, flowering tops, Lamiaceae family): it is possible that this species was the lavender of classical times. The essential oil has a penetrating, camphoraceous lavender scent. The composition is variable; it contains camphor (15–55%), *d*-fenchone (15–50%) and 1,8-cineole (up to 15%) with camphene, α-pinene, small amounts of *l*-linalool and others; sometimes small amounts of linalyl acetate, sometimes not. It might be expected that the oil would have pain-relieving and expectorant actions, but it is rarely used in aromatherapy because of the *d*-fenchone and camphor content. However, it has a long history of use in folk medicine; in Spain and Portugal it was used for strewing the floors of churches and homes on festive occasions, and to make fires on St John's Day, when evil spirits were around; *L. stoechas* was an ingredient of the 'Four Thieves Vinegar' of the Middle Ages; it was used for healing wounds and as an expectorant and antispasmodic. It is used in Unani Tibb medicine for brain disorders such as epilepsy. Research has revealed that the oil has anticonvulsant activity (attributed to its linalool, pinene and linalyl acetate content), and it modulates Ca^{2+} channels.

Galangal (*Alpinia galanga* rhizomes, Zingiberaceae family): the essential oil has a penetrating, fresh, spicy, cineolic, camphoraceous odour, with depth and tenacity; constituents include 1,8-cineole (30%), camphor (up to 14%), β-pinene (10%), α-terpineol (up to 10%), *d*-limonene and others; this would suggest that it has pain-relieving, anti-inflammatory and antimicrobial properties, and is directed to the musculoskeletal and respiratory systems.

Galbanum (*Ferula galbaniflua* oleoresin, Umbelliferae family): the essential oil has a intense, fresh, sharp, green odour, reminiscent of cut green peppers, with coniferous, pine-like, old wood, earthy, musty notes; contains β-pinene (45–60%), δ-3-carene (2–12%), with *d*-limonene, α-pinene, sabinene, β-myrcene and others; analgesic, anti-inflammatory, expectorant, wound-healing actions probable, based on these constituents. The intense green notes can be modified by adding blackcurrant bud, or Roman chamomile. Traditional uses include skin care, the treatment of inflammation, and as a respiratory tonic.

Genet (*Spartium junceum* flowers, Fabaceae family): from the Spanish broom, the absolute has a green-floral scent that is persistent, sweet and warm, with rosy, green, herbaceous and hay notes; complex composition; contains esters such as ethyl myristate, ethyl palmitate, ethyl oleate and linalyl acetate, and alcohols such as linalool, phenyl ethanol. Blends well with mimosa, narcissus, cassie and rose absolutes. The plant is toxic, and safety information regarding the absolute is not available, so it should, in the meantime, be restricted to inhalation and the appreciation of its fragrance.

Ginger lily (*Hedychium spicatum* dried rhizomes, Zingiberaceae family): the essential oil has a pungent, aromatic, green-spicy, woody odour, with faint orris-like, violet notes, it has depth and tenacity, the dryout is myrrh-like; constituents include 1,8-cineole (6–45%), linalool (10–25%) and many others including the unusual T-muurolol, hedycaryol and aromatic esters; may contain the very toxic ascaridole (check with supplier). Restrict use to inhalation for pleasure and relaxation (keep away from children). In India it is known as *kapur-kachri* and it is an ancient and valued incense ingredient.

Ginger lily, white (*Hedychium coronarium* flowers, Zingiberaceae family): the absolute is warm, sweet and honey-like, an indolic floral, with spicy, fruity and balsamic notes; constituents include *l*-linalool (up to 30%), *iso*-eugenol (15–18%), indole (up to 7%), esters such as methyl jasmonate, methyl benzoate, benzyl benzoate, with others including *cis*-jasmone, β-ionone and lactones. The presence of *l*-linalool and *iso*-eugenol (and eugenol at 1.5%) would suggest pain-relieving properties; it can be used for relieving stress and tension, and for relaxation; it is thought to be antidepressant, and has been used as a meditation aid.

Golden rod (*Solidago canadensis*, flowering plant, Asteraceae family): the essential oil has a cut grass-like opening, before soft coniferous, fresh-woody and herbaceous notes emerge; dominated by bornyl acetate (20%), sabinene (19%) and *d*-limonene (18%) with α-phellandrene (12%), β-myrcene (10%), terpinolene, γ-terpinene, β-pinene, borneol, *l*-linalool and others. Although little used, the oil is available and, based on this constituent profile, we might expect analgesic, anti-nociceptive, anti-inflammatory and antimicrobial actions; no apparent cautions or hazards. It will blend well with bornyl acetate-rich, sabinene-rich and *d*-limonene-rich essential oils and can impart a sense of meadows and 'the great outdoors' to blends.

Greek sage (*Salvia triloba* leaves, Greece, Turkey, Crete, Lamiaceae family): the essential oil is dominated by 1,8-cineole, with *d*-limonene (38%), camphor (15%), α-terpineol and borneol (7%), α- and β-thujone (6–7%) and α- and β-pinene (5–6%); expectorant, mucolytic and wound-healing actions. The camphor and thujone content presents a hazard (seizure), therefore check composition with supplier, and use with caution. *S. triloba* is sometimes classed as *S. libanotica* (see Lebanese sage).

Green mallee (*Eucalyptus viridis* leaves and twigs, Myrtaceae family): sweet, fresh and cineolic; very similar to eucalyptus blue gum oil in terms of constituents and actions.

Guaiacwood (*Bulnesia sarmientoi* wood, Zygophyllaceae family): the essential oil has a soft, sweet, clean, tea rose, woody and balsamic scent; it is dominated by bulnesol (40%) with guaicol, eudesmol and elemol. Information regarding its therapeutic properties or the actions of the constituents was not available; however, the scent is appealing and can be used to enhance rosy notes in blends containing geranium, rose, immortelle, or to impart soft rosy-wood elements to spicy and woody blends.

Guava leaf (*Psidium guajava*, Myrtaceae family): the essential oil has a fresh, green, cut grass-like odour, with lemon-like and pepper notes; contains *d*-limonene, β-caryophyllene, α- and β-pinene, aromadendrene and β-bisabolene; both *d*-limonene and aromadendrene have cancer-suppressing actions; anti-inflammatory and pain-relieving actions are possible. The inhibition zones of guava leaf *extract* were greater than those of tea tree oil for *P. acnes*, and equal for staphylococci; possible use for acne.

Gully-gum or Smith's gum (*Eucalyptus smithii*, leaves and twigs, Myrtaceae family): fresh and cineolic; contains 1,8-cineole (76–78%), with β-eudesmol and others; some varieties may also contain substantial amounts of phellandrene.

Hay (*Hierochloe alpina* (alpine sweetgrass), or *Anthoxanthum odoratum* (vanilla grass, holy grass, buffalo grass) dried leaves, Poaceae family): related to sweetgrass (*H. odorata*), which is used in Native American ceremonies and rituals. The absolute has a rich, warm, sweet, green, hay-like aroma, with vanilla-like notes;

contains coumarin and benzoic acid (no contraindications for skin or inhalation). The essential oil of *A. odoratum* is called flouve, which is sweet and hay-like and reminiscent of mimosa; hay absolute is often described as having a 'happy smell', and can be used for its uplifting, comforting aroma; create an aromatherapeutic version of a cut grass perfume (*foin coupé*) by combining hay absolute with bergamot, lavender and clary sage essential oils or absolutes, oakmoss absolute and trace amounts of wintergreen or sweet birch.

Hemp (*Cannabis sativa* aerial parts of flowering plant, Cannabaceae family): the essential oil contains β-myrcene (33%), *trans*-β-ocimene (15%), terpinolene, β-caryophyllene and caryophyllene oxide (1.4%); good analgesic and anti-inflammatory potential, a 5-LOX inhibitor; good potential for treating inflammatory and dry skin disorders; could be used in conjunction with the fixed oil.

Hiba wood (*Thujopsis dolobrata*, *T. dolobrata* var. *hondai* wood, Cupressaceae family): the essential oil is woody, intense and pungent; little information could be accessed regarding its composition and safety; contains thujopsene and cedrol; probably best used by inhalation; for mood modification only.

Hops (*Humulus lupus* dried strobiles (catkins, cones), Moraceae family): the essential oil has a rich, heady, sweet and spicy scent, with pleasant beer-like notes emerging at drydown; dominant constituents are α- and β-caryophyllene (47%), β-myrcene (25%), with γ- and δ-cadinene, α-humulene, geraniol, sabinene and others. Traditional uses were for the nerves; it was widely used as a sedative, an aphrodisiac and as a flavour in beers and tobacco; the constituent profile would suggest anti-inflammatory, pain-relieving and possibly antimicrobial actions.

Hyssop (*Hyssopus officinalis* leaves and flowering tops, Lamiaceae family): the essential oil has a strong, sweet, camphoraceous, warm, spicy odour; the linalool chemotype is less likely to present a hazard than the pinocamphone type (up to 80% *iso*- and pinocamphones); dominated by *d*-linalool (50%), with 1,8-cineole (12–15%), *d*-limonene (5%) and others including α-pinene, camphene, β-myrcene and sabinene, with *iso*-pinocamphone (1.5%) and pinocamphone (up to 1%), suggestive of pain-relieving, anti-inflammatory, expectorant, mucolytic and possibly antitussive actions; historically associated with cleansing and purification.

Inula (*Inula graveolens* flowering tops, Asteraceae family): the essential oil has a penetrating, slightly camphoraceous and pine-like, sweet and herbaceous odour; dominated by bornyl acetate (46%) and borneol (15–16%), with camphene, β-caryophyllene, γ-cadinene, α-terpineol and others; bornyl acetate is noted for its analgesic and anti-inflammatory actions and affinity with the respiratory system; borneol is antimicrobial, also with anti-inflammatory action and wound-healing activity; noted as a powerful mucolytic when administered by inhalation.

Jabara (*Citrus jabara* peel, Rutaceae family): a rare oil, jabara is a 'sour citrus', indigenous to Wakayama in Japan, related to yuzu; jabara extract is used in phytocosmeceuticals as a soothing, anti-allergenic ingredient; contains β-myrcene (47%), with *d*-limonene (28%) and γ-terpinene (15%).

Japanese cedar (*Cryptomeria japonica* needles and twigs, Cupressaceae family): the essential oil has a fresh, sweet, coniferous, woody scent, completely lacking in any harsh, 'disinfectant' notes; constituents include α-pinene, sabinene, α-kaurene, elemol, terpinen-4-ol (figures not available); antioxidant, anti-inflammatory (inhibits pro-inflammatory cytokines and mediators – NO, PGE_2, TNF-α, IL-1β, IL-6), antimicrobial. Excellent antibacterial activities against *P. acnes* and *S. epidermidis*, including drug-susceptible and drug-resistant strains; a potential acne-mitigating candidate for skin health. In Nepal it is known as tsugi pine, and it is burned as incense.

Kanuka or **Kunzea** (*Kunzea ericoides* leaves and twigs, Myrtaceae family): this New Zealand essential oil has a medicated scent, reminiscent of tea tree; constituents (variable according to source) include α-pinene (50–55%), with viridiflorol or aromadendrene (7–8%), 1,8-cineole, *d*-limonene, *para*-cymene and others; it has analgesic, anti-inflammatory and antimicrobial properties; often used in combination with manuka oil.

Labdanum (*Cistus ladaniferus* and *C. creticus* oleoresin (gum), Cistaceae family): steam-distilled essential oil (absolute also available); rich, sweet, soft balsamic, ambra (recalling ambergris – complex, rich, musty, musky, earthy and ambery) with woody, herbaceous notes; complex and variable composition, including α-pinene (up to 45%), camphene (up to 7%), and very many others including *para*-cymene, sabinene, α-terpineol, bornyl acetate, borneol, terpinen-4-ol; many unusual phenols, lactones and acids; acetopheneone and its derivatives, dihydroambrinol, α-ambrinol, drimenone – this would suggest pain-relieving and anti-inflammatory actions, an affinity with the respiratory system, antimicrobial activity (possibly against dermatophytes). The aroma of the oil can enhance many blends. Labdanum is mentioned in the writings of all the ancient cultures; it was an ingredient (known as *onycha*) in the holy incense of Moses, it was widely used by the Egyptians as incense and in cosmetics, and it was probably sacred to Aphrodite and burned at her altars on Cyprus, her 'birthplace'. Dioscorides mentions labdanum in the ingredients of the 'Royal Unguent'.

Lavandin (*Lavandula × intermedia* flowering tops, Lamiaceae family): a cross between true lavender and spike lavender; the essential oil has a lavender-like aroma, but more penetrating and fresher, less fruity than true lavender, and less camphoraceous than spike; varieties include 'Abrialis', 'Grosso' and 'Super'. Constituents vary according to variety; linalyl acetate (25–44%), *l*-linalool (23–33%), camphor (5–30%; 'Super' has only 5%), 1,8-cineole (3–11%; 'Abrialis'

11%), borneol (2–4%), and others; anti-nociceptive and anxiolytic actions; caution with anticoagulant medication and bleeding disorders.

Lebanese sage (*Salvia libanotica* leaves, East Mediterranean, Lamiaceae family): the essential oil has a camphor-like odour. It belongs in Group III. The composition is very variable; however, notable consituents include 1,8-cineole (can be up to 50%), α-terpineol, linalyl acetate and camphor; α- and β-thujone may also be present. Camphor and thujone present a risk (seizure), so check with supplier and use with caution. The essential oil has antiproliferative and apoptosis-inducing actions. The herb has a very long history of use, as early as 1400 BCE. Nowadays it is estimated that most of the imported sage in the United States is *S. libanotica* rather than *S. officinalis*. It is used in the Middle East to treat colds and abdominal pain; in Lebanon, Syria and Jordan, herbal practitioners regard it as a panacea, but its notable uses include treating headaches, sore throats and abdominal pains, treating depression, and as a tranquilliser and sedative. This species was formerly known as *S. triloba* because of its leaves, which have the appearance of three lobes, and it is sometimes still called Greek or Cretan sage.

Lemon myrtle (*Backhousia citriodora* leaves, Myrtaceae family): the essential oil has a strong, harsh, lemon-like odour; dominated by citral (geranial 45–60% and neral 30–40%), this very high citral content warrants caution because of the potential for skin sensitisation and drug interaction. The oil has good antimicrobial actions; it displays significant activity against *Staphylococcus aureus*, MRSA, *Escherichia coli*, *Pseudomonas aerugionosa*, *Candida albicans*, *Klebsiella pneumoniae* and *Propionibacterium acnes*; it could be used, with care, in low concentrations as an antiseptic and for acne; a product containing 1% essential oil showed low toxicity to human skin cells and fibroblasts. Citral has relaxing and antidepressant properties; it is likely that the essential oil will have these actions too.

Lemon-scented eucalyptus (*Eucalyptus citriodora* leaves and twigs, Myrtaceae family): the essential oil has a strong, fresh rosy-citronella odour; contains a minimum of 70% citronellal. The citronellal content probably confers anti-nociceptive, anti-inflammatory, anti-oxidant, antibacterial (*P. acnes*), sedative and sleep-inducing properties.

Lemon-scented ironbark (*Eucalyptus staigeriana* leaves and twiglets, Myrtaceae family): the essential oil has a sweet, fresh, fruity-lemon, verbena-like scent; constituents include *l*-limonene (30%), geranial and neral (18%), β-phellandrene (6–7%), geranyl acetate (4%), geraniol (4%), and others; this suggests anti-inflammatory and pain-relieving actions, and probable antifungal action.

Lemon-scented tea tree (*Leptospermum petersonii* leaves and twiglets, Myrtaceae family): the essential oil has a distinctive lemony, pungent, diffusive odour; constituents include geranial (45%), neral (30%), α-pinene, citronellol, geraniol, and others; this suggests probable antimicrobial, antifungal and anti-inflammatory actions, with relaxing, sedative effects.

Linden blossom (*Tilea vulgaris* dried flowers, Tiliaceae family): the absolute has a fresh, delicate, green-floral aroma, with notes of honey, broom, white lilac, lily of the valley, lily and hay; dominated by farnesol; farnesol has anti-inflammatory action (it is an inhibitor of 5-LOX). In herbalism, linden flowers are used for migraine, cramps, hypertension and as a sedative; will blend well with farnesol-containing oils for skin care, and could be blended with mimosa, hops, golden rod, hay and mastic to produce a relaxing, agrestic-style therapeutic perfume.

Long pepper (*Piper longum* dried fruits, Piperaceae family): the essential oil has an aroma very similar to black pepper – dry, spicy, woody and warm; contains β-caryophyllene at 18% and piperine. Has analgesic (counter-irritant), anti-inflammatory actions (and can reduce oedema associated with inflammation), also anti-asthmatic actions; however, it also has anti-fertility actions at 1gm/kg, and so should be avoided in pregnancy.

Lotus, pink (*Nelumbo nucifera* flowers, Nelumbonaceae family): an aquatic perennial; there are several cultivars, but they all have similar scents; the absolute has a rich, sweet, aromatic floral aroma, with fruity, herbaceous, leathery, powdery, spicy, earthy and medicinal notes; lotus absolute needs to mature in order to develop its fragrance. Complex composition – constituents include caryophyllene oxide, β-caryophyllene, *cis*-jasmone, 1,4-dimethoxybenzene. *White* lotus is rich, sweet, aromatic and floral, but has an animalic and herbaceous dryout; *N. lutea* is the yellow-flowering American lotus, and it has a more pronounced jasmine note. Buddhists adopted the lotus as a symbol of *dharma*; the Buddha is often depicted as sitting on the flower. The pink lotus is very much associated with Kuan Yin, who represents the principle of compassion; the flowers symbolise immortality, resurrection and trancendence.

Mace (*Myristica fragrans*, aril surrounding the nutmeg (seed), Myristaceae family): the East Indian essential oil has an odour similar to that of nutmeg, but it is less pine-like in the top note; dominated by α- and β-pinene (up to 46%), sabinene (12–15%), terpinen-4-ol, γ-terpinene and others; and, like nutmeg, contains safrole (up to 2%) and methyleugenol (traces), so requires caution. Constituents suggest pain-relieving and anti-inflammatory actions; reputed to be psychtropic.

Mandarin petitgrain (*Citrus reticulata* leaf, Rutaceae family): the essential oil has a mild, floral, sweet, orange-citrus scent; contains dimethyl anthranilate (40–52%), γ-terpinene (24–29%), with *d*-limonene (up to 12%), *para*-cymene, α- and β-pinene, β-caryophyllene, α-thujene; constituents suggest pain-relieving and anti-inflammatory actions, also possible anti-atherosclerosis activity because of high γ-terpinene content; to augment γ-terpinene, consider blending with mandarin, yuzu and narcissus absolute.

Manuka (*Leptospermum scoparium* leaves, Myrtaceae family): the essential oil has a distinctive medicinal, tea tree-like odour; composition is variable; contains leptospermone (up to 20%), with sesquiterpenes and their oxygenated derivatives;

leptospermone is a cyclic ketone, which is said to inactivate hyalarodinase, an enzyme that increases diffusion of toxins in the tissues, and so can act as an anti-venom-spreading agent. Used in traditional Maori medicine, and widely regarded as an antibacterial and antifungal essential oil; it also has virucidal activity against HSV1, including drug-resistant isolates; best used on its own, or in combination with kanuka, for antiseptic topical applications.

Mastic (*Pistacia* var. *chia* gum resin, Anacardiaceae family): the essential oil has a fresh, balsamic scent, with mild, sweet coniferous notes; dominated by α-pinene (up to 78%), with β-myrcene, *d*-limonene, *l*-linalool, β-pinene, verbenone, terpinen-4-ol and others; the essential oil has a strong lipid-lowering action. An important resin in the ancient world, where it was burned as incense.

May chang (*Litsea cubeba* small fruits, Lauraceae family): also called tropical verbena; the essential oil has a fresh, sweet, intense, sharp lemon-like odour, with fruity notes; it has a moderate tenacity and can contribute lemon notes to the heart of a blend; dominated by citral (geranial 40%, neral 34%), also *d*-limonene (up to 23%) and others, including methyl heptenone, β-myrcene, *l*-linalool, geraniol, sabinene. Because of the citral content, the oil might have use in the management of pain that involves superficial sensory nerves and the skin – such as allodynia or itching; it has anti-nociceptive activity, and can also reduce induced oedema and inflammation.

Mimosa (*Acacia dealbata* flowers, Mimosaceae family): the absolute has a soft, sweet, delicate green-floral scent, with woody, waxy, honey and hawthorn blossom notes; a complex compositon – most sources indicate that farnesol is a dominant constituent, with others such as phenylethanol, aldehydes C_9 and, *cis*-3-hexenyl acetate, benzaldehyde, ethyl benzoate, linalool, anethole, *cis*-jasmone, anisaldehyde and 2-*trans*-6-*cis*-nonadien-1-al; however, Tisserand and Young (2014) give lupenone (20%), lupeole (7.8%) and *cis*-heptadec-8-ene (6%). Farnesol has anti-inflammatory action (it is an inhibitor of 5-LOX); mimosa blends well with farnesol-containing oils such as linden blossom, cassie and golden champaca for skin care; also indicated for stress, tension and anxiety.

Mojito mint (*Mentha* × *villosa* leaves, Lamiaceae family): rarely available; the essential oil has therapeutic potential; contains two identified active constituents, piperitone oxide and rotundifolone (63%); the oil has hypotensive, vasodilating, vasorelaxing and antispasmodic actions.

Monarda (*Monarda fistulosa* var. *menthaefolia* (wild bergamot or horsemint), *M. didyma* (bee balm, red bergamot), flowering plant, Lamiaceae family):

> *Wild bergamot* essential oil has a sweet, rosy floral odour with lemon-like and terpene notes; it is characterised by geraniol (up to 93%) with *l*-linalool, neral, geranial, γ-terpinene and others.

Bee balm has a softer, woody-floral, herbal scent with lemon-like, pine-like and slight camphoraceous notes; it is characterised by *l*-linalool (up to 75%), with bornyl acetate, germacrene D, γ-terpinene, sabinene and others.

Inhalation of monarda (species not identified) essential oil can reduce the cholesterol content in the aorta and atherosclerotic plaques, but without affecting blood cholesterol; may have a role in the prevention of atherosclerosis; consider blending with mastic and lavender for this purpose.

Moroccan thyme, borneol CT (*Thymus saturoides*, flowering herb, Lamiaceae family): borneol (20%), with carvacrol (20%) and thymol (10%), also α-terpineol, *l*-linalool, camphene, *para*-cymene, β-caryophyllene, bornyl acetate and others. Use with caution due to 30% phenol content; phenol rule applies. Antimicrobial, analgesic, anti-inflammatory, probably broncholytic, antitussive, expectorant, antispasmodic; indicated for muscular pain, arthritis, respiratory congestion, coughs.

Myrtle (*Myrtus communis* leaves, Myrtaceae family): the essential oil has a pleasant, fresh, camphoraceous, floral-herbaceous odour, with resinous undertones; a degree of variability in composition depending on source. Contains α-pinene (20–55%), 1,8-cineole (20–40%), myrtenyl acetate (up to 20%), *d*-limonene (up to 12%), *l*-linalool (up to 10%), α-terpinyl acetate (up to 5%), α-terpineol (up to 4%), geranyl acetate, linalyl acetate and others; 'red myrtle' is the 1,8-cineole CT; 'green myrtle' is the myrtenyl acetate/linalool CT; may contain traces of methyleugenol and methyl chavicol (check with supplier). Anti-inflammatory, expectorant, antifungal; renowned in many cultures for its scent and beauty; the theme of myrtle being sacred to gods and important in worship, or appearing in prophesies, recurs across time and cultures.

Nagarmotha (*Cyperus scariosus* dried rhizomes, Cyperaceae family): also known as cyperus, nagarmotha essential oil has a persistent, rich, deep, smoky, woody, peppery, earthy odour; a complex composition and unusual constituents, such as cyperene, cyperenol, cyperone, with *iso*-patchoulenone, patchouli alcohol and patchoulenone, corymbolone, rotundone, and many others including the familiar 1,8-cineole, camphene, *d*-limonene. No known hazards; the essential oil has antibacterial, antifungal, analgesic, anti-nociceptive, antispasmodic and antidepressant actions. In perfumery it has been used as a substitute for patchouli; *Cyperus* species (aromatic flatsedges) were important incense ingredients in ancient cultures; the scent is highly appropriate for meditative practice and creates a peaceful ambience.

Narrow-leaved (black) peppermint (*E. radiata* leaves and twigs, Myrtaceae family): an 'industrial eucalypt'; contains 1,8-cineole (60–65%) with α-terpineol, *cis*-piperitol, *d*-limonene, piperitone, geraniol and others; some varieties contain substantial amounts of phellandrene; intrinsic synergy for 'colds and flu', that is, the monoterpene:terpene alcohol:1,8-cineole ratio.

Niaouli (the 'five-veined paperbark', *Melaleuca quinquenervia* CT cineole, CT viridiflorol, CT nerolidol and CT linalool leaves, Myrtaceae family): the essential oil has a strong, sweet and camphoraceous/cineolic odour; the composition is very variable and depends on the chemotype – but typically 1,8-cineole (40%), viridiflorol (traces to 45%), *trans*-nerolidol (5–92%), *l*-linalool (0–24%). Used in French aromatic medicine; noted for its antiseptic properties; the constituents of the cineole chemotype reflect the 'cold and flu synergy' (the monoterpene:terpene alcohol:1,8-cineole ratio); has anti-allergic, pain-relieving and expectorant actions.

Opoponax (*Commiphora guidottii*, *C. erythraea* oleo-gum resin, Burseraceae family): the essential oil has a sweet, balsamic, resinous, warm and slightly spicy scent, floral, woody, olibanum-like (frankincense-like), and lacking the slightly medicinal character of myrrh essential oil; the composition is complex and variable; contains β-ocimene (33%), *cis*-α-bisabolene (22%), α-santalene (16%), and also furanodiene and others. Possibly has anti-inflammatory action; the main species of 'myrrh' of the ancient world, which would have been used in incenses, unguents and perfumes. Best used at around 0.5% in a blend or for evaporation; excellent mood enhancement potential, relaxing, and blends well with many oils.

Osmanthus (*Osmanthus fragrans* flowers, Oleaceae family): the absolute has a sweet, rich, complex, fruity-floral aroma, with notes of honey and dried fruit (raisins, plums, apricots); the scent can vary according to type. The flowers range from silvery white to reddish orange; the golden-orange-yellow flowers are regarded as having the best scent. Constituents include β-ionone (up to 34%) and dihydro-β-ionone (up to 16%), γ-decalactone (up to 12%) and related lactones, *l*-linalool (traces to 10%), nerol, geraniol and α-ionone. The scent is activating and antidepressant. In China it is known as *kweiha* and it is one of their ten traditional flowers. Can be used in antidepressant blends where a fruity-floral element is desired, and also in therapeutic perfumes, where it blends well with pink lotus; however, its delicacy and complexity and unique floral-fruity balance mean that it does not need to be blended (indeed it is challenging to work with as a perfume ingredient) – it is a complete perfume as it stands.

Palo santo, holy wood (*Bursera graveolens* wood, Burseraceae family): the essential oil has a penetrating woody odour with fresh mint-like notes, a faint medicinal quality, and balsamic, caramel notes; contains *d*-limonene, α-terpineol, β-bisabolene, *l*-carvone and others – these constituents would suggest anti-inflammatory, anti-nociceptive, wound-healing and antimicrobial (antifungal) actions. The small tree is an endangered species. Widely used in shamanic ceremony and ritual to clear negative energy and purify the spirit; it is a good oil for scenting a space for meditation, or alternatively as the focus of a meditation.

Perilla (*Perilla frutescens* leaves, Lamiaceae family): the essential oil has a complex and pleasant odour – fresh, green and peppery, with nuances of apple seed, basil, cumin, caraway and cinnamon. Seven chemotypes have been identified

– perillaldehyde (the most common), perilla ketone, elsholtzia ketone, citral, perillene, piperitenone and phenylpropanopid; a 'typical' essential oil contains *l*-perillaldehyde (87%), perillyl alcohol (5.5%) and *l*-linalool (1.5%), and based on these constituents we could expect analgesic, anti-inflammatory, anti-oxidant, antimicrobial and anti-cancer (apoptosis-inducing) actions; the essential oil has antidepressant actions. It is challenging to blend with other oils because of the odour, but if used in small amounts it is compatible with floral oils such as rose, jasmine, ylang ylang, also geranium, basil, spice and citrus oils.

Petitgrain 'bigarade' (*Citrus* × *aurantium* leaf, Rutaceae family): the essential oil has a mild, floral sweet, orange-citrus scent; petitgrain 'Paraguay' has a stronger, sweet, woody-floral aroma; contains linalyl acetate (50–70%), *l*-linalool (up to 25%), *d*-limonene (up to 8%), and others including geraniol, α-terpineol, geranyl acetate, β-pinene, neryl acetate, β-ocimene, β-myrcene; the constituents suggest pain-relieving and anti-inflammatory properties. A useful addition to blends where you would like to augment linalyl acetate and *l*-linalool; you might also consider orange, mandarin or lemon petitgrain essential oils. Petitgrain bigarade is a ingredient in most eaux de Cologne formulae.

Pink pepper (*Schinus molle* dried fruits, Anacardiaceae family): the essential oil has a spicy, warm, penetrating odour, reminiscent of black pepper but less dry, with soft citrus and woody notes; constituents include β-myrcene (up to 20%), also α-phellandrene, *para*-cymene, *d*-limonene and β-phellandrene; these constituents indicate analgesic activity – and no hazards or known contraindications; it also has anti-inflammatory and antispasmodic actions. The *molle* was the sacred tree of the Incas; the rubber that exudes from the trunk was used for embalming.

Pomelo (*Citrus maxima* peel, Rutaceae family): the essential oil is similar to grapefruit, characterised by *d*-limonene, citral and 3,3-dimethyl-1-hexene; it has considerable anti-oxidant activity. Use in conjunction with grapefruit.

Poplar bud or balsam poplar (*Populus balsamifera* buds, Salicaceae family): the absolute has a tenacious, sweet, cinnamon-like, balsamic odour, with resinous and grass/hay notes. Poplar bud absolute has strong inhibitory activity against human leukocyte elastase; it could be used in skin care formulations to improve the appearance of sun damage and to improve skin texture and elasticity. An essential oil is available; this is dominated by *d*-α-bisabolol (25–30%), with *trans*-nerolidol, δ-cadinene, γ-curcumene and others; these constituents are strongly suggestive of anti-inflammatory activity, and perhaps antiproliferative activity. In traditional medicine, the resin from the sticky buds was used as a salve; poplar bud is also used in contemporary herbal medicine as an expectorant.

Ravintsara (*Cinnamomum camphora* CT 1,8-cineole leaves, Madagascar, Lauraceae family): the essential oil has a fresh, clean, cineolic scent; contains 1,8-cineole (53–68%), sabinene (12–15%), α- and β-pinene (up to 10%), β-myrcene (1–2%), camphor (0%-traces); antiviral and antimicrobial; said to be an immunostimulant, often indicated for flu and asthma; constituents also suggest analgesic, anti-inflammatory and expectorant qualities; possible synergy with saro.

Red spruce (*P. rubens* needles and twigs, cones, Pinaceae family); in comparison with black spruce, the essential oil has a lighter, fresher coniferous aroma, with underlying citrus rather than green notes; contains 15–17% bornyl acetate, α-pinene (15–16%), camphene (13%), β-pinene (12%) and *d*-limonene (12%) with δ-3-carene, β-myrcene and β-phellandrene (<5%); this profile of constituents is similar to that of hemlock and black spruce, but bornyl acetate does not dominate; it would be reasonable to suggest that red spruce has analgesic and anti-inflammatory actions. It could also be used in conjunction with these bornyl acetate-rich oils.

Rosalina (*Melaleuca ericifolia* leaves and twigs, Myrtaceae family): the essential oil has a soft, pine-like, earthy odour and is dominated by monoterpenoids, but the composition is highly variable and dependent on the geographical source: type 1 oils from the northern coastal regions of Australia are linalool-rich and cineole-poor; type 2 oils from the far south coastal areas are cineole-rich and linalool-poor. Typical constituents are linalool (35–55%), 1,8-cineole (15–25%), with α-pinene, *d*- and *l*-aromadendrene, *d*-limonene, γ-terpinene, α-terpineol, terpinen-4-ol and *para*-cymene; this profile would suggest anti-nociceptive, pain-relieving, anti-inflammatory, antimicrobial and expectorant properties; aromadendrene and *d*-limonene have cancer-suppressing actions.

Rosewood (*Aniba rosaeodora* wood, Lauraceae family): the essential oil has a soft, mild, sweet woody odour, with rosy notes; a racemic mix of *d*- and *l*-linalool dominates (85%), with α-terpineol (3–5%) and *cis*- and *trans*-linalool oxide (3%); based on these constituents it should have anti-nociceptive, anti-inflammatory, anti-oxidant, antimicrobial and anxiolytic actions.

Sardinian sage (*Salvia desoleana* leaves, Lamiaceae family): the main constituents are linalyl acetate, α-terpinyl acetate, *l*-linalool and 1,8-cineole; this would place the Sardinian sage in Group II, and with low toxicity; strong antifungal activity, active against most dermatophytes; may be of value for immunocompromised individuals. This species is indigenous to Sardinia, where it is used in folk medicine to treat menstrual, central nervous system and digestive disorders, much like the traditional uses of other sage species; limited availability, but very good aromatherapeutic potential.

Saro (*Cinnamomosma fragrans* leaves, Canallaceae family): the essential oil has a clean, fresh, penetrating, medicinal aroma that is reminiscent of eucalyptus, ravintsara and tea tree; constituents include 1,8-cineole (45–55%), α- and β-pinene (10–16%), terpinen-4-ol, α-terpineol, *d*-limonene, *l*-linalol and others; the constituent profile suggests analgesic, anti-inflammatory and expectorant properties; reputed to be an immunostimulant.

Silver birch bud (*Betula pendula* buds, Betulaceae family): used in traditional medicine for urinary tract disorders, skin diseases, infections and inflammation, and as a flavouring for food and both alcoholic and non-alcoholic beverages; the essential oil is rare, but has a pleasant fragrance and therapeutic potential; the main components are α-copaene, germacrene D (11–18%) and δ-cadinene (11–15%).

Somalian sage, wild (*Salvia somalensis* leaves, Lamiaceae family): the essential oil has a pleasant herbal, resinous aroma; characterised by bornyl aceate and an absence of α- and β-thujone; anti-inflammatory, anti-oxidant; no known hazards; can be used to combat oxidative stress in the skin, therefore may be useful in anti-ageing formulae; limited availability at time of writing, but has good aromatherapeutic potential.

Spanish marjoram (*Thymus mastichina* flowering herb, Lamiaceae family): the essential oil is dominated by 1,8-cineole (45–60%), with camphor (up to 10%), and α- and β-pinene, camphene, borneol, α-terpineol, *l*-linalol, sabinene, terpinen-4-ol, and others; this is suggestive of pain-relieving, anti-inflammatory and antimicrobial actions, and perhaps an affinity with the respiratory system; cautions apply because of the 1,8-cineole content (children) and the camphor content (neurotoxicity – however check level with supplier).

Spanish oreganum (*Thymus capitatus*, flowering herb, Lamiaceae family): the essential oil often contains very high levels of carvacrol (70–85%); check composition with supplier. Anti-oxidant and anti-hypertensive actions; cautions apply; in blending, the phenol rule applies.

Spanish sage or lavender-leaved sage (*Salvia lavandulaefolia*, flowering herb, Lamiaceae family): camphor can be present at 11–36%, with 1,8-cineole from 10 to 30% and traces of thujones; however, it also contains *cis*-sabinyl acetate, which has abortifacient actions. The essential oil can increase alertness, but not necessarily enhance cognitive functioning or memory. Contraindicated in pregnancy and breastfeeding; camphor content (check with supplier) carries risk of neurotoxicity; cautions apply; suggested maximum dermal limit is high, at 12.5%, based on camphor content.

Spanish thyme (*Thymus zygis*, flowering herb, Lamiaceae family): thymol, carvacrol, thymol/carvacrol and linalool chemotypes are available – it is suggested that the linalool chemotype is used; *l*-linalool (70–80%), linalyl acetate (up to 9%), low levels of thymol (up to 4%) and carvacrol (1%), with α-terpineol, borneol, *para*-cymene, β-caryoplyllene, β-myrcene, camphene; pain-relieving and anti-inflammatory actions.

Spearmint (*Mentha spicatum*, *M. viridis*, *M. crispa* aerial parts, Lamiaceae family): the essential oil has a sweet, warm, minty, green aroma with herbaceous notes; dominated by *l*-carvone (55–68%), with *l*-limonene (9–14%), β-myrcene (up to 5%), and others including *cis*-dihydrocarvone, 1,8-cineole and menthone;

anti-nociceptive, antispasmodic, decongestant and mucolytic. The essential oil has an affinity with the digestive system (spasm) and the respiratory system; often described as 'cooling'.

Spike lavender (*Lavandula latifolia*, *L. spica* subsp. *fragrans*, flowering tops, Lamiaceae family): the essential oil is lavender-like and penetrating, but camphoraceous and lacking the soft, fruity nuances of true lavender; dominated by *l*-linalool (28–44%) with 1,8-cineole (up to 35%) and camphor (up to 23%) and others including borneol, α- and β-pinenes, β-caryophyllene. Linalyl acetate is absent, and thus the oil does not have anxiolytic action; the constituent profile suggests pain-relieving, anti-inflammatory and expectorant actions; caution due to camphor content (check with supplier).

Spikenard (*Nardostachys jatamansi* rhizomes, Valerianaceae family): the essential oil has a pungent, earthy, valerian-like odour; the top note is sweet, woody and spicy, the body is heavy, animalic, woody and spicy, and the dryout is woody and spicy. Widely differing reports of constituents: Lawless (1992) includes bornyl acetate, *iso*-bornyl valerianate, borneol, patchouli alcohol, terpinyl valerianate, α-terpineol, eugenol and pinenes; Tisserand and Young (2014) cite Mahalwal and Ali (2002), who found that the principal component was nardol (10.1%) and an isomer, with formic acid, α-selinene and an isomer, dihydro-β-ionone, propionic acid, β-caryophyllene, and others at less than 3%. The oil, when inhaled, has sedative effects, and anticonvulsant actions have been noted. Its pungent, aromatic rhizomes have been used since early times, when it was known as 'the root of nard', or sometimes locally as 'muskroot'; in India it was widely used as incense, and the smoke was believed to drive away evil; in Ayurvedic medicine spikenard is used to balance all three doshas, and promote awareness and strength of mind; in ancient Rome it was an important perfume ingredient, used in several formulations such as *Foliatum* and *Natron*, both of which were also used to encourage hair growth, and *Regalium*, the 'Royal Unguent'.

Star anise (*Illicium verum* dried fruits, Illiciaceae family): the essential oil has a sweet, anisic aroma, warm, spicy and reminiscent of liquorice; *trans*-anethole (70–90%), *l*-limonene (up to 5%), methyl chavicol (trace–6.5%); similar in actions to sweet fennel; cautions apply.

Sweet birch (*Betula lenta* bark, Betulaceae family): the essential oil has a sweet, woody, wintergreen-like odour; contains methyl salicylate at around 90%; it is an anti-inflammatory that can be used in very low doses on intact skin. Methyl salicylate can inhibit blood clotting and interfere with some medications, so use with caution; avoid in pregnancy.

Szechuan pepper (*Zanthoxylum piperitum* dried fruits, Rutaceae family): the essential oil has a fresh, vibrant, citrus (lemon) aroma, with a warm, spicy aspect and green notes; dominated by *d*-limonene (around 40–45%) and has a significant β-myrcene content; this suggests analgesic activity, with no hazards other than potential sensitisation if an oxidised product is used; it has established anti-oxidant activity, suggesting use in phytocosmeceuticals, and prokinetic actions that would indicate it for gut dysfunction.

Tachibana (*Citrus tachibana* peel, Rutaceae family): related to mandarin and associated with Japan, where it is cultivated at shrines and is used as a motif at New Year or coming of age celebrations; the essential oil has a sweet, green, citrus, 'juicy' aroma; it is dominated by *d*-limonene and also contains linalool.

Tarragon, estragon (*Artemisia dracunculus* leaves, Asteraceae family): the essential oil has a sweet, anisic, spicy-green, basil-like odour; dominated by methyl chavicol (75–87%), with *cis*- and *trans*-β-ocimene, *d*-limonene, α-pinene and traces of methyl eugenol; similar in composition to exotic basil, and the same cautions apply; tarragon has anticonvulsant and antiplatelet activity.

Tea tree (*Melaleuca alternifolia* leaves, Myrtaceae family): the essential oil has a very distinctive odour, spicy and aromatic, with cardamom, nutmeg and sweet marjoram-like notes; more suited to local applications and inhalation rather than in massage; the 'ISO standard type' composition is terpinen-4-ol (30–48%), γ-terpinene (10–28%), 1,8-cineole (traces–15%), α-terpinene (5–13%), *para*-cymene (0.5–8%), α-pinene (1–6%), with terpinolene, sabinene, *d*-aromadendrene, δ-cadinene, *d*-limonene, globulol and viridifloral all at less than 5%; anti-nociceptive, analgesic (peripheral), anti-inflammatory, anti-allergic (reduces histamines, cytokines), anti-oxidant, LDL anti-oxidant, anti-cancer, wide spectrum antimicrobial actions (some *Pseudomonas* species may be resistant), antiviral potential, antispasmodic, bronchodilator; indicated for infection control, oropharyngeal candidiasis, allergic responses, respiratory infections, bronchial spasm, pain and inflammation; potential synergy with lavender for dermatophyte infection; potential synergy between terpinen-4-ol in tea tree and eugenol in clove bud.

Texas cedarwood (*Juniperus ashei* wood, Cupressaceae family): the rectified essential oil has a sweet, woody, balsamic aroma; dominated by thujopsene (up to 45%), α-cedrene (up to 30%) and cedrol (up to 20%); it is without hazard, and given its similarities with Virginian cedarwood, will possibly share its actions.

Tobacco (*Nicotiana tabacum*, semi-dried, cured leaves, Solanaceae family): tobacco absolute has an intense, rich, warm, mellow tobacco odour; it must be used in dilution, and there may be solubility problems in oily bases. It can be used for relaxation and stress relief, and blends very well with vanilla, heavy or indolic florals such as tuberose and honeysuckle, also guaiacwood, sandalwood and patchouli.

Tuberose (*Polianthus tuberosa* flowers, Agavaceae family): the absolute has a heavy, honey-like, sweet-caramel, floral aroma, with a slight camphor-like note; very complex composition, including *trans*-methyl isoeugenol (32%), methyl salicylate

(8%) and other esters such as methyl benzoate, methyl anthranilate, benzyl benzoate, also nerol, *trans-trans*-farnesol, geraniol, benzyl alcohol, isoeugenol, tuberone and traces of indole. The heavy, heady scent of tuberose is said to have narcotic properties; it is used to promote relaxation and sleep. Across the world it is one of the most important flowers in garlands; in Hawaii it is used in leis, and in India it is very important in culture and used at wedding ceremonies, traditional rituals, in garlands and decorations; in India all of its names refer to its fragrance, such as the Bengali name *rajoni-ghanda*, meaning 'scent of the world'.

Valerian (*Valeriana officinalis* roots, Valerianaceae family): the essential oil has a warm, earthy, green-woody, balsamic odour; contains bornyl acetate (up to 35%), valerianol (up to 34%), and related valeranone and valeranal, with numerous others including camphene, *d*-limonene, α-pinene, borneol, β-caryophyllene, patchouli alcohol. Possible anti-inflammatory action; does not stimulate sympathetic activity; the constituent profile may also suggest an affinity with the respiratory system and wound-healing actions; the herb is widely used as a sedative and soporific agent; has sedative effects when used in combination with lemon balm; for soporific effects also consider combining with hops, vetiver, lavender, patchouli, spikenard.

Vanilla (*Vanilla planifolia* cured vanilla pods, Orchidaceae family): the absolute has a strong vanillic, balsamic, sweet, rich and warm scent with notes of wood and tobacco; the Bourbon type is considered to be the best from the aroma perspective. Complex composition is variable; vanillin (85%), other constituents include hydroxybenzaldehyde (8–9%), acetic acid, *iso*-butyric acid, caproic acid, eugenol and furfural. Vanilla has therapeutic uses – medicinal preparations are said to be tonic, cephalic, diuretic, decongestant; a blood purifier, a digestive aid, and stimulant of childbirth; the scent is also therapeutic; can be used for relaxation and stress relief.

Violet leaf (*Viola odorata* leaves, Violaceae family): the absolute has an intense green, diffusive odour, with leafy (crushed green leaves), peppery, floral/violet, woody and earthy notes; the scent is best experienced in high dilution. A very complex composition, constituents include 2-*trans*-6-*cis*-nonadien-1-al (up to 20%) and 9,12-octadecadienoic acid. Violet leaf absolute can inhibit HLE; may have applications on sun-damaged skin, and as an anti-ageing absolute. Its intense green note is difficult to work with, but it can be used in trace amounts with rose, ylang ylang, osmanthus, mimosa, linden blossom, tagetes, blackcurrant bud, clary sage absolute and lavender absolute; often recommended for those who have been traumatised and need to 'let go'.

Virginian cedarwood (*Juniperus virginiana* wood, Cupressaceae family): the essential oil has a mild, dry, light, fresh woody aroma, reminiscent of pencil shavings, with oily, resinous, balsamic and earthy notes; α-cedrene (20–40%), thujopsene (20–25%), cedrol (12–24%), β-cedrene (8–10%), and others. Anti-inflammatory, wound-healing; often recommended in blends for arthritis, bronchitis, respiratory congestion. Blends well with cypress, lavender, geranium, immortelle, sweet marjoram, rosemary, juniperberry, hemp, patchouli, sandalwood, rose, poplar bud; possible synergy with lavender for the treatment of bacterial (respiratory) infections and thrush; consider also Texas cedarwood, which is very similar.

West Indian bay (*Pimenta racemosa* leaves, Myrtaceae family): contains up to 56% eugenol, and many other constituents which are associated with pain-relieving and anti-inflammatory actions (such as β-myrcene at up to 25%). This could also be considered as an alternative to holy basil for musculoskeletal system applications, but it too merits caution as it also contains small amounts of methyl eugenol.

White spruce (*P. alba*, *P. glauca*, needles, twigs, cones, Pinaceae family): the essential oil is dominated by β-pinene (23.0%) and α-pinene (17%), with bornyl acetate (14%) and *d*-limonene (13%); it does not have an aromatherapeutic tradition of use, and research concerning its actions was not found; it could be reasonably expected that it will share the properties of red and black spruce oils; it is said to have a liberating effect on the senses; Holmes (2001) describes white spruce as having a 'delicious salty undertow that drifts you away to the open sea...' (p.34).

Wild thyme (*Thymus serpyllum*, flowering herb, Lamiaceae family): two chemotypes are produced – limonene (*d*-limonene (24%), with thymol (28%) and carvacrol (20%)); and the more common thymol/carvacrol (carvacrol (26%), thymol (26%), with γ-terpinene, β-caryophyllene, *para*-cymene, and many others). Antimicrobial, analgesic, anti-inflammatory; cautions apply (drug interactions, blood clotting, bleeding disorders); dermal limit 1%; 'phenol rule' applies.

Wintergreen (*Gaultheria procumbens* leaves, pre-treated by warm aqueous maceration, Ericaceae family): the essential oil has a very strong, intense, sweet, penetrating, medicinal, wintergreen odour, with woody and fruity notes; dominated by methyl salicylate (99%). Anti-inflammatory; traditionally used in liniments for pain relief, and for treating arthritis; must be used with caution and in very low doses; contraindicated with anticoagulant medication and bleeding disorders.

Yarrow (*Achillea millefolium* dried aerial parts, Asteraceae family): the essential oil has a green, herbaceous scent with woody and camphoraceous notes; composition is variable and several chemotypes exist (it is recommended that the camphor chemotype is avoided); the chamazulene chemotype is dominated by sabinene (25–26%), chamazulene (up to 20%), with many others including β-myrcene, α- and β-pinene, germacrene D, β-caryophyllene, camphene, β-phellandrene, camphor, borneol, bornyl acetate, 1,8-cineole and others. The composition suggests anti-inflammatory, pain-relieving and antifungal actions, perhaps an affinity with the respiratory system.

AFTERWORD

This book is peppered with questions designed to aid reflection and stimulate discussion. These are all questions that I have asked myself over the years, and I have found that the responses change as my experience and understanding develops; this is to be expected as time progresses, and as we continue to flourish both personally and professionally. Sometimes we meet individuals who help us look at things in different ways – we might embrace this, or resist it. Some ideas will resonate with us, whilst others will meet with resistance. Some practitioners will inspire us, and others will not really make a difference! Always, we need to ask why? Reflection is very important indeed. So, rather than write a formal conclusion to this book, it feels better to end with some personal reflection. You might agree with some of this, or you might not – either way, I would welcome your comments and insights, which can reach me via the publisher, Singing Dragon.

WHAT CAN WE LEARN FROM THIS EXPLORATION?

I learned that:

* Much, but not all, of our traditional understanding of essential oil actions can be supported by contemporary research.

* There are many oils which have enormous aromatherapeutic potential that have yet to become part of 'mainstream' practice – and I have had the real pleasure of featuring them in this book.

* Scientific research still tends to focus on 'active constituents', sometimes at the expense of the whole essential oil. However, change is in the air – de Mendonça Rocha *et al.* (2012) made the following comment that is very relevant to aromatherapy:

> The inherent activity of an oil may be related to its chemical composition, the proportions of the components and the interactions between them. Some studies have concluded that the oils as a whole have much greater [antibacterial] activity than a mixture of the major components, which suggests that minor components are critical for this activity and may have a synergistic or potentiating influence. (p.12024)

This is very encouraging; indeed, it completely supports our argument for synergistic blending.

HOW HAS IT CHANGED ME –
PERSONALLY AND PROFESSIONALLY?

Writing this book has changed me at a deeply personal level:

* Many, many laboratory animals, mostly rodents, have suffered, and continue to suffer in experiments. The published papers all carry the statement that strict welfare standards were adhered to in the research; and I do not doubt this. However, using animals for experimentation is not acceptable to me, because I do not believe that we have any right to cause suffering and death in sentient beings. This is just my own, personal opinion; you may hold a different view. Now, I am doing what I can to raise awareness of animal-free research methodologies, and support organisations that advocate the ethical and compassionate treatment of animals (see 'Resources'). The process of conducting the literature search for this book has certainly fuelled my desire to make a difference in this respect. Yes, I have changed – from a vegetarian to a vegan lifestyle.

* I have formed relationships with oils that are not often used in aromatherapy practice, from the agrestic and lively hops, to the deeply smoky nagarmotha – which is the closest I can get to the profound effect that burning agarwood had on me at Alec Lawless' artisan perfumery course in 2012. Many of these unusual oils have traditional uses that are backed up by contemporary research, and they deserve a place in our practice – I do hope that you will explore these, and let your fellow therapists know of your experiences.

* I have not been in practice for several years now, and so my current experience of essential oils is mostly via olfaction and meditation, and as a recipient of aromatherapy. It is tempting to think that their main benefits will be on my psyche, and indeed I do benefit from them on a virtually daily basis – when I write, there is inevitably a neat row of aromatics on blotters for sniffing and sometimes inhaling. (Today it is Szechuan pepper that is talking to me.) I cannot imagine living or working without them, my fragrant friends. However, as I research and read, it becomes clear that even 'just' inhalation can make profound and beneficial changes at a very 'physical' level. We might not yet realise it, but some of these volatile aromatics could well be part of future preventative medical practices, and the full implications of metabonomics studies have yet to be explored.

* I have become acutely and embarrassingly aware of personal preferences and bias in terms of the scents of essential oils. Try as I might, I find it hard to work with German chamomile, and also the medicinal aromas of, for example, tea tree and the cineole-rich eucalypts. It is not that I dislike these aromas *per se* – I just find it hard to incorporate them in blends! Give me the spicy fenugreek or sensual patchouli any day! If you too have a particular negative bias (and it would be most unusual if you loved all scents equally),

I think it is best to acknowledge the situation, and use these oils when the situation cries out for them, perhaps 'solo' or in very simple blends, rather than trying to make them something they are not, under the influence of other oils!

THE PRESENCE OF THE PAST

I would like to conclude with just one more thought. Aromatic plants have been around for thousands of years. Their scents are unchanging; when we smell a lily or a rose, or saffron or cloves, we are having the same olfactory experience that our distant ancestors would have had. Fragrance is a paradox – a transient but permanent link with the past; indeed, it brings the past into the present moment. It is hugely evocative; it carries its messages across millennia. We should remain aware of the wisdom of our predecessors, and harness their knowledge into our aromatherapy practice wherever possible.

We live in exciting and enlightening times; the future of aromatherapy is very bright indeed if we embrace traditional aromatic knowledge in the light of contemporary understanding.

It has been such a privilege and a pleasure. Thank you.

GLOSSARY

Adrenergic system and noradrenergic system: the neurotransmitters adrenalin and noradrenalin are responsible for the 'fight or flight' response. Cyclic AMP (cyclic adenosine monophosphate) is used as a messenger. The receptors are α receptors, which mediate excitation – for example, in vascular smooth muscle – and β receptors, which mediate relaxation (except in the heart). So we have a sympathetic nervous system response – an 'accelerator' for fight and flight; and a parasympathetic response – a 'brake' for rest and relaxation. Adrenalin and noradrenalin belong to the monoamine group of neurotransmitters.

Agonist: a substance that behaves like another substance, thus stimulating an action; for example, when a substance binds to a receptor and elicits a response.

ar- (prefix): *ar-* denotes 'aromatic', that is, a phenyl ring is present in the molecular structure – for example, *ar*-turmerone is 2-methyl-6-(4-methylphenyl)-2-hepten-4-one, a benzenoid sesquiterpenoid alkene ketone (Tisserand and Young 2014, p.644).

Chirality: or 'handedness'; refers to the configuration of an optically active molecule; some molecules exist as 'mirror images' of each other, or symmetrical opposites.

Cholinergic system: cholinergic systems stimulate the production of acetylcholine, a molecule which is released at the neuromuscular junction and causes contraction, but it has a wider role as a stimulant of the autonomic nervous system, as a vasodilator and cardiac depressant. Cholinergic receptors in the cortex of the brain are implicated in cognitive functioning; modulation of the cholinergic system is thought to be beneficial in cognitive functioning.

Cosmeceuticals: cosmetic, personal skin care products such as moisturisers that contain biologically active ingredients which offer clinical benefits, including the prevention of UV damage, reducing free radical formation, improving the skin lipid barrier, improving skin tone and appearance, improving texture and reducing pore size.

Dopaminergic system: dopamine is a neurotransmitter that belongs to the monoamine group; dopaminergic systems act via dopamine. It is associated with reward-motivated behaviour, and some disorders such as Parkinson's disease and schizophrenia are noted for their altered levels of dopamine. Outside of the nervous system, dopamine acts as a vasodilator and a diuretic, and it can reduce gut motility and decrease the activity of lymphocytes (amongst other activities).

Downregulation and upregulation: *upregulation* is an increase in response to a stimulus, resulting in an increase of a cellular component; for example, the increase in cellular response to a molecular stimulus as a result of the increase in the number of receptors on the cell surface. *Downregulation* is where the cellular receptors decrease, in response to, for example, receptor agonists, and the cell becomes less responsive to a molecular stimulus.

GABA (gamma-aminobutyric acid): fast signalling inhibition – an 'off switch'. Drugs such as benzodiazepines work by affecting GABA – they enhance GABAergic function and produce anxiolysis.

GABAergic system: gamma-aminobutyric acid (GABA) is the main inhibitory neurotransmitter in the central nervous system; some substances, including essential oils and their components, can modulate GABAergic transmission.

Glutamate: an amino acid, a neurotransmitter with many physiological functions; fast signalling and excitation; glutamate receptors (AMPA, kainate, NMDA) are found in the brain and neurons and glia in the spinal cord. Glutamate uptake is decreased in Alzheimer's disease.

Glutamergic system: receptors are found in both the central and the peripheral nervous system and they mediate most of the excitatory neurotransmissions. Some essential oil constituents such as *l*-linalool modulate glutamergic neurotransmission, possibly via NDMA receptor interactions. Dysfunction in the system has profound effects, such as mood disorders.

Glycation: the binding of sugars such as fructose and glucose with proteins or lipids, leading to the formation of advanced glycation end products (AGEs), which, in the presence of free radicals, are involved in further cross-linking with proteins. This causes hardening of the tissue (e.g. cardiovascular structures and also collagen in the skin). AGEs are implicated in many diseases such as cancers, cardiovascular disease, Alzheimer's and peripheral neuropathy, and of course textural changes in the skin – loss of elasticity because of hardened collagen. Causes of glycation can be exogenous – for example, where sugars are cooked with fats at high temperatures, forming carcinogenic and inflammatory acrylamides, and then consumed – or endogenous, where, if there is a high blood sugar level, absorbed simple sugars form AGEs. To reduce the risk of glycation it is recommended that, for example, barbecued and fatty/sugary foods that have been cooked at high temperatures, and also excess sugar in the diet are avoided.

Hedonic mechanism: where the effects of an odour depend on the subject's state of pleasure or displeasure with that odour.

Indolic: indole is a cyclic imine – a nitrogen-containing molecule – and is a trace constituent in the volatile oil of some white flowers. It is very important in their aroma, but in higher concentration it is highly unpleasant and can be perceived as the odour of putrefaction; but trace amounts can impart a jasmine-like effect. Jasmine, sambac, gardenia (very scarce), honeysuckle (very scarce), white champaca, orange blossom, white ginger lily and tuberose are all examples of indolic scents.

Isomer: An isomer is one of two or more compounds where the molecular formula is identical, but the atoms are arranged differently – for example, α- and β-pinenes are identical apart from the position of a double bond; γ-terpinene is isomeric with α- and β-terpinenes. *Cis-* and *trans*-isomerism is a type of geometrical isomerism; *cis*-isomers have groups of similar atoms on one side of a double bond, *trans*-isomers have the same groups of atoms on the opposite side of a double bond. An example is geraniol (*cis-*) and nerol (*trans-*). Optical isomerism describes the situation where the molecule of one form is the mirror image of the other form – for example, *d*- and *l*-limonene and *d*- and *l*-carvone.

Metabonomics: the study of the metabolic responses elicited by, for example, exposure to the aerial diffusion of essential oils; specifically the changes in metabolic markers such as carbohydrates, neurotransmitters, amino acids and fatty acids in tissues and body fluids.

Monoamine oxidase: abbreviated to MAO, an enzyme that breaks down the neurotransmitters serotonin, dopamine, adrenalin and noradrenalin (and others). Some essential oils and their components (such as myristicin and eugenol) are thought to inhibit MAO, hence their antidepressant actions.

Monoaminergic systems: these include the serotoninergic, noradrenergic and dopaminergic systems of the brain and CNS – monoamines effectively reduce the availability and uptake of serotonin and noradrenalin.

Nitrergic system: neuronal nitric oxide synthase has a role in non-synaptic interneuronal communications; it is a messenger and neurotoxicant.

NMDA: N-methyl-D-aspartate; NMDA antagonists have antidepressant properties.

Noradrenergic system and adrenergic system: see **Adrenergic system and noradrenergic system**.

Opioid system: receptors are found in the brain and spinal cord, and in the digestive system. Morphine is an agonist, so can block pain; naloxone is an antagonist that reverses the effects of morphine overdose. The opioid system can affect body weight; binge eating (which is an evolutionary trait) releases endorphins.

Phenol rule: devised by Guba (2000), the 'phenol rule' applies up to a 10% concentration, and relates to dermal use only; the ratio of phenolic oils to non-irritant oils should not exceed 1:9, and the total concentration of phenolic oils should not exceed 1% of the blend. The exception is when cinnamon bark (*Cinnamomum zeylanicum*) or cassia (*C. cassia* or *C. aromaticum*), both rich in cinnamaldehyde, are to be used – then the concentration should not exceed 5%, *and* they can be used in conjunction with oils such as clove bud that have a high eugenol content, or oils with a high *d*-limonene content. This is because eugenol and *d*-limonene can quench the sensitising potential of cinnamaldehyde (Guin *et al.* 1984).

Phenylethanol: 2-phenylethyl alcohol is the main commercial alcohol apart from ethyl alcohol, and the most used fragrance ingredient in the perfumes and cosmetics industry. It is a minor constituent in narcissus, hyacinth, geranium Bourbon, and *Alep* pine, rose and jasmine flowers; up to 60% in rose absolute, and 35% in golden champaca. It has a sweet, honey, rose-like aroma.

Placebo/expectation mechanism: if an individual is told that a certain odour will have a specific effect, and this becomes a belief, then the chances are that the odour will indeed elicit the expected effect.

Prostaglandins: lipids with hormone-like effects; they have a wide-ranging role in physiology, including the contraction and relaxation of smooth muscle; they are also produced at sites of injury.

Semantic mechanism: we usually experience smells in the context of life situations, and smells, memory and associations quickly and irreversibly become linked. Each odour thus carries an emotional memory, the impact of which can lead to physiological changes, such as an increase in heart rate or blood adrenalin.

Serotonin: also known as 5-hydroxytrypyamine (5-HT), serotonin is derived from *l*-tryptophan, and is found in the brain and also the gut, where it is involved in the regulation of intestinal movements; in the brain, serotonin modifies mood and contributes to feelings of wellbeing.

Upregulation: see **Downregulation and upregulation**.

APPENDIX

FIXED PLANT AND MACERATED HERBAL OILS IN AROMATHERAPY

Carrier oil	Characteristics and properties
Almond (*Prunus amygdalus* var. *dulcis*)	Fairly thick, not rapidly absorbed. Moisturising and emollient; soothing, antipruritic.
Aloe (*Aloe barbadensis, A. capensis, A. vera*)	Although not a fixed oil, aloe is becoming increasingly popular as a carrier medium for essential oils. It is used in traditional medicine for skin disorders and infections (including *Staphylococcus aureus* and various dermatophytes); it is virucidal and used to treat *herpes simplex*. It is a COX inhibitor; increases collagen biosynthesis and degradation in granulation tissue; and is topically applied for radiation-induced dermatitis and ulcers, frostbite, burns, infections and cold sores, pruritis, pain, psoriasis and contact dermatitis. It is contraindicated in pregnancy and lactation (Thornfeldt 2005).
Apricot kernel (*Prunus armeniaca*)	Light texture, readily absorbed. For dry and sensitive skins, emollient and antipruritic.
Argan kernel (*Argania spinosa*)	Pleasant, rapidly absorbed oil that is useful for skin with pimples, juvenile acne, scarring, and can help reduce appearance of wrinkes and alleviate dry skin conditions; contains Vitamin E (anti-oxidant), sterols, fatty acids (principally oleic and linoleic) and triacylglycerols (Charrouf and Guillaume 2008).
Avocado (*Persea gratissima*)	Fairly thick; good skin penetration and feel. Promotes cell regeneration; can increase skin hydration, indicated for sun damage, inflammation, ageing skin.
Black caraway (or cumin) seed (*Nigella sativa*)	Anti-oxidant – add to other carriers to enhance stability and offer protection against free radical damage.
Blackcurrant seed (*Ribes nigrum*)	Contains gamma-linolenic acid (11–17%), and is a good source of essential fatty acids, tocopherols and phytosterols (Bakowska, Schieber and Kolodziejczyk 2009).
Borage seed (*Borago officinalis*)	Use at up to 10% with other carriers. Soothing, moisturising, regenerating and firming.
Camellia (*Camellia sinensis*)	Light texture, readily absorbed, good slippage for massage. Skin restructuring and moisturising properties, helps reduce appearance of scars, or prevent scarring. *Camellia sinensis* has 5α-reductase inhibitory and anti-inflammatory actions (Azimi *et al.* 2012).

Coconut (*Cocos nucifera*)	Several products are available, including fractionated, and light. The unrefined product is solid at cool temperatures, gives good lubrication and leaves a slightly greasy film on the skin. The fractionated product is a slightly viscous liquid and has skin-softening properties. Unrefined product has skin- and hair-coating properties; soothing, moisturising.
Comfrey (*Symphytum officinale*)	Anti-inflammatory, traditionally used for breaks and sprains. Oral consumption can be fatal (it contains hepatotoxic pyrriolizidine alkaloids); it is carcinogenic and contraindicated in pregnancy (Thornfeldt 2005). Extracts of comfrey root, and allantoin, have anti-inflammatory, antioxidant and soothing keratolytic actions, and can induce epidermal cell proliferation; topical comfrey-based products are used to treat wounds, ulcers, burns, dermatitis, psoriasis, impetigo and acne (Thornfeldt 2005).
Cranberry seed (*Vaccinium macrocarpon*)	Contains around 22% α-linolenic acid, an anti-oxidant that can be added to other carriers to enhance stability and offer protection against free radical damage. May have anti-inflammatory properties.
Evening primrose (*Oenothera biennis*)	Unsuitable as a lubricant on its own, but useful in combination with other carriers at up to 20%. Treatment of eczema and psoriasis. Useful on dry, scaly skin. May improve skin elasticity and accelerate healing.
Gotu kola (*Centella asiatica*)	Dermatitis and the healing of superficial wounds – surgical wounds and burns. It may improve circulation. Stimulates skin regeneration and helps with loss of elasticity.
Grapeseed (*Vitis vinifera*)	Good slippage. Prevents moisture loss, emollient. Grapeseed extract has anti-oxidant, anti-inflammatory and antimicrobial actions, and it can reduce induced pigmentation (Fowler *et al.* 2010). It contains anti-oxidant proanthocyanidins, flavonoids, querticin glucosides, stilbebes, tocopherols, essential fatty acids. Topical application can improve cutaneous photoprotection to UVB, inhibit histamine synthesis, promote wound healing and reduce vascular engorgement (Thornfeldt 2005).
Hazelnut (*Corylus americana*)	Good lubricant, very good penetration and skin feel. Nourishing to the skin, slightly astringent, stimulates circulation. Emollient, restructuring properties and also prevents dehydration. Potential sun filter.
Hemp seed (*Cannabis sativa*)	Contains around 19% α-linolenic acid, an anti-oxidant oil that can be added to other carriers to enhance stability and offer protection against free radical damage. Also contains γ-linolenic acid, which contributes to its good skin feel and ease of absorption. Indicated for dry skin conditions and eczema. Anti-inflammatory and analgesic.
Holy basil (*Ocimum sanctum*) seed	Anti-inflammatory (α-linolenic acid).

Jojoba (*Simmondsia chinensis*)	Very compatible with the skin, temperature-sensitive (wax when cold) and good slippage/skin feel. Protective, anti-inflammatory, treatment for eczema, dandruff, sun damage and acne. In aromatherapy, used on both dry and oily skins (sebum control).
Kukui nut (*Aleurite moluccans*)	Very well absorbed and excellent skin feel. Possibly one of the most useful carriers. Treatment of superficial skin injuries and burns, slows down moisture loss, emollient (treatment of psoriasis and eczema). Antipruritic. Also used in cancer care (radiation treatment). Possibly anti-ageing.
Lime (linden) blossom (*Tilia cordata*) infused oil	Emollient and antipruritic; used for wrinkles.
Linseed (*Linum usitatissimum*)	Anti-inflammatory (α-linolenic acid).
Lucuma nut (*Pouteria lucuma*)	Regenerating; wound-healing potential. Major components include linolenic acid, oleic acid, palmitic acid, steraric acid and γ-linolenic acids; the oil decreases nitric oxide production, promotes tissue regeneration and significantly accelerates cutaneous wound closure (Rojo *et al.* 2010).
Macadamia nut (*Macadamia integrifolia*)	Good penetration and slippage. Nourishing, moisturising and restructuring. Useful on mature skin.
Marigold (*Calendula officinalis*) macerated oil	Anti-inflammatory and vulnerary. Can be used for broken capillaries, varicose veins, bruises and eczema. Antibacterial activity; could be useful for skin infections.
Olive (*Olea europaea*)	Heavy and sticky, pronounced odour. Soothing, anti-inflammatory and emollient – used on burns, sprains, bruises, dermatitis and insect bites.
Passion flower seed (*Passiflora incarnata*)	Light texture, readily absorbed, not greasy. Moisturising and emollient. Passion flower oil is used in treatment of burns; anti-inflammatory. Said to be relaxing.
Peach kernel (*Prunus persica*)	Light texture, but more body than apricot kernel oil. Moisturising, emollient and antipruritic; used for skin protection, regeneration, anti-ageing and antipruritic.
Rosehip seed oil (*Rosa canina*)	Too rich for massage, but good in combination at 10–50%. Skin regeneration – used on scarring. May also help burns, wounds and eczema heal. Tissue regeneration – also improves skin texture and discolouration. Useful on wrinkles. Very effective in combination with gotu kola (*Centella asiatica*) (Kusmirek 2002). Has potential in the management of eczema, trophic ulcers and neurodermatitis (Chrubasik *et al.* 2008).
Safflower (*Carthamus tinctorius*)	Inexpensive and light, but poor keeping qualities. Emollient, moisturising.

Sesame seed (*Sesame indicum*)	Sticky skin feel – however, suitable in combinations at up to 20%. Skin restructuring, moisturising and emollient. Improves resilience and skin integrity. Free radical scavenger.
St John's Wort (*Hypericum perforatum*) macerated oil	In Turkish traditional medicine an olive oil extract of the flowering aerial parts is used to heal wounds, cuts and burns. It is anti-inflammatory, and useful if nerve pain e.g. sciatica, neuralgia, is present; also has notable wound-healing activity. (Phototoxic – avoid direct sunlight.)
Sunflower seed (*Helianthus annuus*)	Sticky skin feel but reasonable slippage. Emollient and moisturising.
Tamanu (*Calophylum inophyllum*)	Thick and sticky with strong odour, so not very suitable for massage unless in combination. Healing and protective; analgesic, anti-inflammatory and cicatrisant. Increases local blood circulation. Not suitable for massage but topical applications are very effective – especially for relieving the pain of shingles (50:50 tamanu with ravintsara). Tamanu stimulates phagocytosis (Schnaubelt 1999).
Walnut (*Juglans regia*)	Excellent, medium weight, good texture and skin feel for massage, fairly slow rate of absorption. Highly emollient, reduces moisture loss; regenerative and anti-ageing qualities. Used in treatment of eczema.
Wild carrot seed (*Daucus carota*)	Contains 80% oleic acid; a useful anti-oxidant; tonic, cicatrisant and antipruritic; indicated for eczema and psoriasis.

Table compiled and adapted from Kusmirek (2002), Price (1999), Schnaubelt (1999) and others (where cited).

A note on fatty acids

For some time it has been recognised that some fatty acids have anti-oxidant, free radical-scavenging, anti-inflammatory and antihyperlipidemic activities. These have been harnessed in medicine – for example, evening primrose oil (which contains *cis*-linoleic acid, or γ-linoleic acid) has been used as an anti-inflammatory in rheumatoid arthritis. Others with notable anti-inflammatory actions are linseed and holy basil seed, both containing α-linolenic acid (Beg *et al.* 2011). Yu, Zhou and Parry (2005) highlighted the potentially therapeutic anti-oxidant properties of cold-pressed black caraway, cranberry and hemp seed oils, which contain substantial amounts of α-linolenic acid, and wild carrot seed, which has 80% oleic acid and is low in total saturated fatty acids.

Hemp seed oil is said to have a 'perfect balance' in its 3:1 ratio of linoleic and linolenic acids – at least in regard to its nutritional value. The presence of γ-linolenic acid also makes it of value in skin care products; these fatty acids are known for their high penetration into the skin (Oomah *et al.* 2002).

Fixed oils in dermatological preparations

Several fixed oils have been used in dermatological treatments, and in preparations for the treatment of acne (Kanlayavattanakul and Lourith 2011). These include *Helianthus annuus* (sunflower seed) and *Cucurbita pepo* (pumpkin seed), *Prunus armeniaca* (American plum kernel), *Argania spinosa* (argan), *Persea gratissima* (avocado), *Adansonia digitata* (baobab), *Ribes nigrum* (blackcurrant seed), *Vaccinium macrocarpon* (American cranberry or bearberry), *Zea mays* (corn), *Oenothera biennis* (evening primrose), *Vitis vinifera* (grapeseed), *Corylus americana* (hazelnut), *Schinziophyton rautanenii* (mongongo kernel), *Moringa oleiferea* (ben nut), *Elaeis guineensis* (African palm), *Papaver orientale* (poppy seed), *Brassica napus* (rapeseed), *Rubus ideaus* (raspberry seed), *Oryza sativa* (rice bran), *Carthamus tinctorius* (safflower), *Sesame indicum* (sesame seed), *Glycine soya* (soya), *Prunus amygdalus* (almond kernel) and *Juglans regia* (walnut).

REFERENCES

Aazza, S., Lyoussi, B., Megias, C., Cortés-Giraldo, I., Figueiredo, A.C. and Miguel, M.G. (2014) 'Anti-oxidant, anti-inflammatory, and anti-proliferative activities of Moroccan commercial essential oils.' *Natural Product Communications 9*, 4, 587–594.

Abad, M.J., Ansuategui, M. and Bermejo, P. (2007) 'Active antifungal substances from natural sources.' *ARKIVOC 7*, 116–145.

Abdel-Fattah, A.M., Matsumoto, K. and Watanabe, H. (2000) 'Anti-nociceptive effects of *Nigella sativa* oil and its major component, thymoquinone, in mice.' *European Journal of Pharmacology 400*, 89–97.

Abu-Darwish, M.S., Cabral, C., Ferreira, I.V., Gonçalves, M.J., Cavaleiro, C., Cruz, M.T. *et al.* (2013) 'Essential oil of common sage (*Salvia officinalis* L.) from Jordan: Assessment of safety in mammalian cells and its antifungal and anti-inflammatory potential.' *Biomed Research International.* doi: 101155/2013/538940. Available at www.ncbi.nlm.nih.gov/pubmed/24224168, accessed on 7 April 2015.

Adams, S. and Thrash, T.P. (2010) 'Methods for wound treatment and healing using limonene-based compositions.' International Application Published under the Patent Cooperation Treaty, WO2010/062933 A1. Cited by Süntar, I., Tumen, I., Ustün, O., Keleş, H. and Akkol, E.K. (2012) 'Appraisal on the wound-healing and anti-inflammatory activities of the essential oils obtained from the cones and needles of *Pinus* species by *in vivo* and *in vitro* experimental models.' *Journal of Ethnopharmacology 139*, 2, 533–540.

Adorjan, B. and Buchbauer, G. (2010) 'Biological properties of essential oils: an updated review.' *Flavour and Fragrance Journal 25*, 407–426.

Agnew, T., Leach, M. and Segal, L. (2013) 'The clinical impact and cost-effectiveness of essential oils and aromatherapy for the treatment of acne vulgaris: a protocol for a randomised controlled trial.' *Journal of Alternative and Complementary Medicine 20*, 399–405.

Ahmad, H., Tijerina, M. and Tobola, A. (1997) 'Preferential over-expression of a class MU glutathione S-transferase subunit in mouse liver by myristicin.' *Biochemical and Biophysical Research Communications 236*, 825–828. Cited by Edris, A.E. (2007) 'Pharmaceutical and therapeutic potentials of essential oils and their individual volatile constituents: a review.' *Phytotherapy Research 21*, 308–323.

Akhlaghi, M., Shabanian, G., Rafieian-Kopaei, M., Parvin, M. and Saadat, M. (2011) '*Citrus aurantium* blossom and preoperative anxiety.' *Brazilian Journal of Anesthesiology 61*, 6, 702–712.

Akkol, E.K., Güvenc, A. and Yesilada, E. (2009) 'A comparative study on the anti-nociceptive and anti-inflammatory activities of five *Juniperus* taxa.' *Journal of Ethnopharmacology 125*, 2, 330–336.

Alaoui-Ismaïli, O., Vernet-Maury, E., Dittmar, A., Delhomme, G. and Chanel, J. (1997) 'Odor hedonics: connection with emotional response estimated by autonomic parameters.' *Chemical Senses 22*, 237–248.

Albuquerque, A.A., Sorenson, A.L. and Leal-Cardoso, J.H. (1995) 'Effects of essential oil of *Croton zehntneri*, and of anethole and estragole on skeletal muscles'. *Journal of Ethnopharmacology 49*, 1, 41–49. Cited by Bowles, E.J. (2003) *The Chemistry of Aromatherapeutic Oils.* (3rd edition.) Crows Nest, NSW: Allen and Unwin.

Albuquerque, E.L.D., Lima, J.K.A., Souza, F.H.O., Silva, I.M.A. *et al.* (2013) 'Insecticidal and repellence activity of the essential oil of *Pogostemon cablin* against urban ants species.' *Acta Tropica 127*, 181–186.

Alenzi, F.Q., El-Bolkini, Y.S. and Salem, M.L. (2010) 'Protective effects of *Nigella sativa* oil and thymoquinone against toxicity induced by the anticancer drug cyclophosphamide.' *British Journal of Biomedical Science 67*, 20–28.

Ali, B. and Blunden, G. (2003) 'Pharmacological and toxicological properties of *Nigella sativa.*' *Phytotherapy Research 17*, 4, 299–305.

Allahverdiyev, A., Duran, N., Ozguven, M. and Koltas, S. (2004) 'Antiviral activity of the volatile oils of *Melissa officinalis* L. against *Herpes simplex* type-2.' *Phytomedicine 11*, 7–8, 657–661. Cited by Edris, A.E. (2007) 'Pharmaceutical and therapeutic potentials of essential oils and their individual volatile constituents: a review.' *Phytotherapy Research 21*, 308–323.

Almeida, R.N., Hiruma, C.A. and Barbosa-Filho, J.M. (1996) 'Analgesic effect of rotundifolone in rodents.' *Fitoterapia 67*, 334–338. Cited by de Sousa, D.P., Júnior, E.V.M., Oliveira, F.S., de Almeida, R.N., Nunes, X.P. and Barbosa-Filho, J.M. (2007) 'Anti-nociceptive activity of structural analogues of rotundifolone: structure activity relationship.' *Z. Naturforsch 62c*, 39–42.

Altaei, D.T. (2012) 'Topical lavender oil for the treatment of recurrent apthous ulceration.' *American Journal of Dentistry 25*, 1, 39–43.

Amber, K., Aijaz, A., Immaculata, X., Luqman, K.A. and Nikhat, M. (2010) 'Anticandidal effect of *Ocimum sanctum* essential oil and its synergy with fluconazole and ketoconazole.' *Phytomedicine 17*, 12, 921–925. Cited by Lang, G. and Buchbauer, G. (2012) 'A review on recent research results (2008–2010) on essential oils as antimicrobials and antifungals. A review.' *Flavour and Fragrance Journal 27*, 13–39.

Ammar, A.H., Bouajila, J., Lebrihi, A., Mathieu, F., Romdhane, M. and Zagrouba, F. (2012) 'Chemical composition and *in vitro* antimicrobial and antioxidant activities of *Citrus aurantium* L. flowers essential oil (Neroli oil).' *Pakistani Journal of Biological Science 15*, 21, 1034–1040.

Anthony, J.C., Breitner, J.C.S., Zandi, P.P., Meyer, M.R., Jurasova, I., Norton, M.C. *et al.* (2000) 'Reduced prevalence of AD in users of NSAIDS and H2 receptor agonists: the cache county study.' *Neurology 54*, 2066–2071. Cited by Okonogi, S. and Chaiyana, W. (2012) 'Enhancement of anti-cholinesterase activity of *Zingiber cassumunar* essential oil using a microemulsion technique.' *Drug Discoveries and Therapeutics 6*, 5, 249–255.

Arambewela, L.S.R., Arawwawala, L.D.A.M. and Ratnasooriya, W.D. (2004) 'Antinociceptive activities of aqueous and ethanolic extracts of Alpinia calcarata rhizomes in rats.' *Journal of Ethnopharmacology 95*, 2–3, 311–316.

Arawwawala, L.D.A.M., Arambewela, L.S.R. and Ratnasooriya, W.D. (2012) '*Alpinia calcarata* Roscoe: a potent anti-inflammatory agent'. *Journal of Ethnopharmacology 139*, 3, 889–892.

Aris, S.R.S., Taib, M.N. and Murat, Z. (2011) 'Effect of *Citrus hystrix* aroma on human cognition via emotive responses.' UiTM report. Available at ir.uitm.edu.my/7155, accessed on 7 April 2015.

Arora, R.B., Sharma, P.L. and Kapila, K. (1958) 'Antiarrhymic and anticonvulsant activity of jatamansone.' *Indian Journal of Medical Research 46*, 782–791. Cited by de Almeida, R.N., Agra, M.F., Maior, F.N.S. and de Sousa, D.P. (2011) 'Essential oils and their constituents: anticonvulsant activity.' *Molecules 16*, 2726–2742.

Asgary, S., Naderi, G.A., Shams Ardekani, M.R., Sahebkar, A., Airin, A., Aslani, S. *et al.* (2013) 'Chemical analysis and biological activities of *Cupressus sempervirens* var. *horizontalis* essential oils.' *Pharmaceutical Biology 51*, 2, 137–144.

Astani, A., Reichling, J. and Schnitzler, P. (2010) 'Comparative study on the antiviral activity of selected monoterpenes derived from essential oils.' *Phytotherapy Research 24*, 5, 673–679. Cited by Adorjan, B. and Buchbauer, G. (2010) 'Biological properties of essential oils: an updated review.' *Flavour and Fragrance Journal 25*, 407–426.

Athikomkulchai, S., Watthanachaiyingcharoen, R. and Tunvichien, S. (2008) 'The development of anti-acne products from *Eucalyptus globulus* and *Psidium guajava* oil.' *Journal of Health Research 22*, 3, 109–113.

Atsumi, T. and Tonosaki, K. (2007) 'Smelling lavender and rosemary increases free radical scavenging activity and decreases cortisol level in saliva.' *Psychiatry Research 150*, 89–96.

Aupaphong, V., Ayudhya, T.D.N. and Koontongkaew, S. (2013) 'Inhibition of lipopolysaccharide-induced expression of cyclooxygenase–2 by *Zingiber cassumunar* Roxb. constituents in human dental pulp cells.' *Journal of Medicinal Plants Research 7*, 33, 2451–2458.

Awadh Ali, N.A., Wurster, M., Arnold, N., Lindequist, U. and Wessjohan, L. (2009) 'Chemical composition and biological activities of essential oils from the oleogum resins of three endemic Soqotraen *Boswellia* species.' *Records of Natural Products 2*, 1, 6–12. Cited by Hussain, H., Al-Harrasi, A., Al-Rawahi, A. and Hussain, J. (2014) 'Chemistry and biology of essential oils of genus *Boswellia.*' *Evidence Based Complementary and Alternative Medicine.* doi: 10.1155/2013/140509.

Azanchi, T., Shafaroodi, H. and Asgarpanah, J. (2014) Anticonvulsant activity of *Citrus aurantium* blossom essential oil (neroli): involvement of the GABAergic system. *Natural Product Communications 9*, 11, 1615–1618.

Azimi, H., Fallah-Tafti, M., Khakshur, A.A. and Abdollahi, M. (2012) 'A review of the treatment of acne vulgaris: perspective of new pharmacological treatments.' *Fitoterapia 83*, 8, 1306–1317.

Azizi, Z., Ebrahimi, S., Saadatfar, E., Kamalinejad, M. and Majlessi, N. (2012) 'Cognitive-enhancing activity of thymol and carvacrol in two rat models of dementia.' *Behavioural Pharmacology 23*, 3, 241–249.

Bagetta, G., Morrone, L. A., Rombolà, L., Amatea, D. *et al.* (2010) 'Neuropharmacology of the essential oil of bergamot.' *Fitoterapia 81*, 6, 453–461.

Bakowska, A.M., Schieber, A. and Kolodziejczyk, P. (2009) 'Characterization of Canadian black currant (*Ribes nigrum* L.) seed oils and residues.' *Journal of Agricultural and Food Chemistry 57*, 24, 11528–11536.

Balacs, T. (1995) 'The psychopharmacology of essential oils.' *Aroma '95 Conference Proceedings*. Brighton: Aromatherapy Publications.

Baldwin, H.E. (2006) 'Tricks for improving compliance with acne therapy.' *Dermatologic Therapy 19*, 224–236.

Ballard, C.G., O'Brien, C.T., Reichelt, K. and Perry, E.K. (2002) 'Aromatherapy as a safe and effective treatment for the management of agitation in severe dementia: the results of a double-blind, placebo-controlled trial with melissa.' *Journal of Clinical Psychiatry 63*, 553–558.

Barkat, S., Le Berre, E., Coureaud, G., Sicard, G. and Thomas-Danguin, T. (2012) 'Perceptual blending in odor mixtures depends on the nature of odorants and human olfactory expertise.' *Chemical Senses 37*, 159–166.

Barocelli, E., Calcina, F., Chiavarini, M., Impicciatore, M. *et al.* (2004) 'Anti-nociceptive and gastroprotective effects of inhaled and orally administered *Lavandula hybrida* Reverchon "Grosso" essential oil.' *Life Science 76*, 213–223.

Barra, A., Coroneo, V., Dessi, S., Cabras, P. and Angioni, A. (2010) 'Chemical variability, antifungal and anti-oxidant activity of *Eucalyptus camadulensis* essential oil from Sardinia.' *Natural Products Communication 5*, 329–335.

Barreto, R.S.S., Albuquerque-Júnior, R.L.C., Araújo, A.A.S., Almeida, J.R.G.S. *et al.* (2014) 'A systematic review of the wound-healing effects of monoterpenes and iridoid derivatives.' *Molecules 19*, 846–862.

Bastos, J.F., Moreira, I.J., Ribeiro, T.P., Medeiros, I.A. *et al.* (2010) 'Hypotensive and vasorelaxant effects of citronellol, a monoterpene alcohol, in rats.' *Basic and Clinical Pharmacology and Toxicology 106*, 4, 331–337.

Batista, P.A., Werner, M.F., Oliveira, E.C., Burgos, L. *et al.* (2008) 'Evidence for the involvement of ionotropic glutamatergic receptors on the anti-nociceptive effect of (–)-linalool in mice.' *Neuroscience Letters 440*, 299–303.

Batista, P., Harris, E., Werner, M., Santos, A. and Story, G. (2011) 'Inhibition of TRPA1 and NMDA channels contributes to anti-nociception induced by (–)-linalool. *Journal of Pain 12*, 30. Cited by Guimarães, A.G., Quintans, J.S.S. and Quintans-Júnior, L.J. (2013) 'Monoterpenes with analgesic activity – a systematic review.' *Phytotherapy Research 27*, 1, 1–15.

Baumann, L.S. (2003) 'Cosmeceutical critique: chamomile.' *Skin and Allergy News* 2003, 39–43. Cited by Thornfeldt, C. (2005) 'Cosmeceuticals containing herbs: fact, fiction and future.' *Dermatologic Surgery 31*, 873–880.

Baumann, L.S. (2007a) 'Less-known botanical cosmeceuticals.' *Dermatologic Therapy 20*, 330–342.

Baumann, L.S. (2007b) 'German chamomile and cutaneous benefits.' *Journal of Drugs in Dermatology 6*, 11, 1084–1085.

Baylac, S. and Racine, P. (2003) 'Inhibition of 5-lipoxygenase by essential oils and other natural fragrant extracts.' *International Journal of Aromatherapy 13*, 2/3, 138–142.

Baylac, S. and Racine, P. (2004) 'Inhibition of human leukocyte elastase by natural fragrant extracts of aromatic plants.' *International Journal of Aromatherapy 14*, 4, 179–182.

Beg, S., Swain, S., Hasan, H., Barkat, M.A. and Hussain, M.S. (2011) 'Systematic review of herbals as potential anti-inflammatory agents: recent advances, current clinical status and future perspectives.' *Pharmacognosy Reviews 5*, 10, 120–137.

Begrow, F., Engelbertz, J., Feistel, B., Lehnfeld, R., Bauer, K. and Verspohl, E.J. (2010) 'Impact of thymol in thyme extracts on their antispasmodic action and ciliary clearance.' *Planta Medica 76*, 4, 311–318.

Behra, O., Rakotoarison, C. and Harris, R. (2001) 'Ravintsara vs. ravensara: a taxonomic clarification.' *International Journal of Aromatherapy 11*, 1, 4–7.

Behrendt, H.J, Germann, T., Gillen, C., Hatt, H. and Jostock, R. (2004) 'Characterisation of the mouse cold-menthol receptor TRPM8 and vanilloid receptor type-1 VR1 using a fluorimetric imaging plate reader (FLIPR) assay.' *British Journal of Pharmacology 141*, 737–745. Cited by Guimarães, A.G., Quintans, J.S.S. and Quintans-Júnior, L.J. (2013) 'Monoterpenes with analgesic activity: a systematic review.' *Phytotherapy Research 27*, 1, 1–15.

Bensouilah, J. (2005) 'The history and development of modern British aromatherapy.' *International Journal of Aromatherapy 15*, 3, 134–140.

Bensouilah, J. and Buck, P. (2006) *Aromadermatology: Aromatherapy in the Treatment of Skin Conditions.* Oxford: Radcliffe Publishing.

Berger, H. (1929) 'Über das Elektrenkephalogramm des Menschen.' *Archiv für Psychiatrie und Nervenkrankheiten 87*, 527–570. Cited by Bagetta, G., Morrone, L.A., Rombolà, L., Amatea, D. *et al.* (2010) 'Neuropharmacology of the essential oil of bergamot.' *Fitoterapi 81*, 453–461.

Bhalla, Y., Gupta, V.K. and Jaitak, V. (2013) 'Anticancer activity of essential oils: a review.' *Journal of the Science of Food and Agriculture 93*, 3643–3653.

Bhardwaj, P., Garg, P.K., Maulik, S.K., Saraya, A., Tandon, R.K. and Acharya, S.K.A. (2009) 'Randomised controlled trial of anti-oxidant supplementation for pain relief in patients with chronic pancreatitis.' *Gastroenterology 136*, 149–159.

Bhatt, D., Sachan, A.K., Jain, S. and Barik, R. (2011) 'Studies on inhibitory effect of eucalyptus oil on sebaceous glands for the management of acne.' *Indian Journal of Natural Products and Resources 2*, 3, 345–349.

Bhwang, K., Kumar, S.S., Lalit, S., Sharmistha, M. and Tanuja, S. (2013) '*Cyperus scariosus* – a potential medicinal herb.' *International Research Journal of Pharmacy 4*, 6, 17–20.

Blanco, M.M., Costa, C.A.R.A., Freire, A.O., Santos, J.G. Jr. and Costa, M. (2009) 'Neurobehavioural effect of essential oil of *Cymbopogon citratus* in mice.' *Phytomedicine 16*, 2–3, 265–270. Cited by de Almeida, R.N., Agra, M.F., Maior, F.N.S. and de Sousa, D.P. (2011) 'Essential oils and their constituents: anticonvulsant activity.' *Molecules 16*, 2726–2742.

Bloom, W. (2011) *The Power of Modern Spirituality.* London: Piatkus.

Bodake, H., Panicker, K., Kailaje, V. and Rao, V. (2002) 'Chemopreventative effect of orange oil on the development of hepatic preneoplastic lesions induced by N-nitrosodiethylamine in rats: an ultrastructural study.' *Indian Journal of Experimental Biology 40*, 245–251. Cited by Edris, A.E. (2007) 'Pharmaceutical and therapeutic potentials of essential oils and their individual volatile constituents: a review.' *Phytotherapy Research 21*, 4, 308–323.

Boddeke, H.W., Best, R. and Boeijinga, P.H. (1997) 'Synchronous 20 Hz rhythmic activity in hippocampal networks induced by activation of metabotropic glutamate receptors *in vitro*.' *Neuroscience 76*, 653–658. Cited by Bagetta, G., Morrone, L.A., Rombolà, L., Amatea, D. *et al.* (2010) 'Neuropharmacology of the essential oil of bergamot.' *Fitoterapia 81*, 453–461.

Boskabady, M.H., Kiani, S. and Rakhshandah, H. (2006) 'Relaxant effects of *Rosa damascena* on guinea pig tracheal chains and its possible mechanism(s).' *Journal of Ethnopharmacology 106*, 3, 377–382.

Boskabady, M.H., Mohsenpoor, N. and Takaloo, L. (2010) 'Antiasthmatic effect of *Nigella sativa* in airways of asthmatic patients.' *Phytomedicine 17*, 10, 707–713. Cited by Khan, M.A., Chen, H., Tania, M. and Zhang, D. (2011) 'Anticancer activities of *Nigella sativa* (black cumin).' *African Journal of Traditional, Complementary and Alternative Medicines 8*, 5, 226–232.

Bouayed, J., Rammal, H. and Soulimani, R. (2009) 'Oxidative stress and anxiety relationship and cellular pathways.' *Oxidative Medicine and Cellular Longevity 2*, 2, 63–67. Cited by Zhang, Y., Wu, Y., Chen, T., Yao, L. *et al.* (2013) 'Assessing the metabolic effects of aromatherapy in human volunteers.' *Evidence-Based Complementary and Alternative Medicine*. Available at http://dx.doi.org/10.1155/2013/356381, accessed on 7 April 2015.

Boukhatem, M.N., Kameli, A., Ferhat, M.A., Saidi, F. and Mekarnia, M. (2013) 'Rose geranium essential oil as a source of new and safe anti-inflammatory drugs.' *Libyan Journal of Medicine 8*, 22520. Available at http://dx.doi.org/10.3402/ljm.v8i0.22520, accessed on 7 April 2015.

Boukhatem, M.N., Ferhat, M.A., Kameli, A., Saidi, F. and Kebir, H.T. (2014) 'Lemon grass (*Cymbopogon citratus*) essential oil as a potent anti-inflammatory and antifungal drugs.' *Libyan Journal of Medicine 9*, 25431. 7 April 2015 Available at http://dx.doi.org/10.3402/ljm.v9.25431, accessed on 7 April 2015.

Bounihi, A., Hajjaj, G., Alnamer, R., Cherrah, Y. and Zellou, A. (2013) '*In vivo* potential anti-inflammatory activity of *Melissa officinalis* L. essential oil.' *Advances in Pharmacological Sciences*. doi: 10.1155/2013/101759. Available at www.ncbi.nim.nlh.gov/pmc/articles/PMC3870089, accessed on 7 April 2015.

Boussaada, O. and Chemli, R. (2006) 'Chemical composition of essential oils from flowers, leaves and peel of *Citrus aurantium* L. var. *amara* from Tunisia.' *Journal of Essential Oil Bearing Plants 9*, 133–139.

Bowe, W.P., Leyden, J.J., Crerand, C.E., Sarwer, D.B. and Margolis, D.J. (2007) 'Body dysmorphic disorder symptoms among patients with acne vulgaris.' *Journal of the American Academy of Dermatology 57*, 222–230.

Bowe, W.P. and Shalita, A.R. (2008) 'Effective over-the-counter acne treatments.' *Seminars in Cutaneous Medicine and Surgery 27*, 170–176.

Bowles, E.J. (2003) *The Chemistry of Aromatherapeutic Oils*. (3rd edition.) Crows Nest, NSW: Allen and Unwin.

Boyd, E.M. and Pearson, G.L. (1946) 'The expectorant action of volatile oils.' *American Journal of Medical Science 211*, 602–610. Cited by Van Toller, S. and Dodd, G.H. (eds) (1988) *Perfumery: The Psychology and Biology of Fragrance*. London: Chapman & Hall.

Braden, R., Reichow, S. and Halm, M.A. (2009) 'The use of the essential oil of lavandin to reduce preoperative anxiety in surgical patients.' *Journal of PeriAnesthesia Nursing 24*, 6, 348–355. Cited by Dobetsberger, C. and Buchbauer, G. (2011) 'Actions of essential oils on the central nervous system: an updated review.' *Flavour and Fragrance Journal 26*, 300–316.

Brand, C., Townley, S., Finlay-Jones, J. and Hart, P. (2002) 'Tea tree oil reduces histamine-induced oedema in murine ears.' *Inflammation Research 51*, 283–289.

Brito, R.G., Guimarães, A.G. and Quintans, J.S.S. (2012) 'Citronellol, a monoterpene alcohol, reduces nociceptive and inflammatory activities in rodents.' *Journal of Natural Medicine 66*, 4, 637–644.

Brophy, J.J. and Doran, J.C. (2004) 'Geographic variation in oil characteristics in Melaleuca ericifolia.' *Journal of Essential Oil Research 16*, 1, 4–8.

Brophy, J.J., Fookes, C.J.R. and Lassak, E.V. (1991) 'Constituents of *Santalum spicatum* (R.Br.) A. DC. wood oil.' *Journal of Essential Oil Research 3*, 6, 381–385.

Bua-in, S. and Paisooksantivatana, Y. (2009) 'Essential oil and anti-oxidant activity of cassumunar ginger (Zingiberaceae: *Zingiber montanum* (Koenig) Link ex Dietr.) collected from various parts of Thailand.' *Kasetsart Journal (Natural Science) 43*, 467–475.

Burfield, T. (2002) 'Cedarwood oils.' *The Cropwatch Series*. Available at www.cropwatch.org, accessed on 30 November 2011.

Burr, C. (2007) *The Perfect Scent*. New York: Picador.

Busse, D., Kudella, P., Grüning, N.M., Gisselmann, G. *et al.* (2014) 'A synthetic sandalwood odorant induces would-healing processes in human keratinocytes via the olfactory receptor OR2AT4.' *Journal of Investigative Dermatology*. doi: 10.1038/jid.2014.273.

Butt, M.S., Pasha, I., Sultan, M.T., Randhawa, M.A., Saeed, F. and Ahmed, W. (2013) 'Black pepper and health claims: a comprehensive treatise. *Critical Reviews in Food Science and Nutrition 53*, 9, 875–886.

Cai, J., Lin, P., Zhu, X. and Su, Q. (2006) 'Comparative analysis of clary sage (*S. sclarea* L.) oil volatiles by GC–FTIR and GC–MS. *Food Chemistry 99*, 401–407.

Calcabrini, A., Stringaro, A., Toccacieli, L., Meschini, S. *et al.* (2004) 'Terpinen-4-ol, the main component of *Melaleuca alternifolia* (tea tree) oil, inhibits the *in vitro* growth of human melanoma cells.' *Journal of Investigative Dermatology 122*, 349–360.

Caldecott, T. (2006) *Ayurveda, the Divine Science of Life*. London: Mosby Elsevier.

Camarda, L., Dayton, T., Di Stefano, V., Pitonzo, R. and Schillaci, D. (2007) 'Chemical composition and antimicrobial activity of some oleogum resin essential oils from *Boswellia* species (Burseraceae).' *Annali di Chimica 97*, 9, 837–844. Cited by Hussain, H., Al-Harrasi, A., Al-Rawahi, A. and Hussain, J. (2014) 'Chemistry and biology of essential oils of genus *Boswellia*.' *Evidence-Based Complementary and Alternative Medicine*. doi: 10.1155/2013/140509.

Caplin, J.L., Allan, I. and Hanlon, G.W. (2009) 'Enhancing the *in vitro* activity of *Thymus* essential oils against *Staphylococcus aureus* by blending oils from specific cultivars.' *International Journal of Essential Oil Therapeutics 3*, 35–39.

Carrasco, F.R., Schmidt, G., Romero, A.L., Sartoretto, J.L. *et al.* (2009) 'Immunomodulatory activity of *Zingiber officinale* Roscoe, *Salvia officinalis* L. and *Syzygium aromaticum* L. essential oils: evidence for humor- and cell-mediated responses.' *Journal of Pharmacy and Pharmacology 61*, 7, 961–967.

Carson, C.F., Hammer, K.A. and Riley, T.V. (2006) '*Melaleuca alternifolia* (tea tree) oil: a review of antimicrobial and other medicinal properties.' *Clinical Microbiology Reviews 19*, 50–62.

Carvalho-Freitas, M.I.R. and Costa, M. (2002) 'Anxiolytic and sedative effects of extracts and essential oil from *Citrus aurantium* L.' *Biological and Pharmaceutical Bulletin 25*, 1629–1633. Cited by de Almeida, R.N., Agra, M.F., Maior, F.N.S. and de Sousa, D.P. (2011) 'Essential oils and their constituents: anticonvulsant activity.' *Molecules 16*, 2726–2742.

Casetti, F., Wölfle, U., Gehring, W. and Schempp, C.M. (2011) 'Dermocosmetics for dry skin: a new role for botanical extracts.' *Skin Pharmacology and Physiology 24*, 6, 289–293.

Casetti, F., Bartelke, S., Biehler, K., Augustin, M., Schempp, C.M. and Frank, U. (2012) 'Antimicrobial activity against bacteria with dermatological relevance and skin tolerance of the essential oil from *Coriandrum sativum* L. fruits.' *Phytotherapy Research 26*, 3, 420–424.

Cassella, S., Cassella, J.P. and Smith, I. (2002) 'Synergistic antifungal activity of tea tree (*Melaleuca alternifolia*) and lavender (*Lavandula angustifolia*) essential oils against dermatophyte infection.' *International Journal of Aromatherapy 12*, 1, 2–15.

Cavalieri, E., Mariotto, S., Fabrizi, C., de Prati, A.C. *et al.* (2004) 'α-Bisabolol, a non-toxic natural compound, strongly induces apoptosis in glioma cells.' *Biochemical and Biophysical Research Communications 315*, 589–594.

Ceccarelli, I., Masi, F., Fiorenzani, P. and Aloisi, A.M. (2002) 'Sex differences in the citrus lemon essential oil-induced increase of hippocampal acetylcholine release in rats exposed to a persistent painful stimulation.' *Neuroscience Letters 330*, 25–28. Cited by Bagetta, G., Morrone, L.A., Rombolà, L., Amatea, D. *et al.* (2010) 'Neuropharmacology of the essential oil of bergamot.' *Fitoterapia 81*, 453–461.

Cermelli, C., Fabio, A., Fabio, G. and Quaglio, P. (2008) 'Effect of eucalyptus essential oil on respiratory bacteria and viruses.' *Current Microbiology 56*, 1, 89–92.

Ch, M.M. and Smitha, P.V. (2011) 'Phytochemical composition and antimicrobial activity of three plant preparations used in folk medicine and their synergistic properties.' *Journal of Herbs, Spices and Medicinal Plants 17*, 4, 339–350.

Chaiwongsa, R., Ongchai, S., Boonsong, P., Kongtawelert, P., Panthong, A. and Reutrakul, V. (2013) 'Active compound of Zingiber cassumunar Roxb. down-regulates the expression of genes involved in joint erosion in a human synovial fibroblast cell line.' *African Journal of Traditional Complementary and Alternative Medicine 10*, 1, 40–48. Available at http://dx.doi.org/10.4314/ajtcam.v10i1.7, accessed on 19 June 2015.

Chang, S.Y. (2008) 'Effects of aroma hand massage on pain, state anxiety and depression in hospice patients with terminal cancer.' *Taehan Kanho Hakhoe Chi 38*, 493–502. (Article in Korean.) Cited by Dobetsberger, C. and Buchbauer, G. (2011) 'Actions of essential oils on the central nervous system: an updated review.' *Flavour and Fragrance Journal 26*, 300–316.

Chaouki, W., Leger, D.Y., Liagre, B., Beneytout, J.L. and Hmamouchi, M. (2009) 'Citral inhibits cell proliferation and induces apoptosis and cycle arrest in MCF-7 cells.' *Fundamental and Clinical Pharmacology 23*, 549–556. Cited by Guimarães, A.G., Quintans, J.S.S. and Quintans-Júnior, L.J. (2013) 'Monoterpenes with analgesic activity – a systematic review.' *Phytotherapy Research 27*, 1, 1–15.

Charrouf, Z. and Guillaume, D. (2008) 'Argan oil: occurrence, composition and impact on human health.' *European Journal of Lipid Science and Technology 110*, 7, 632–636.

Chauhan, K., Solanki, R., Patel, A., Macwan, C. and Patel, M. (2011) 'Phytochemical and therapeutic potential of *Piper longum* Linn.: a review.' *International Journal of Research in Ayurveda and Pharmacy 2*, 1, 157–161.

Chen, N., Sun, G., Yuan, X., Hou, J. *et al.* (2014) 'Inhibition of lung inflammatory responses by bornyl acetate is correlated with regulation of myeloperoxidase activity.' *Journal of Surgical Research 186*, 1, 436–445.

Chen, S.W., Min, L., Li, W.J., Kong, W.X., Li, J.F. and Zhang, Y.J. (2004) 'The effects of angelica essential oil in three murine tests of anxiety.' *Pharmacology Biochemistry and Behaviour 79*, 2, 377–382.

Chen, Y., Zhou, C., Ge, Z., Liu, Y. *et al.* (2013) 'Composition and potential anticancer activities of essential oils obtained from myrrh and frankincense.' *Oncology Letters 6*, 4, 1140–1146.

Chen, Y.-J., Cheng, F., Shih, Y., Chang, T.-M., Wang, M.-F., and Lan, S.-S. (2008) 'Inhalation of neroli essential oil and its anxiolytic effects.' *Journal of Complementary and Integrative Medicine 5*, 1, 18. Cited by Dobetsberger, C. and Buchbauer, G. (2011) 'Actions of essential oils on the central nervous system: an updated review.' *Flavour and Fragrance Journal 26*, 300–316.

Cheng, J., Chang, G. and Wu, W. (2001) 'A controlled clinical study between hepatic arterial infusion with embolized *curcuma* aromatic oil and chemical drugs in treating primary liver cancer.' *Zhongguo Zhong Xi Yi Jie He Za Zhi (Chinese Journal of Integrative Traditional Western Medicine) 21*, 165–167. Cited by Edris, A.E. (2007) 'Pharmaceutical and therapeutic potentials of essential oils and their individual volatile constituents: a review.' *Phytotherapy Research 21*, 4, 308–323.

Chi, T., Ji, X., Xia, M., Rong, Y., Qiu, F. and Zou, L. (2009) 'Effect of six extractions from Wuhu decoction on isolated tracheal smooth muscle in guinea pig.' *Zhongguo Shiyan Fangjixue Zazhi 15*, 52–55. Cited by de Casia da Silveira e Sá, R., Andrade, L.N., de Oliveira, R. and de Sousa, D.P. (2014) 'A review on the anti-inflammatory activity of phenylpropanoids found in essential oils.' *Molecules 19*, 1459–1480.

Chioca, L.R., Antunes, V.D.C., Ferro, M.M., Losso, E.M. and Andreatini, R. (2013) 'Anosmia does not impair the anxiolytic-like effects of lavender essential oil inhalation in mice.' *Life Sciences 92*, 971–975.

Chiranthanut, N., Hanprasertpong, N. and Teekachunhatean, S. (2014) 'Thai massage and Thai herbal compresses versus oral ibuprofen in symptomatic treatment of osteoarthritis of the knee: a randomised controlled trial.' *BioMed Research International* Article ID 490512. Available at http://dx.doi.org/10.1155/2014/490512, accessed on 7 April 2015.

Choi, S.Y., Kang, P., Lee, H.S., Seol, G.H. (2014) 'Effects of inhalation of essential oil of Citrus aurantium L. var. amara on menopausal symptoms, stress, and estrogen in postmenopausal women: a randomized controlled trial.' *Evidence-Based Complementary and Alternative Medicine.* http://dx.doi.org/10.1155/2014/796518.

Chotjumlong, P. (2005) 'Effect of plai (*Zingiber cassumunar* Roxb.) extract on the levels of hyaluronan, glycosaminoglycan and matrix metalloproteases from oral fibroblast and epithelial cells.' MSc thesis, Chiang Mai University. Abstract available at http://thaiherbinfo.com/en/herb_in_product.php?id_pro=3693, accessed on 7 April 2015.

Chrea, C., Grandjean, D., Delplanque, S., Cayeux, I. *et al.* (2009) 'Mapping the semantic space for the subjective experience of emotional responses to odours.' *Chemical Senses 34*, 49–62.

Chrubasik, C., Roufogalis, B.D., Müller-Ladner, U. and Chrubasik, S. (2008) 'A systematic review on the *Rosa canina* effect and efficacy profiles.' *Phytotherapy Research 22*, 6, 725–733.

Clerc, O. (1995) 'Portraits in oils.' *International Journal of Aromatherapy 7*, 1, 15–17.

Cooke, B. and Ernst, E. (2000) 'Aromatherapy: a systematic review.' *British Journal of General Practice 50*, 493–496.

Cosentino, M., Luini, A., Bombelli, R., Corasaniti, M.T., Bagetta, G. and Marino, F. (2014) 'The essential oil of bergamot stimulates reactive oxygen species production in human polymorphonuclear leukocytes.' *Phytotherapy Research 28*, 8, 1232–1239.

Costa, C.A., Kohn, D.O., De Lima, V.M., Gargano, A.C., Flório, J.C and Costa, M. (2011) 'The GABAergic system contributes to the anxiolytic-like effect of essential oil from *Cymbopogon citratus* (lemongrass).' *Journal of Ethnopharmacology 137*, 1, 828–836.

Cornwall, P.A. and Barry, B.W. (1994) '456 sesquiterpene components of volatile oils as skin penetration enhancers for the hydrophilic permeant 5 fluorouracil.' *Journal of Pharmacy and Pharmacology 46*, 4, 261–269.

Dalgard, F., Gieler, U., Holm, J.Ø., Bjertness, E. and Hauser, S. (2008) 'Self-esteem and body satisfaction among late adolescents with acne: results from a population survey.' *Journal of the American Academy of Dermatology 59*, 746–751.

Dalton, P. (1996) 'Cognitive aspects of perfumery.' *Perfumer and Flavorist 21*, 13–20.

Dandlen, S.A., Lima, A.S., Mendes, M.D., Miguel, M.G. *et al.* (2010) 'Anti-oxidant activity of six Portuguese thyme species essential oils.' *Flavour and Fragrance Journal 25*, 150–155.

Danh, L., Han, L., Triet, N., Zhao, J., Mammucari, R. and Foster, N. (2013) 'Comparison of chemical composition, anti-oxidant and antimicrobial activity of lavender (*Lavandula angustifolia* L.) essential oils extracted by supercritical CO_2, hexane and hydrodistillation.' *Food and Bioprocess Technology 6*, 3481–3489.

Daniel, A.N., Sartoretto, S.M., Schmidt, G., Caparroz-Assef, M., Bersani-Amado, C.A. and Cuman, R.K.N. (2008) 'Antinflammatory and antinociceptive activities of eugenol essential oil in experimental animal models.' *Brazilian Journal of Pharmacognosy 19*, 212–217.

Davies, S.J., Harding, L.M. and Baranowski, A.P. (2002) 'A novel treatment for postherpetic neuralgia using peppermint oil.' *Clinical Journal of Pain 18*, 200–202. Cited by Guimarães, A.G., Quintans, J.S.S. and Quintans-Júnior, L.J. (2013) 'Monoterpenes with analgesic activity: a systematic review.' *Phytotherapy Research 27*, 1, 1–15.

de Almeida, R.N., Agra, M.F., Maior, F.N.S. and de Sousa D.P. (2011) 'Essential oils and their constituents: anticonvulsant activity.' *Molecules 16*, 2726–2742.

de Cássia da Silveira e Sá, R., Andrade, L.N., de Oliveira, R. and de Sousa, D.P. (2014) 'A review on the anti-inflammatory activity of phenylpropanoids found in essential oils.' *Molecules 19*, 1459–1480.

Delaquis, P.J., Stanich, K., Girard, B. and Mazza, G. (2002) 'Antimicrobial activity of individual and mixed fractions of dill, cilantro, coriander and eucalyptus essential oils.' *International Journal of Food Microbiology 74*, 101–109.

de Mendonça Rocha, P.M., Rodilla, J.M., Díez, D., Elder, H. *et al.* (2012) 'Synergistic antibacterial activity of the essential oil of Aguaribay (*Schinus molle* l.).' *Molecules 17*, 12023–12036.

de Pradier, E. (2006) 'A trial of a mixture of three essential oils in the treatment of postoperative nausea and vomiting.' *International Journal of Aromatherapy 16*, 1, 15–20.

de Rapper, S., Kamatou, G., Viljoen, A. and van Vuuren, S. (2013) 'The *in vitro* antimicrobial activity of *Lavandula angustifolia* essential oil in combination with other aroma-therapeutic oils.' *Evidence-based Complementary and Alternative Medicine* 2013: 852049. Available at www.hindawi.com/journals/ecam/2013/852049, accessed on 7 April 2015.

de Rapper, S., Van Vuren, S.F., Kamatou, G.P., Viljoen, A.M. and Dagne, E. (2012) 'The additive and synergistic antimicrobial effects of select frankincense and myrrh oils – a combination from the ancient pharaonic pharmacopoeia.' *Letters in Applied Microbiology 54*, 4, 352–358.

de Sousa, A., Alviano, D., Blank, A., Alves, P., Alviano, C. and Gattass, C. (2004) '*Melissa officinalis* L. essential oil: antitumoural and anti-oxidant activities.' *Journal of Pharmacy and Pharmacology 56*, 677–681. Cited by Edris, A.E. (2007) 'Pharmaceutical and therapeutic potentials of essential oils and their individual volatile constituents: a review.' *Phytotherapy Research 21*, 4, 308–323.

de Sousa, D.P. (2012) 'Anxiolytic essential oils.' *Natural Products Chemistry and Research* 1, e102. doi: 10.4172/npcr.1000e102

de Sousa, D.P., Júnior, E.V.M., Oliveira, F.S., de Almeida, R.N., Nunes, X.P. and Barbosa-Filho, J.M. (2007) 'Anti-nociceptive activity of structural analogues of rotundifolone: structure–activity relationship.' *Zeitschrift für Naturforschung C 62*, 39–42.

de Sousa, D.P., Júnior, G.A., Andrade, L.N., Calasans, F.R. *et al.* (2008) 'Structure and spasmolytic activity relationships of monoterpene analogues found in many aromatic plants.' *Zeitschrift für Naturforschung C 63*, 11–12, 808–812.

Díaz, C., Quesada, S., Brenes, O., Aguilar, G. and Cicció, J.F. (2008) 'Chemical composition of *Schinus molle* essential oil and its cytotoxic activity on tumour cell lines.' *Natural Products Research 22*, 17, 1521–1534.

Dictionary.com. n.d. *Synergy* [Online]. Random House, Inc. Available at http://dictionary.reference.com/browse/synergy, accessed on 28 September 2014.

Diego, M.A., Jones, N.A., Field, T., Hernandez-Reif, M. *et al.* (1998) 'Aromatherapy positively affects mood, EEG patterns of alertness and math computations.' *International Journal of Neuroscience 96*, 217–224.

Dozmorov, M.G., Yang, Q., Wu, W., Wren, J. *et al.* (2014) 'Differential effects of selective frankincense (Ru Xiang) essential oil versus non-selective sandalwood (Tan Xiang) essential oil on cultured bladder cancer cells: a microarray and bioinformatics study.' *Chinese Medicine 9*, 18.

Dréno, B., Layton, A., Zouboulis, C., López-Estebaranz, J. *et al.* (2012) 'Adult female acne: a new paradigm.' *Journal of the European Academy of Dermatology and Venereology 27*, 1063–1070.

Du, J.R., Bai, B., Yu, Y., Wang, C.Y. and Qian, Z.M. (2005) 'The new progress of the study about volatile oil of the angelica.' *Zhongguo Zhong Yao Za Zhi 30*, 18, 1400–1406. (Article in Chinese.)

Edris, A.E. (2007) 'Pharmaceutical and therapeutic potentials of essential oils and their individual volatile constituents: a review.' *Phytotherapy Research 21*, 4, 308–323.

Edris, A.E. (2009) 'Anti-cancer properties of *Nigella* spp. essential oils and their major constituents, thymoquinone and elemene.' *Current Clinical Pharmacology 4*, 43–46. Cited by Bhalla, Y., Gupta, V.K. and Jaitak, V. (2013) 'Anticancer activity of essential oils: a review.' *Journal of the Science of Food and Agriculture 93*, 3643–3653.

Edwards-Jones, V., Buck, R., Shawcross, S.G., Dawson, M.M. and Dunn, K. (2004) 'The effect of essential oils on methicillin-resistant *Staphylococcus aureus* using a dressing model.' *Burns 30*, 8, 772–777.

Elliot, M.S.J., Abuhamdah, S., Howes, M-J.R., Lees, G. *et al.* (2007) 'The essential oils from *Melissa officinalis* L. and *Lavandula angustifolia* Mill. as potential treatment for agitation in people with severe dementia.' *International Journal of Essential Oil Therapeutics 1*, 4, 143–152.

Emamghoreishi, M., Khasaki, M. and Aazam, M.F. (2005) '*C. sativum*: evaluation of its anxiolytic effects in the elevated plus-maze.' *Journal of Ethnopharmacology 96*, 3, 365–370.

Emami, S.A., Asili, J., Rahimizadeh, M., Fazly-Bazzaz, B.S. and Hassanzadeh-Khayyat, M. (2006) 'Chemical and antimicrobial studies of *Cupressus sempervirens* L and *C. horizontalis* Mill. essential oils.' *Iranian Journal of Pharmaceutical Sciences 2*, 103–108.

Enshaieh, S., Jooya, A., Siadat, A.H. and Iraji, F. (2007) 'The efficacy of 5% topical tea tree oil gel in mild to moderate acne vulgaris: a randomized, double-blind, placebo-controlled study.' *Indian Journal of Dermatology, Venereology and Leprosy 73*, 1, 22–25.

Ersan, S., Bakir, S., Ersan, E.E. and Dogan, O. (2006) 'Examination of free radical metabolism and anti-oxidant defence system elements in patients with obsessive-compulsive disorder.' *Progress in Neuropsychpharmacology and Biological Psychiatry 30*, 6, 1039–1042. Cited by Zhang, Y., Wu, Y., Chen, T., Yao, L. *et al.* (2013) 'Assessing the metabolic effects of aromatherapy in human volunteers.' *Evidence-Based Complementary and Alternative Medicine*. Available at http://dx.doi.org/10.1155/2013/356381, accessed on 7 April 2015.

Fabbrocini, G., Padova, M., Cacciapuoti, S. and Tosti, A. (2012) 'Acne.' In Tosti, A., Grimes, P.E. and De Padova, M.P. (eds) *Color Atlas of Chemical Peels.* Berlin/Heidelberg: Springer.

Farrer-Halls, G. (2014) *The Spirit in Aromatherapy.* London: Singing Dragon.

Faturi, C.B., Leite, J.R., Alves, P.B., Canton, A.C. and Teixeira-Silva, F. (2010) 'Anxiolytic-like effect of sweet orange aroma in Wistar rats.' *Progress in Neuro-psychopharmacology and Biological Psychiatry 34*, 4, 605–609.

Fernández, L.F., Palomino, O.M. and Frutos, G. (2014) 'Effectiveness of *Rosmarinus officinalis* essential oil as antihypotensive agent in primary hypotensive patients and its influence on health-related quality of life.' *Journal of Ethnopharmacology 151*, 1, 509–516.

Fewell, F., McVicar, A., Gransby, R. and Morgan, P. (2007) 'Blood concentration and uptake of *d*-limonene during aromatherapy massage with sweet orange oil: a pilot study.' *International Journal of Essential Oil Therapeutics 1*, 97–102.

Fidelis, C.H.V., Augusto, F., Sampaio, P.T.B., Krainovic, P.M. and Barata, L.E.S. (2012) 'Chemical characterization of rosewood (*Aniba rosaeodora* Duke) leaf essential oil by comprehensive two-dimensional gas chromatography coupled with quadrupole mass spectrometry.' *Journal of Essential Oil Research 24*, 3, 245–251.

Field, T., Cullen, C., Largie, S., Diego, M., Schanberg, S. and Kuhn, C. (2008) 'Lavender bath oil reduces stress and crying and enhances sleep in very young infants.' *Early Human Development 84*, 399. Cited by Dobetsberger, C. and Buchbauer, G. (2011) 'Actions of essential oils on the central nervous system: an updated review.' *Flavour and Fragrance Journal 26*, 300–316.

Fowler, J.F., Woolery-Lloyd, H., Waldorf, H. and Saini, R. (2010) 'Innovations in natural ingredients and their use in skin care.' *Journal of Drugs in Dermatology 9*, 6, 72–81.

Franchomme, P. and Pénoël, D. (1990) *L'aromathérapie Exactement.* Limoges: Jallois.

Frank, M.B., Yang, Q., Osban, J., Azzarello, J.T. *et al.* (2009) 'Frankincense oil derived from *Boswellia carteri* induces tumour cell specific cytotoxicity.' *BMC Complementary and Alternative Medicine 9* (Article 6). Available at www.biomedcentral.com/1472-6882/9/6, accessed on 7 April 2015.

Frawley, D. and Lad, V. (1986) *The Yoga of Herbs.* Twin Lakes, WI: Lotus Press.

Freire, C.M.M., Marques, M.O.M. and Costa, M. (2006) 'Effects of seasonal variation on the central nervous system activity of *Ocimum gratissimum* L. essential oil.' *Journal of Ethnopharmacology 105*, 1–2, 161–166. Cited by de Almeida, R.N., Agra, M.F., Maior, F.N.S. and de Sousa, D.P. (2011) 'Essential oils and their constituents: anticonvulsant activity.' *Molecules 16*, 2726–2742.

Freyberg, R. and Ahren, M.-P. (2011) 'A preliminary trial exploring perfume preferences in adolescent girls.' *Journal of Sensory Studies 26*, 3, 237–243.

Fu, Y.-J., Zu, Y.-G., Chen, L.-Y., Shi, X.-G. *et al.* (2007) 'Antimicrobial activity of clove and rosemary essential oils alone and in combination.' *Phytotherapy Research 21*, 10, 989–994.

Fujiwara, R., Komori, T. Noda, Y., Kuraoka, T. *et al.* (1998) 'Effects of a long-term inhalation of fragrances on the stress-induced immunosuppression in mice.' *Neuroimmunomodulation 5*, 318–322. Cited by Trellakis, S., Fischer, C., Rydleuskaya, A., Tagay, S. *et al.* (2012) 'Subconscious olfactory influences of stimulant and relaxant odours on immune function.' *European Archives of Otorhinolaryngology 269*, 1909–1916.

Fukumoto, S., Morishita, A., Furutachi, K., Terashima, T., Nakayama, T. and Yokogoshi, H. (2007) 'Effect of flavour components in lemon essential oil on physical or psychological stress.' *Stress and Health 24*, 1, 3–12. Cited by Dobetsberger, C. and Buchbauer, G. (2011) 'Actions of essential oils on the central nervous system: an updated review.' *Flavour and Fragrance Journal 26*, 300–316.

Funk, J.L., Frye, J.B., Oyarzo, J.N., Zhang, H. and Timmermann, B.N. (2010) 'Anti-arthritic effects and toxicity of the essential oils of turmeric (*Curcuma longa L.*).' *Journal of Agricultural and Food Chemistry 58*, 2, 842–849.

Garozzo, A., Timpanaro, R., Bisignano, B., Furneri, P.M., Bisignano, G. and Castro, A. (2009) '*In vitro* antiviral activity of *Melaleuca alternifolia* essential oil.' *Letters in Applied Microbiology 49*, 6, 806–808.

Geiger, J.L. (2005) 'The essential oil of ginger, *Zingiber officinale*, and anaesthesia.' *International Journal of Aromatherapy 15*, 1, 7–14.

Giordani, R., Regli, P., Kaloustian, J., Mikail, C., Abou, L. and Portugal, H. (2004) 'Antifungal effect of various essential oils against *Candida albicans*. Potentiation of antifungal action of amphotericin B by essential oil from *Thymus vulgaris*.' *Phytotherapy Research 18*, 12, 990–995. Available at http://dx.doi.org/10.1002/ptr.1594, accessed on 7 April 2015.

Glišić, S.B., Svetomir, Ž., Milojević, S.Z., Dimitrijrvić, S.I., Orlović, A.M. and Skala, D.U. (2007) 'Antimicrobial activity of the essential oil and different fractions of *Juniperus communis* L. and a comparison with some commercial antibiotics.' *Journal of the Serbian Chemistry Society 72*, 4, 311–320.

Gobel, H., Schmidt, G. and Soyka, D. (1994) 'Effect of peppermint and eucalyptus oil preparations on neurophysiological and experimental algesimetric headache parameters.' *Cephalagia 14*, 228–234. Cited by Guimarães, A.G., Quintans, J.S.S. and Quintans-Júnior, L.J. (2013) 'Monoterpenes with analgesic activity: a systematic review.' *Phytotherapy Research 27*, 11–15.

Goes, T.C., Antunes, F.D., Alves, P.B. and Teixeira-Silva, F. (2012) 'Effect of sweet orange aroma on experimental anxiety in humans.' *Journal of Alternative and Complementary Medicine 18*, 8, 798–804.

Grassmann, J., Hippeli, S., Vollmann, R. and Elstner, F. (2003) 'Antioxididative properties of the essential oil from *Pinus mugo*.' *Journal of Agricultural and Food Chemistry 51*, 7576–7582.

Grassmann, J., Hippeli, S., Spitzenberger, R. and Elstner, F. (2005) 'The monoterpene terpinolene from the oil of *Pinus mugo* L. in concert with α-tocopherol and beta carotene effectively prevents oxidation of LDL.' *Phytomedicine 12*, 6–7, 416–423.

Gray, R. (2011) 'Why your special perfume is a very personal choice.' *Sunday Telegraph,* 9 October.

Greenway, F.L., Frome, B.M., Engels, T.M. and McLellan, A. (2003) 'Temporary relief of postherpetic neuralgia pain with topical geranium oil.' *American Journal of Medicine 115*, 7, 586–587.

Grieve, M. (1992) *A Modern Herbal*. London: Tiger Books International. (Original work published in 1931.)

Grosjean, N. (1992) *Aromatherapy from Provence*. Saffron Walden: C.W. Daniel Co. Ltd.

Guba, R. (2000) 'Toxicity myths: the actual risks of essential oil use.' *International Journal of Aromatherapy 10*, 1/2, 37–49.

Guedes, D.N., Silva, D.F., Barbosa-Filho, J.M. and de Medeiros, I.A. (2004a) 'Calcium antagonism and the vasorelaxation of the rat aorta induced by rotundifolone.' *Brazilian Journal of Medical and Biological Research 37*, 1881–1887.

Guedes, D.N., Silva, D., Barbosa-Filho, J. and de Medeiros, I. (2004b) 'Endothelium-dependent hypotensive and vasorelaxant effects of the essential oil from aerial parts of *Mentha × villosa* in rats.' *Phytomedicine 11*, 6, 490–497.

Guimarães, A.G., Quintans, J.S.S. and Quintans-Júnior, L.J. (2013) 'Monoterpenes with analgesic activity: a systematic review. *Phytotherapy Research 27*, 1, 1–15.

Guin, J.D., Meyer, B.N., Drake, R.D. and Haffley, P. (1984) 'The effect of quenching agents on contact urticaria caused by cinnamic aldehyde.' *Journal of the American Academy of Dermatology 10*, 45–51. Cited by Tisserand, R. and Young, R. (2014) *Essential Oil Safety.* (2nd edition.) Edinburgh: Churchill Livingstone.

Gulfraz, M., Mehmood, S., Minhas, N., Jabjeen, N. *et al.* (2008) 'Composition and antimicrobial properties of essential oil of *Foeniculum vulgare.*' *African Journal of Biotechnology 7*, 24, 4364–4368.

Hadji-Mingalou, F. and Bolcato, O. (2005) 'The potential role of specific essential oils in the replacement of dermacorticoid drugs.' *International Journal of Aromatherapy 15*, 2, 66–73.

Halvorsen, J. A., Stern, R.S., Dalgard, F. and Thoresen, M. (2011) 'Suicidal ideation, mental health problems and social impairment are increased in adolescents with acne: a population based survey.' *Journal of Investigative Dermatology 131*, 363–370.

Hanstock, T.L. and O'Mahony, J.F. (2002) 'Perfectionism, acne and appearance concerns.' *Personality And Individual Differences 32*, 1317–1325.

Harris, R. (2002) 'Synergism in the essential oil world.' *International Journal of Aromatherapy 12*, 179–186.

Harvala, C., Menounos, P. and Argyriadou, N. (1987) 'Essential oil from Salvia triloba.' *Fitoterapia 58*, 5, 353–356.

Hassan, J., Grogan, S., Clark-Carter, D., Richards, H. and Yates, V.M. (2009 'The individual health burden of acne: appearance-related distress in male and female adolescents and adults with back, chest and facial acne.' *Journal of Health Psychology 14*, 1105–1118.

Hatano, V.Y., Torricelli, A.S., Giassi, A.C., Coslope, L.A. and Vianna, M.B. (2012) 'Anxiolytic effects of repeated treatment, with an essential oil from *Lippia alba* and (R)-(+)-carvone in the elevated T-maze.' *Brazilian Journal of Medical and Biological Research 45*, 238–243.

Haug, T.T., Mykletun, A. and Dahl, A.A. (2002) 'Are anxiety and depression related to gastrointestinal symptoms in the general population?' *Scandinavian Journal of Gastroenterology 37*, 3, 294–298. Cited by Zhang, Y., Wu, Y., Chen, T., Yao, L. *et al.* (2013) 'Assessing the metabolic effects of aromatherapy in human volunteers.' *Evidence-Based Complementary and Alternative Medicine.* Available at http://dx.doi.org/10.1155/2013/356381, accessed on 7 April 2015.

Hayes, A.J. and Markovic, B. (2002) 'Toxicity of Australian essential oil *Backhousia citriodora* (lemon myrtle). Part 1. Antimicrobial activity and *in vitro* cytotoxicity.' *Food Chemistry and Cytotoxicology 40*, 535–543. Cited by Azimi, H., Fallah-Tafti, M., Khakshur, A.A. and Abdollahi, M. (2012) 'A review of the treatment of acne vulgaris: perspective of new pharmacological treatments.' *Fitoterapia 83*, 8, 1306–1317.

Haze, S., Sakai, K. and Gozu, Y. (2002) 'Effects of fragrance inhalation on sympathetic activity in normal adults.' *Japanese Journal of Pharmacology 90*, 247–253.

Heinrich, M., Barnes, J., Gibbons, S. and Williamson, E.M. (2004) *Fundamentals of Pharmacognosy and Phytotherapy.* Edinburgh: Churchill Livingstone.

Heuberger, E., Hongratanaworakit, T., Bohm, C., Weber, R. and Buchbauer, G. (2001) 'Effects of chiral fragrances on human autonomic nervous system parameters and self-evaluation.' *Chemical Senses 26*, 281–292.

Heuberger, E., Hongratanaworakit, T. and Buchbauer, G. (2006) 'East Indian sandalwood and α-santalol odor increase physiological and self-rated arousal in humans.' *Planta Medica 72*, 9, 792–800.

Heuskin, S., Godin, B., Leroy, P., Capella, Q. *et al.* (2009) 'Fast gas chromatography characterisation of purified semiochemicals from essential oils of *Matricaria chamomilla* L. (Asteraceae) and *Nepeta cataria* L. (Lamiaceae).' *Journal of Chromatography A 1216*, 2768–2775.

Hicks, A., Hicks, J. and Mole, P. (2011) *Five Elements Constitutional Acupuncture.* London: Elsevier.

Him, A., Ozbek, H., Turel, I. and Oner, A.C. (2008) 'Antinociceptive activity of alpha-pinene and fenchone.' *Pharmacologyonline 3*, 363–369. Cited by Guimarães, A.G., Quintans, J.S.S. and Quintans-Júnior, L.J. (2013) 'Monoterpenes with analgesic activity – a systematic review.' *Phytotherapy Research 27*, 1, 1–15.

Hinde, J. and Hozzel, M. (2015) Personal communication.

Hirota, R., Roger, N.N., Nakamura, H., Song, H.-S., Sawamura, M. and Suganuma, N. (2010) 'Anti-inflammatory effects of limonene from yuzu (*Citrus junos* Tanaka) essential oil on eosinophils.' *Journal of Food Science 75*, 87–92.

Hirsch, A., Ye, Y., Lu, Y. and Choe, M. (2007) 'The effects of the aroma of jasmine on bowling score.' *International Journal of Essential Oil Therapeutics 1*, 79–82.

Höferl, M., Stoilova, I., Schmidt, E., Wanner, J. *et al.* (2014) 'Chemical composition and anti-oxidant properties of juniper berry (*Juniperus communis* L.) essential oil. Action of the essential oil on the anti-oxidant protection of *Saccharomyces cerevisiae* model organism. *Anti-oxidants 3*, 81–98.

Holmes, P. (1996) 'Ginger: warmth and soul strength.' *International Journal of Aromatherapy 7*, 4, 16–19.

Holmes, P. (1997) *Fragrance Energetics: a Working Model of Holistic Aromapharmacology.* Aroma 97 Seminar presentation at warwick University. Brighton: Aromatherapy Publications.

Holmes, P. (1998/1999) 'Energy medicine: aromatherapy past and present.' *International Journal of Aromatherapy 9*, 2, 53–56.

Holmes, P. (2001) *Clinical Aromatherapy.* Boulder, CO: Tigerlily Press Inc.

Hongratanaworakit, T. (2009a) 'Relaxing effects of rose on humans.' *Natural Product Communications 4*, 2, 291. Cited by Dobetsberger, C. and Buchbauer, G. (2011) 'Actions of essential oils on the central nervous system: an updated review.' *Flavour and Fragrance Journal 26*, 300–316.

Hongratanaworakit, T. (2009b) 'Simultaneous aromatherapy massage with rosemary oil on humans.' *Scientica Pharmaceutica 77*, 375–387. Cited by Dobetsberger, C. and Buchbauer, G. (2011) 'Actions of essential oils on the central nervous system: an updated review.' *Flavour and Fragrance Journal 26*, 5, 300–316.

Hongratanaworakit, T. (2010) 'Stimulating effect of aromatherapy massage with jasmine oil.' *Natural Product Communications 5*, 1, 157.

Hongratanaworakit, T. (2011) 'Aroma-therapeutic effects of massage blended essential oils on humans.' *Natural Product Communications 6*, 8, 1199.

Hongratanaworakit, T. and Buchbauer, G. (2004) 'Evaluation of the harmonizing effect of ylang ylang on humans after inhalation.' *Planta Medica 70*, 7, 632–636.

Hongratanaworakit, T. and Buchbauer, G. (2006) 'Relaxing effect of ylang ylang on humans after transdermal absorption.' *Phytotherapy Research 20*, 9, 758–763.

Hongratanaworakit, T. and Buchbauer, G. (2007a) 'Chemical composition and stimulating effect of *Citrus hystrix* oil on humans.' *Flavour and Fragrance Journal 22*, 443–449.

Hongratanaworakit, T. and Buchbauer, G. (2007b) 'Autonomic and emotional responses after transdermal absorption of sweet orange oil in humans: placebo controlled trial.' *International Journal of Essential Oil Therapeutics 1*, 29–34.

Hongratanaworakit, T., Heuberger, E. and Buchbauer, G. (2004) 'Evaluation of the effects of East Indian sandalwood oil and α-santalol on humans after transdermal absorption.' *Planta Medica 70*, 1, 3–7.

Hosseini, M., Rakhsandah, H., Shafieenic, R. and Dolati, K. (2003) 'Analgesic Effect of *Rosa damascena* on Mice.' In *Abstract Book of 16th Iranian Congress of Physiology and Pharmacology.* Cited by Boskabady, M.H., Kiani, S. and Rakhshandah, H. (2006) 'Relaxant effects of *Rosa damascena* on guinea pig tracheal chains and its possible mechanism(s).' *Journal of Ethnopharmacology 106*, 377–382.

Hoya, Y., Matsumura, I., Fujita, T. and Yanaga, K. (2008) 'The use of nonpharmacological interventions to reduce anxiety in patients undergoing gastroscopy in a setting with an optimal soothing environment.' *Gastroenterology Nursing 31*, 6, 395–399. Cited by Dobetsberger, C. and Buchbauer, G. (2011) 'Actions of essential oils on the central nervous system: an updated review.' *Flavour and Fragrance Journal 26*, 300–316.

Hsu, H.C., Yang, W.C., Tsai, W.J., Chen, C.-C., Huang, H.-Y. and Tsai Y.-C. (2006) 'Alpha-bulnesene, a novel PAF receptor antagonist isolated from *Pogostemon cablin.' Biochemical and Biophysical Research Communications 345*, 1033–1038. Cited by Tisserand, R. and Young, R. (2014) *Essential Oil Safety.* Edinburgh: Churchill Livingstone.

Hu, L.F., Li, S.P., Cao, H., Liu, J.J. *et al.* (2006) 'GC-MS fingerprint of *Pogostemon cablin* in China.' *Journal of Pharmaceutical and Biomedical Analysis 42*, 200–206.

Huseini, H.F., Amini, M., Mohtashami, R., Ghamarchehre, M.E. *et al.* (2013) 'Blood pressure lowering effect of *Nigella sativa* L. seed oil in healthy volunteers: a randomised, double-blind, placebo-controlled clinical trial.' *Phytotherapy Research 27*, 12, 1849–1853.

Hussain, H., Al-Harrasi, A., Al-Rawahi, A. and Hussain, J. (2013) 'Chemistry and biology of essential oils of genus *Boswellia*.' *Evidence-Based Complementary and Alternative Medicine.* doi: 10.1155/2013/140509.

Hwang, J.H. (2006) 'The effects of the inhalation method using essential oils on blood pressure and stress responses of clients with essential hypertension.' *Taehan Kanhoe Hakhoe Chi 36*, 7, 1123–1134. (Article in Korean.) Available at www.ncbi.nlm.nih.gov/pubmed/17211115, accessed on 7 April 2015.

Ilhan, A., Gurel, A., Armutcu, F., Kamisli, S. and Iraz, M. (2005) 'Antiepileptogenic and anti-oxidant effects of *Nigella sativa* oil against pentylenetetrazol-induced kindling in mice.' *Neuropharmacology 49*, 456–464. Cited by de Almeida, R.N., Agra, M.F., Maior, F.N.S. and de Sousa, D.P. (2011) 'Essential oils and their constituents: anticonvulsant activity.' *Molecules 16*, 2726–2742.

Ilmberger, J., Heuberger, E., Mahrhofer, C., Dessovic, H., Kowarik, D. and Buchbauer, G. (2001) 'The influence of essential oils on human attention 1: alertness.' *Chemical Senses 26*, 239–245.

Innocenti, G., Dall'Acqua, S., Scialino, G., Banfi, E. *et al.* (2010) 'Chemical composition and biological properties of *Rhododendron anthopogon* essential oil.' *Molecules 15*, 2326–2338.

Ishikawa, J., Shimotoyodome, Y., Chen, S., Ohkubo, K. *et al.* (2012) 'Eucalyptus increases ceramide levels in keratinocytes and improves stratum corneum function.' *International Journal of Cosmetic Science 34*, 17–22.

Ismail, M. (2006) 'Central properties and chemical composition of *Ocimum basilicum* essential oil.' *Pharmaceutical Biology 44*, 619–626. Cited by de Almeida, R.N., Agra, M.F., Maior, F.N.S. and de Sousa, D.P. (2011) 'Essential oils and their constituents: anticonvulsant activity.' *Molecules 16*, 2726–2742.

Itai, T., Amayasu, H., Kuribayashi, M., Kawamura, N. *et al.* (2000) 'Psychological effects of aromatherapy on chronic hemodialysis patients.' *Psychiatry and Clinical Neurosciences 54*, 4 393–397.

Itani, W.S., El-Banna, S.H., Hassan, S.B., Larsson, R.L., Bazarbachi, A. and Gali-Muhtasib, H.U. (2008) 'Anti-colon cancer components from Lebanese sage (*Salvia libanotica*) essential oil.' *Cancer Biology and Therapy 7*, 11, 1765–1773. Cited by Tisserand, R. and Young, R. (2014) *Essential Oil Safety.* (2nd edition.) Edinburgh: Churchill Livingstone.

Jacob, J.N. and Badyal, D.K. (2014) 'Biological studies of turmeric oil, part 3: anti-inflammatory and analgesic properites of turmeric oil and fish oil in comparison with aspirin.' *Natural Product Communications 9*, 2, 225–228.

Jaén, C. and Dalton, P. (2014) 'Asthma and odours: the role of risk perception in asthma exacerbation.' *Journal of Psychosomatic Research 77*, 4, 302–308.

Jaganthan, S.K. and Supriyanto, E. (2012) 'Antiproliferative and molecular mechanism of eugenol-induced apoptosis in cancer cells.' *Molecules 17*, 6290–6304.

Jain, R., Aqil, M., Ahad, A., Ali, A. and Khar, R.K. (2008) 'Basil oil is a promising skin penetration enhancer for transdermal delivery of labetolol hydrochloride.' *Drug Development and Industrial Pharmacy 34*, 4, 384–389. Cited by Adorjan, B. and Buchbauer, G. (2010) 'Biological properties of essential oils: an updated review.' *Flavour and Fragrance Journal 25*, 407–426.

James, A. (2014) Personal communication.

Jamshidi, R., Afzali, Z. and Afzali, D. (2009) 'Chemical composition of hydrodistillation essential oil of rosemary in different origins in iran and comparison with other countries.' *American–Eurasian Journal of Agricultural and Environmental Sciences 5*, 78–81.

Janahmadi, M., Niazi, F., Danyali, S. and Kamalinejad, M. (2006) 'Effects of the fruit essential oil of *Cuminum cyminum* Linn. (Apiaceae) on pentylenetetrazol-induced epileptiform activity in F1 neurones of *Helix aspera*.' *Journal of Ethnopharmacology 104*, 1–2, 278–282.

Jasicka, I., Lipok, J., Nowakowska, E.M., Wieczorek, P.P., Mylnarz, P. and Kafarsli, P.Z. (2004) 'Antifungal activity of the carrot seed oil and its major sesquiterpene compounds.' *Zeitschrift für Naturforschung C 59*, 11–12, 791–796. Cited by Abad, M.J., Ansuategui, M. and Bermejo, P. (2007) 'Active antifungal substances from natural sources.' *ARKIVOC 7*, 116–145.

Jeenapongsa, R., Yoovathaworn, K., Sriwatanakul, K.M., Pongprayoon, U. and Sriwatanakul, K. (2003) 'Anti-inflammatory activity of (E)–1-(1,3,4-dimethoxyphenyl) butadiene from *Zingiber cassumunar* Roxb.' *Journal of Ethnopharmacology 87*, 2–3, 143–148.

Jeong, J.B., Choi, J., Jiang, X. and Lee, S.H. (2013) 'Patchouli alcohol, an essential oil of *Pogostemon cablin*, exhibits anti–tumorigenic activity in human colorectal cancer cells.' *International Immunopharmacology 16*, 2, 184–190.

Jellinek, J.S. (1997) 'Psychodynamic odor effects and their mechanisms.' *Perfumer and Flavorist 22*, 29–41.

Jirovetz, L., Eller, G., Buchbauer, G., Schmidt, E. *et al.* (2006) 'Chemical composition, antimicrobial activities, and odor descriptions of some essential oils with characteristic floral-rosy scent and of their principal aroma compounds.' *Recent Developments in Agronomy and Horticulture 2*, 1–12.

Joint Formulary Committee (2010) *British National Formulary.* [Online]. London. Accessed on 21 April 2010 at http://bnf.org/bnf/bnf/current/6004.htm.

Jorge, A.T.S., Arroteia, K.F., Lago, J.C., de Sá-Rocha, V.M., Gesztesi, J. and Moreira, P.L. (2011) 'A new potent natural anti-oxidant mixture provides global protection against oxidative skin cell damage.' *International Journal of Cosmetic Science 33*, 113–119.

Joseph, D. and Sterling, A. (2009) 'The psychological effects of acne in teenagers.' *Practice Nursing 20*, 232–238.

Kagawa, D., Jokura, H., Ochiai, R., Tokimitsu, I. and Tsubone, H. (2003) 'The sedative effects and mechanism of action of cedrol inhalation with behavioural pharmacological evaluation. *Planta Medica 69*, 637–641.

Kang, P., Han, S.H., Moon, H.K., Lee, J.-M. *et al.* (2013) '*Citrus bergamia* Risso elevates intracellular Ca^{2+} in human vascular endothelial cells due to release of Ca^{2+} from primary intracellular stores.' *Evidence-Based Complementary and Alternative Medicine*, Article ID 759615. Available at http://dx.doi.org/10.1155/2013/759615, accessed on 7 April 2015.

Kanlayavattanakul, M. and Lourith, N. (2011) 'Therapeutic agents and herbs in topical applications for acne treatment.' *International Journal of Cosmetic Science 33*, 4, 289–297.

Kar, K., Puri, V.N., Patnaik, G.K., Sur, R.N., Dhawan, B.N., Kulshrestha, D.K. and Rastogi, R.P. (1975) 'Spasmolytic constituents of Cedrus deodora (Roxb.) Loud: pharmacological evaluation of himachalol.' *Journal of Pharmaceutical Science 64*, 2, 258–262. Cited by Burfield, T. (2002) 'Cedarwood oils.' *The Cropwatch Series*. Available at www.cropwatch.org, accessed on 31 November 2011.

Karimian, P., Kavoosi, G. and Amirghofran, Z. (2014) 'Anti-oxidative and anti-inflammatory effects of *Tagetes minuta* essential oil in activated macrophages'. *Asian Pacific Journal of Tropical Biomedicine 4*, 3, 219–227.

Karpouhtsis, I., Pardali, E., Feggou, E., Kokkini, S., Scouras, Z.G. and Mavragani-Tsipidou, P. (1998) 'Insecticidal and genotoxic activities of oregano essential oils.' *Journal of Agricultural and Food Chemistry 46*, 1111–1115. Cited by Tisserand, R. and Young, R. (2014) *Essential Oil Safety.* (2nd edition.) Edinburgh: Churchill Livingstone.

Kathirvel, P. and Ravi, S. (2012) 'Chemical composition of the essential oil from basil (*Ocimum basilicum* Linn.) and its *in vitro* cytotoxicity against HeLa and Hep-2 human cancer cell lines and NIH 3T3 mouse embryonic fibroblasts.' *Natural Products Research 26*, 1112–1118.

Kennedy, D.O., Little, W., Haskell, C.F. and Scholey, A.B. (2006) 'Anxiolytic effects of a combination of *Melissa officinalis* and *Valeriana officinalis* during laboratory induced stress.' *Phytotherapy Research 20*, 2, 96–102.

Kennedy, D.O., Dodd, F.L., Robertson, B.C., Okello, E.J. *et al.* (2010) 'Monoterpenoid extract of sage (*Salvia lavandulaefolia*) with cholinesterase inhibiting properties improves cognitive performance and mood in healthy adults.' *Journal of Psychopharmacology 25*, 1088.

Khan, A., Ahmad, A., Manzoor, N. and Khan, L.A. (2010) 'Antifungal activities of *Ocimum sanctum* essential oil and its lead molecules.' *Natural Product Communications 5*, 2, 345–349. Cited by Lang, G. and Buchbauer, G. (2012) 'A review on recent research results (2008–2010) on essential oils as antimicrobials and antifungals. A review.' *Flavour and Fragrance Journal 27*, 13–39.

Khan, M.A., Chen, H., Tania, M. and Zhang, D. (2011) 'Anticancer activities of *Nigella sativa* (black cumin).' *African Journal of Traditional, Complementary and Alternative Medicines 8*, 5, 226–232.

Khodabakhsh, P., Shafaroodi, H. and Asgarpanah, J. (2015) 'Analgesic and anti-inflammatory activities of *Citrus aurantium* L. blossoms essential oil (neroli): involvement of the nitric oxide/cyclic-guanosine monophosphate pathway.' *Journal of Natural Medicine 69*, 3, 324–331.

Khondker, L., Rahman, M., Mahmud, M., Khan, M., Khan, H. and Kabir, H. (2012) 'Pattern of *acne vulgaris* in women attending in a tertiary care hospital.' *Journal of Dhaka National Medical College and Hospital 18*, 18–23.

Kim, B.J., Kim, J.H., Kim, H.P. and Heo, M.Y. (1997) 'Biological screening of 100 plant extracts for cosmetic use (II): Anti-oxidative activity and free radical scavenging activity.' *International Journal of Cosmetic Science 19*, 6, 299–307.

Kim, H.M. and Cho, S.H. (1999) 'Lavender oil inhibits immediate-type allergic reaction in mice and rats.' *Journal of Pharmacy and Pharmacology 51*, 221–226. Cited by Tisserand, R. and Young, R. (2014) *Essential Oil Safety.* (2nd edition.) Edinburgh: Churchill Livingstone.

Kim, H.-J., Chen, W., Wu, C., Wang, X. and Chung, H.Y. (2004) 'Evaluation of anti-oxidant activity of Australian tea tree (*Melaleuca alternifolia*) oil and its components.' *Journal of Agricultural and Food Chemistry 52*, 2849–2854.

Kim, I.-H., Kim, C., Seong, K., Hur, M.-H., Lim, H.M. and Lee, M.S. (2012) 'Essential oil inhalation on blood pressure and salivary cortisol levels in prehypertensive and hypertensive subjects.' *Evidence-Based Complementary and Alternative Medicine.* http://dx.doi.org/10.1155/2012/984203.

Kim, J.-H., Choi, D.-K., Lee, S.-S., Choi, S.J. *et al.* (2010) 'Enhancement of keratinocyte differentiation by rose absolute oil.' *Annals of Dermatology 22*, 3, 255–261.

Kim, K., Bu, Y., Jeong, S., Lim, J. *et al.* (2006) 'Memory-enhancing effect of a supercritical carbon dioxide fluid extract of the needles of *Abies koreana* on scopolamine-induced amnesia in mice.' *Bioscience Biotechnology and Biochemistry 70*, 1821–1826.

Kim, K.T., Ren, C.J., Fielding, G.A., Pitti, A. *et al.* (2007) 'Treatment with lavender aromatherapy in the post-anesthesia care unit reduces opioid requirements of morbidly obese patients undergoing laparoscopic adjustable gastric banding.' *Obesity Surgery 17*, 7, 920–925.

Kim, M.-J., Yang, K.-W., Kim, S.S., Park, S.M. *et al.* (2013a) 'Chemical composition and anti-inflammatory effects of essential oil from Hallabong flower.' *EXCLI Journal 12*, 933–942.

Kim, S.H., Lee, S.Y., Hong, C.Y., Gwak, K.S. *et al.* (2013b) 'Whitening and anti-oxidant activities of bornyl acetate and nezukol fractionated from *Cryptomeria japonica* essential oil.' *International Journal of Cosmetic Science 35*, 5, 484–490.

Kim, S.S., Baik, J.S., Oh, T.H., Yoon, W.J., Lee, N.H. and Hyun, C.G. (2008) 'Biological activities of Korean Citrus obovoides and Citrus natsudaidai essential oils against acne-inducing bacteria.' *Bioscience, Biotechnology and Biochemistry 72*, 10, 2507–2513.

King, J.R. (1983) 'Have the scents to relax?' *World Medicine 19*, 29–31.

King, J.R. (1988) 'Anxiety Reduction using Fragrances.' In S. Van Toller and G.H. Dodd (eds) *Perfumery: The Psychology and Biology of Fragrance*. London: Chapman & Hall.

Kirk-Smith, M., Van Toller, S. and Dodd, G.H. (1983) 'Unconscious odour conditioning in human subjects.' *Biological Psychology 17*, 221–231.

Kitikannakorn, N., Chaiyakunapruk, N., Nimpitakpong, P., Dilokthornsakul, P., Meepoo, E. and Kerdpeng, W. (2013) 'An overview of the evidences of herbals for smoking cessation.' *Complementary Therapies in Medicine 21*, 5, 557–564.

Knasko, S., Gilbert, A.N. and Sabini, J. (1990) 'Emotional state, physical well-being, and performance in the presence of feigned ambient odour.' *Journal of Applied Social Psychology 20*, 1345–1357. Cited by Ilmberger, J., Heuberger, E., Mahrhofer, C., Dessovic, H., Kowarik, D. and Buchbauer, G. (2001) 'The influence of essential oils on human attention 1: Alertness.' *Chemical Senses 26*, 239–245.

Koh, K., Pearce, A., Marshama, G., Finlay-Jones, J. and Hart, P. (2002) 'Tea tree oil reduces histamine-induced skin inflammation.' *British Journal of Dermatology 147*, 1212–1217.

Komeh-Nkrumah, S.A., Nanjundaiah, S.M., Rajaiah, R., Yu, H. and Moudgil, K.D. (2012) 'Topical dermal application of essential oils attenuates the severity of adjuvant arthritis in Lewis rats.' *Phytotherapy Research 26*, 1, 54–59.

Komori, T. (2009) 'Effects of lemon and valerian inhalation on autonomic nerve activity in depressed and healthy subjects.' *International Journal of Essential Oil Therapeutics 3*, 1, 3–8.

Komori, T., Matsumoto, T., Yamamoto, M., Motomura, T., Shiroyama, T. and Okazaki, Y. (2006) 'Application of fragrance in discontinuing the long-term use of hypnotic benzodiazepines.' *International Journal of Aromatherapy 16*, 1, 3–7.

Kordali, S., Cakir, A., Mavi, A., Kilic, H. and Yildirim, A. (2005) 'Screening of chemical composition and antifungal and anti-oxidant activities of the essential oils from three Turkish *Artemisia* species.' *Journal of Agricultural and Food Chemistry 53*, 5, 1408–1416.

Kuloglu, M., Atmaca, M., Tezcan, E., Ustundag, B. and Bulut, S. (2002) 'Antioxidant enzyme and malondialdehyde levels in patients with panic disorder.' *Neuropsychobiology 46*, 4, 186–189. Cited by Zhang, Y., Wu, Y., Chen, T., Yao, L., Liu, J., Pan, X., Hu, Y., Zhao, A., Xie, G. and Jia, W. (2013) 'Assessing the metabolic effects of aromatherapy in human volunteers.' Evidence-Based Complementary and Alternative Medicine. Available at http://dx.doi.org/10.1155/2013/356381, accessed on 11 June 2015.

Kumar, A., Panghai, S., Mallapur, S.S., Kumar, M., Ram, V. and Singh, B.K. (2009) 'Anti-inflammatory activity of *Piper longum* fruit oil.' *Indian Journal of Pharmaceutical Science 71*, 4, 454–456.

Kuriyama, H., Watanabe, S., Nakaya, T., Shigemori, I. *et al.* (2005) 'Immunological and psychological benefits of aromatherapy massage.' *eCAM 2*, 2, 179–184.

Kusmirek, J. (2002) *Liquid Sunshine: Vegetable Oils for Aromatherapy*. Glastonbury: Floramicus.

Lagalante, A.F. and Montgomery, M.E. (2003) 'Analysis of terpenoids from hemlock (*Tsuga*) species by solid-phase microextraction/gas chromatography/ion-trap mass spectrometry.' *Journal of Agricultural and Food Chemistry 51*, 2115–2120.

Lahlou, S., Carneira-Leão, R.F.L., Leal-Cardoso, J.H. and Toscano, C.F. (2001) 'Cardiovascular effects of the essential oil of *Mentha × villosa* and its main constituent, piperitenone oxide, in normotensive anaesthetised rats: role of the autonomic nervous system.' *Planta Medica 67*, 7, 638–643.

Lahlou, S., Leal-Cardoso, J.H. and Duarte, G. (2003) 'Anti-hypertensive effects of the essential oil of *Alpinia zerumbet* and its main constituent, terpinen-4-ol, in DOCA-salt hypertensive rats: role of the autonomic nervous system.' *Fundamental and Clinical Pharmacology 17*, 323–330.

Lahlou, S., Interaminense, F., Leal-Cardoso, J., Morais, S. and Duarte, G. (2004) 'Cardiovascular effects of the essential oil of *Ocimum gratissimum* leaves in rats: role of the autonomic nervous system.' *Clinical and Experimental Pharmacology and Physiology 1*, 219–225.

Lam, L.K. and Zeng, B. (1991) 'Effects of essential oils on glutathione S-transferase activity in mice.' *Journal of Agricultural and Food Chemistry 39*, 660–662. Cited by Tisserand, R. and Young, R. (2014) *Essential Oil Safety*. (2nd edition.) Edinburgh: Churchill Livingstone.

Lang, G. and Buchbauer, G. (2012) 'A review on recent research results (2008–2010) on essential oils as antimicrobials and antifungals. A review.' *Flavour and Fragrance Journal 27*, 13–39.

Langeveld, W.T., Veldhuizen, E.J. and Burt, S.A. (2014) 'Synergy between essential oil components and antibiotics: a review.' *Critical Reviews in Microbiology 40*, 1, 76–94.

Lavabre, M. (1990) *Aromatherapy Workbook*. Rochester, VT: Healing Arts Press.

Lawless, A. (2009) *Artisan Perfumery: Or Being Led by the Nose*. Stroud: Boronia Souk Ltd.

Lawless, A. (2010) 'The ordinary mind, perfume and natural health.' Available at http://aleclawless. blogspot.co.uk/2010/10/ordinary-mind-perfume-and-natural.html, accessed on 10 June 2015.

Lawless, J. (1992) *The Encyclopaedia of Essential Oils*. Shaftesbury: Element Books.

Lawless, J. (1994) *Aromatherapy and the Mind*. London: Thorsons.

Lee, B., Kim, J., Jung, J., Choi, J.W. *et al.* (2005) 'Myristicin-induced neurotoxicity in human neuroblastoma SK-N-SH cells.' *Toxicology Letters 157*, 1, 49–56. Cited by Edris, A.E. (2007) 'Pharmaceutical and therapeutic potentials of essential oils and their individual volatile constituents: a review.' *Phytotherapy Research 21*, 4, 308–323.

Lee, Y.L., Wu, Y., Tsang, H.W., Leung, A.Y. and Cheung, W.M. (2011) 'A systematic review on the anxiolytic effects of aromatherapy in people with anxiety symptoms.' *Journal of Alternative and Complementary Medicine 17*, 2, 101–108.

Leelarungrayub, D. and Suttagit, M. (2009) 'Potential antioxidant and anti-inflammatory activities of Thai plai (Zingiber cassumunar Roxb.) essential oil.' *International Journal of Essential Oil Therapeutics 3*, 1, 25–30.

Legault, J. and Pichette, A. (2007) 'Potentiating the effect of beta-caryophyllene on anticancer effects of alpha-humulene, isocaryophyllene and paclitaxel.' *Journal of Pharmacy and Pharmacololgy 59*, 12, 6643–6647. Cited by Adorjan, B. and Buchbauer, G. (2010) 'Biological properties of essential oils: an updated review.' *Flavour and Fragrance Journal 25*, 407–426.

Lenochová, P., Vohnoutová, P., Roberts, S.C., Oberzaucher, E., Grammer, K. and Havlíček, J. (2012) 'Psychology of fragrance use: perception of individual odor and perfume blends reveals a mechanism for idiosyncratic effects on fragrance choice.' *PLoS ONE 7*, 3, e33810, 1–10.

Lertsatitthanakorn, P., Taweechaisupapong, S., Aromdee, C. and Khunkitti, W. (2006) '*In vitro* bioactivities of essential oils used for acne control.' *International Journal of Aromatherapy 16*, 1, 43–49.

Liapi, C., Anifantis, G., Chinou, I., Kourunakis, A.P., Theodosopoulos, S. and Galanopoulou, P. (2007) 'Anti-nociceptive properties of 1,8-cineole and β-pinene, from the essential oil of *Eucalyptus camadulensis* leaves, in rodents.' *Planta Medica 73*, 1247–1254.

Liapi, C., Anifandis, G., Chinou, I., Kourounakis, A.P., Theodosopoulos, S. and Galanopoulou, P. (2008) 'Anti-nociceptive properties of 1,8-cineole and beta-pinene, from the essential oil of *Eucalyptus camaldulensis* leaves, in rodents.' *Planta Medica 74*, 7, 789. Cited by Adorjan, B. and Buchbauer, G. (2010) 'Biological properties of essential oils: an updated review.' *Flavour and Fragrance Journal 25*, 407–426.

Liju, V.B., Jeena, K. and Kuttan, R. (2011) 'An evaluation of anti-oxidant, anti-inflammatory and anti-nociceptive activities of essential oil from *Curcuma longa* L.' *Indian Journal of Pharmacology 43*, 5, 526–531.

Lima, D.F., Brandão, M.S., Moura, J.B., Leitão, J.M. *et al.* (2012a) 'Anti-nociceptive activity of the monoterpene α-phellandrene in rodents: possible mechanisms of action.' *Journal of Pharmacognosy and Phytotherapy 64*, 283–292. Cited by Guimarães, A.G., Quintans, J.S.S. and Quintans-Júnior, L.J. (2013) 'Monoterpenes with analgesic activity: a systematic review.' *Phytotherapy Research 27*, 1, 1–15.

Lima, T.C., Mota, M.M., Barbossa-Filho, J.M., dos Santos, M.R.V. and de Sousa, D.P. (2012b) 'Structural relationships and vasorelaxant activity of monoterpenes.' *DARU Journal of Pharmaceutical Sciences 20, 23*. Available at www.darujps.com/content/20/1/23, accessed on 7 April 2015.

Lima, N.G., de Sousa, D.P., Pimenta, F.C., Alves, M.F. and de Sousa, F.S. (2012c) 'Anxiolytic-like activity and GC-MS analysis of (R)-(+)-limonene fragrance, a natural compound found in foods and plants.' *Pharmacology, Biochemistry and Behavior 103*, 450–454. Cited by de Sousa (2012) 'Anxiolytic essential oils.' *Natural Products Chemistry and Research 1*, e102. doi: 10.4172/npcr.1000e102.

Limwattananon, C., Rattanachotphanit, T., Cheawchanwattana, A., Waleekhachonloet, O. *et al.* (2008) 'Clinical efficacy of plai gel containing 1% plai oil in the treatment of mild to moderate acne vulgaris.' *Indian Journal of Pharmaceutical Sciences 1*, 2, 121–133.

Linck, V.M., da Silva, A.L., Figueiró, M., Caramão, E.B., Moreno, P.R.H. and Elisabetsky, E. (2010) 'Effects of inhaled linalool in anxiety, social interaction and aggressive behaviour in mice.' *Phytomedicine 17*, 8–9, 679–683.

Lodén, M., Buraczewska, I. and Halvarsson, K. (2007) 'Facial anti-wrinkle cream: influence of product presentation on effectiveness: a randomised and controlled study.' *Skin Research and Technology 13*, 189–194.

Loizzo, M.R., Saab, A.M., Tundis, R., Statti, G.A. *et al.* (2008a) 'Phytochemical analysis and *in vitro* antiviral activities of the essential oils of seven Lebanon species.' *Chemistry and Biodiversity 5*, 3, 461–470. Cited by Adorjan, B. and Buchbauer, G. (2010) 'Biological properties of essential oils: an updated review.' *Flavour and Fragrance Journal 25*, 407–426.

Loizzo, M.R., Saab, A.M., Tundis, R., Statti, G.A. *et al.* (2008b) 'Phytochemical analysis and *in vitro* evaluation of the biological activity against herpes simplex virus type 1 (HSV–1) of *Cedrus libani* A. Rich.' *Phytomedicine 15*, 1–2, 79–83.

Lorenzi, V., Muselli, A., Bernardini, A.F., Berti, L. *et al.* (2009) 'Geraniol restores antibiotic activities against multidrug-resistant isolates from Gram-negative species.' *Antimicrobial Agents and Chemotherapy 53*, 5, 2209–2211.

Loupattarakasem, W., Kowsuwon, W., Loupattarakasem, P. and Eungpinitpong, W. (1993) 'Efficacy of *Zingiber cassumunar* Roxb. (Plygesal) in the treatment of ankle sprain.' *Srinagarind Medical Journal 8*, 3, 159–164.

Luangnarumitchai, S., Lamlertthon, S. and Tiaboonchai, W. (2007) 'Antimicrobial activity of essential oils against five strains of Propionibacterium acnes.' *Mahidol University Journal of Pharmaceutical Sciences 34*, 1–4, 60–64.

Lv, X.N., Liu, Z.J., Zhang, H.J. and Tzeng, C.M. (2013) 'Aromatherapy and the central nerve system (CNS): therapeutic mechanisms and associated genes.' *Current Drug Targets 14*, 872–879.

Machado, D.G., Kaster, M.P., Binafaré, R.W., Dias, M. *et al.* (2007) 'Antidepressant-like effect of the extract from the leaves of *Schinus molle* in mice: evidence for the involvement of the monoaminergic system.' *Progress in Neuropsychopharmacology Biology and Psychiatry 31*, 2, 421–428.

Machado, D.G., Bettio, L.E., Cunha, M.P., Capra, J.C. *et al.* (2009) 'Antidepressant-like effect of the extract of *Rosmarinus officinalis* in mice: involvement of the monoaminergic system.' *Progress in Neuropsychopharmacology Biology and Psychiatry 33*, 4, 642–650.

Magin, P., Adams, J., Heading, G., Pond, D. and Smith, W. (2006) 'Psychological sequelae of *acne vulgaris*: results of a qualitative study.' *Canadian Family Physician 52*, 979–1005.

Magin, P., Adams, J., Heading, G., Pond, D. and Smith, W. (2008) 'Experiences of appearance-related teasing and bullying in skin diseases and their psychological sequelae: results of a qualitative study.' *Scandinavian Journal of Caring Sciences 22*, 430–436.

Mahalwal, V.S. and Ali, M. (2002) 'Volatile constituents of the rhizomes of *Nardostachys jatamansi* DC.' *Journal of Essential Oil Bearing Plants 5*, 83–89. Cited by Tisserand, R. and Young, R. (2014) *Essential Oil Safety.* (2nd edition.) Edinburgh: Churchill Livingstone.

Mahboubi, M. and Ghazian Bidgoli, F. (2010) '*In vitro* synergistic efficacy of combination of amphotericin B with *Myrtus communis* essential oil against clinical isolates of *Candida albicans*.' *Phytomedicine 17*, 10, 771–774. Cited by Lang, G. and Buchbauer, G. (2012) 'A review on recent research results (2008–2010) on essential oils as antimicrobials and antifungals. A review.' *Flavour and Fragrance Journal 27*, 13–39.

Mahendra, P. and Bischt, S. (2011) 'Anti-anxiety activity of *Coriandrum sativum* assessed using different experimental anxiety models.' *Indian Journal of Pharmacology 43*, 5, 574.

Mailhebiau, P. (1995) *Portraits in Oils.* Saffron Walden: C.W. Daniel Co. Ltd.

Maleki, N.A., Maleki, S.A. and Bekhradi, R. (2013) 'Supressive effects of *Rosa damascena* essential oil on naloxone-precipitated morphine withdrawal signs in male mice.' *Iranian Journal of Pharmaceutical Research 12*, 3, 357–361.

Mallon, E., Newton, J.N., Klassen, A., StewartBrown, S.L., Ryan, T.J., and Finlay, A.Y. (1999) 'The quality of life in acne: a comparison with general medical conditions using generic questionnaires.' *British Journal of Dermatology 140*, 672–676.

Manosroi, J., Dhumtanom, P. and Manosroi, A. (2006) 'Anti-proliferative activity of essential oil extracted from Thai medicinal plants on KB and P388 cell lines.' *Cancer Letters 235*, 114–120.

Mansour, M., Ginawi, O., El-Hadiyah, T., El-Khatib, A., Al-Shabanah, O. and Al-Sawaf, H. (2001) 'Effects of volatile oil constituents of *Nigella sativa* on carbon tetrachloride-induced hepatotoxicity in mice: evidence for anti-oxidant effects of thymoquinone.' *Research Communications in Molecular Pathology and Pharmacology 110*, 239–251. Cited by Edris, A.E. (2007) 'Pharmaceutical and therapeutic potentials of essential oils and their individual volatile constituents: a review.' *Phytotherapy Research 21*, 4, 308–323.

Marongiu, B., Porcedda, A.P.S., Casu, R. and Pierucci, P. (2004) 'Chemical composition of the oil and supercritical CO_2 extract of *Schinus molle* L.' *Flavour and Fragrance Journal 19*, 554–558.

Marozzi, F.J., Kocialski, A.B. and Malone, M.H. (1970) 'Studies on the antihistaminic effects of thymoquinone, thymohydroquinone and quercitin'. *Arzneimittelforschung 20*, 1574–1577. Cited by Tisserand, R. and Young, R. (2014) *Essential Oil Safety.* (2nd edition.) Edinburgh: Churchill Livingstone.

Martinez, A.L., González-Trujano, M.E., Pellicer, F., López-Muñoz, F.J. and Navarrete, A. (2009) 'Antinocicpetive effect and GC/MS analysis of Rosmarinus officinalis L. essential oil from its aerial parts.' *Planta Medica 75*, 5, 508–511.

Martino, L., Feo, V., Fratianni, F. and Nazarro, F. (2010) 'Chemistry, anti-oxidant, antibacterial and antifungal activities of essential oils and their components.' *Natural Product Communications 5*, 1741–1750.

Martins, M.R., Arantes, S., Candeias, F., Tinoco, M.T. and Cruz-Morais, J. (2014) 'Anti-oxidant, antimicrobial and toxicological properties of *Schinus molle* L. essential oils.' *Journal of Ethnopharmacology 151*, 1, 485–492.

Maruyama, N., Ishibashi, H., Hu, W., Morofuji, S. and Yamaguchi, H. (2006) 'Suppression of carrageenan and collagen induced inflammation in mice by geranium oil.' *Mediators of Inflammation 3*, 1–7.

Maruyama, N., Takizawa, T. and Ishibashi, H. (2008) 'Protective activity of geranium oil and its component, geraniol, in combination with vaginal washing against vaginal candidiasis in mice.' *Biological and Pharmaceutical Bulletin 31*, 1501–1506.

Mastelic, J., Jerkovic, I., Blazevic, I., Poljak-Blaži, M. *et al.* (2008) 'Comparative study on the anti-oxidant and biological activities of carvacrol, thymol, and eugenol derivatives.' *Journal of Agricultural and Food Chemistry 56*, 11, 3989–3996.

Matsubara, E., Fukagawa, M., Okamoto, T., Ohnuki, K., Shimizu, K. and Kondo, R. (2011a) '(–)-Bornyl acetate induces autonomic relaxation and reduces arousal level after visual display terminal work without any influences of task performance in low-dose condition.' *Biomedical Research 32*, 2, 151–157.

Matsubara, E., Fukagawa, M., Okamoto, T., Fukida, A. *et al.* (2011b) 'Volatiles emitted from the leaves of *Laurus nobilis* L. improve vigilance performance in visual discrimination task.' *BiOmedical Research 32*, 1, 19–28.

Matsubara, E., Fukagawa, M., Okamoto, T., Ohnuki, K., Shimizu, K. and Kondo, R. (2011c) 'The essential oil of *Abies sibirica* (Pinaceae) reduces arousal levels after visual display terminal work.' *Flavour and Fragrance Journal 26*, 204–210.

Maury, M. (1989) *Marguerite Maury's Guide to Aromatherapy. The Secret of Life and Youth: A Modern Alchemy.* Saffron Walden: C.W. Daniel Co. Ltd. (Original work published in English in 1961.)

Maxia, A., Marongi, B., Piras, A., Porcedda, S. *et al.* (2009) 'Chemical characterisation and biological activity of essential oils from *Daucus carota* L. subsp. *carota* growing wild on the Mediterranean coast and on the Atlantic coast.' *Fitoterapia 80*, 1, 57–61. Cited by Lang, G. and Buchbauer, G. (2012) 'A review on recent research results (2008–2010) on essential oils as antimicrobials and antifungals. A review.' *Flavour and Fragrance Journal 27*, 13–39.

McEvoy, B., Nydegger, R. and Williams, G. (2003) 'Factors related to patient compliance in the treatment of acne vulgaris.' *International Journal of Dermatology 42*, 274–280.

McGeever, M. (2014) 'Is there a Role for the Client in the Selection of Essential Oils in Aromatherapy for a Positive Outcome in Treatment?' Dissertation, Edinburgh Napier University.

McKay, D.L. and Blumberg, J.B. (2006) 'A review of the bioactivity and potential health benefits of chamomile tea (*Matricaria recutita* L.).' *Phytotherapy Research 20*, 7, 519–530.

McMahon, C. (2011) Monograph: 'Frangipani (*Plumeria alba*).' Accessed on 3 December 2011 at www. whitelotusblog.com/2011/07monograph-frangipani-plumeria-alba.html

Medina-Holguin, A.L., Holguin, F.O., Micheletto, S., Goehle, S., Simon, J.A. and O'Connell, M.A. (2008) 'Chemotypic variation of essential oils in the medicinal plant, *Anemopsis californica*.' *Phytochemistry 69*, 4, 919–927. Cited by Adorjan, B. and Buchbauer, G. (2010) 'Biological properties of essential oils: an updated review.' *Flavour and Fragrance Journal 25*, 407–426.

Meghwal, M. and Goswami, T.K. (2013) 'Piper nigrum and piperine: an update.' *Phytotherapy Research 27*, 8, 1121–1130.

Meister, A., Bernhardt, G., Christoffel, V. and Buschauer, A. (1999) 'Antispasmodic activity of *Thymus vulgaris* extract on the isolated guinea-pig trachea: discrimination between drug and ethanol effects.' *Planta Medica 65*, 512–516.

Melo, F.H., Venâncio, E.T., de Sousa, D.P., de França Fonteles, M.M. and de Vasconcelos, S.M. (2010b) 'Anxiolytic-like effect of carvacrol (5-isopropyl–2-methylphenol) in mice: involvement with the GABAergic system.' *Fundamentals of Clinical Pharmacology 24*, 437–443.

Melo, M.S., Sena, L.C.S., Barreto, F.J.N., Bonjardim, L.R. *et al.* (2010a) 'Anti-nociceptive effects of citronellal in mice.' *Pharmaceutical Biology 48*, 411–416.

Mesfin, M., Asres, K. and Shibeshi, W. (2014) 'Evaluation of anxiolytic activity of the essential oil of the aerial part of *Foeniculum vulgare* Miller in mice.' *BMC Complementary and Alternative Medicine 14*, 310. Available at www.biomedcentral.com/1472-6882/14/310, accessed on 10 June 2015.

Miguel, M.G. (2010) 'Anti-oxidant and anti-inflammatory activities of essential oils: a short review.' *Molecules 15*, 9252–9287.

Milinski, M. and Wedekind, C. (2001) 'Evidence for MHC-correlated perfume preferences in humans.' *Behavioural Ecology 12*, 2, 140–149.

Mills, S.Y. (1991) *The Essential Book of Herbal Medicine*. Harmondsworth: Penguin Arkada.

Minami, M., Kita, M., Nakaya, T., Yamamoto, T., Kuriyama, H. and Imanishi, J. (2003) 'The inhibitory effects of essential oils on herpes simplex type-1 replication *in vitro*.' *Microbiology and Immunology 47*, 681–684. Cited by Edris, A.E. (2007) 'Pharmaceutical and therapeutic potentials of essential oils and their individual volatile constituents: a review.' *Phytotherapy Research 21*, 4, 308–323.

Mitoshi, M., Kuriyama, I., Nakayama, H., Miyazato, H. *et al.* (2014) 'Suppression of allergic and inflammatory responses by essential oils derived from herbal plants and citrus fruits.' *International Journal of Molecular Medicine 33*, 1643–1651.

Miyazawa, M., Shindo, M. and Shimada, T. (2002) 'Metabolism of (+)- and (−)-limonenes to respective carveols and perillyl alcohols by CYP2C9 and CYP2C19 in human liver microsomes.' *Drug Metabolism and Disposition 30*, 602–607. Cited by Lima, T.C., Mota, M.M., Barbossa-Filho, J.M., dos Santos, M.R.V. and de Sousa, D.P. (2012b) 'Structural relationships and vasorelaxant activity of monoterpenes.' *DARU Journal of Pharmaceutical Sciences 20*, 23. Available at www.darujps.com/content/20/1/23, accessed on 10 June 2015.

Miyazawa, M., Watanabe, H. and Kameoka, H. (1997) 'Inhibition of acetylcholinesterase activity by monoterpenoids with a p-menthane skeleton.' *Journal of Agricultural and Food Chemistry 45*, 677–679.

Mohamad, R.H., El-Bastawesy, A.M., Abdel-Monem, M.G., Noor, A.M., Al-Mehdar, H.A.R., Sharawy, S.M. and El-Merzabani, M.M. (2011) 'Antioxidant and anticarcinogenic effects of methanolic extract and volatile oil of fennel seeds (Foeniculum vulgare).' *Journal of Medicinal Food 14*, 986–1001.

Mojay, G. (1996) *Aromatherapy for Healing the Spirit*. London: Gaia Books.

Morita, T., Jinno, K., Kawagishi, H., Arimoto, Y., Suganuma, H., Inakuma, T., Sugiyama, K. (2003) 'Hepatoprotective effect of myristicin from nutmeg (Myristica fragrans) on lipopolysaccharide/d-galactosamine-induced liver injury.' *Journal of Agricultural and Food Chemistry 51*, 1560–1565. Cited by Edris, A.E. (2007) 'Pharmaceutical and therapeutic potentials of essential oils and their individual volatile constituents: a review.' *Phytotherapy Research 21*, 308–323.

Morris, E.T. (1984) *Fragrance: The Story of Perfume from Cleopatra to Chanel*. New York: Charles Scribner's Sons.

Morris, N., Birtwistle, S. and Toms, M. (1995) 'Anxiety reduction.' *International Journal of Aromatherapy 7*, 2, 33–39.

Morrone, L.A., Rombola, L., Corasaniti, M.T., Zappettini, S. *et al.* (2007) 'The essential oil of bergamot enhances the levels of amino acid neurotransmitters in the hippocampus of rat: implication of monoterpene hydrocarbons.' *Pharmacology Research 55*, 255–262. Cited by Bagetta, G., Morrone, L.A., Rombolà, L., Amatea, D. *et al.* (2010) 'Neuropharmacology of the essential oil of bergamot.' *Fitoterapia 81*, 453–461.

Moss, L., Rouse, M., Wesnes, K.A. and Moss, M. (2010) 'Differential effects of the aromas of *Salvia* species on memory and mood.' *Human Psychopharmacology 25*, 5, 388–396.

Moss, M., Cook, J., Wesnes, K. and Duckett, P. (2003) 'Aromas of rosemary and lavender essential oils differentially affect cognition and mood in healthy adults.' *International Journal of Neuroscience 113*, 15–38.

Moss, M., Hewitt, S. and Moss, L. (2008) 'Modulation of cognitive performance and mood by aromas of peppermint and ylang ylang'. *International Journal of Neuroscience 118*, 59–77.

Moss, M., Howarth, R., Wilkinson, L. and Wesnes, K. (2006) 'Expectancy and the aroma of Roman chamomile influence mood and cognition in healthy volunteers.' *International Journal of Aromatherapy 16*, 2, 63–73.

Moss, M. and Oliver, L. (2012) 'Plasma 1,8-cineole correlates with cognitive performance following exposure to rosemary essential oil aroma.' *Therapeutic Advances in Psychopharmacology 2*, 3, 103–113.

Muchtaridi, M., Subarnas, A., Apriyantono, A. and Mustarichie, R. (2010) 'Identification of compounds in the essential oil of nutmeg seeds (*Myristica fragrans* Houtt.) that inhibit locomotor activity in mice.' *International Journal of Molecular Science 11*, 4771–4781.

Mulder, M.M.S., Sigurdsson, V., Van Zuuren, E.J., Klaassen, E.J. *et al.* (2001) 'Psycholosical impact of acne vulgaris: evaluation of the relation between a change in clinical acne severity and psychosocial state.' *Dermatology 203*, 124–130.

Munekage, M., Kitagawa, H., Ichikawa, K., Watanabe, J. *et al.* (2011) 'Pharmacokinetics of Daikenchuto, a traditional Japanese medicine (Kampo), after single oral administration to healthy Japanese volunteers.' *Drug Metabolism and Disposition 39*, 10, 1784–1788.

Muthaiyan, A., Martin, E.M., Natesan, S., Crandall, P.G., Wilkinson, B.J. and Ricke, S.C. (2012a) 'Antimicrobial effect and mode of action of terpeneless cold pressed Valencia orange essential oil on methicillin-resistant *Staphylococcus aureus.' Journal of Applied Microbiology 112*, 5, 1020–1033.

Muthaiyan, A., Biswas, D., Crandall, P.G., Wilkinson, B.J. and Ricke, S.C. (2012b) 'Application of orange essential oil as an antistaphylococcal agent in a dressing model.' *BMC Complementary and Alternative Medicine 16*, 12, 125. Available at www.biomedcentral.com/1472-6882/12/125, accessed on 7 April 2015.

Nagai, H., Nakagawa, M., Nakamura, M., Fujii, W., Inui, T. and Asakura, Y. (1991) 'Effects of odours on humans (II) Reducing effects of mental stress and fatigue.' *Chemical Senses 16*, 198.

Nakamura, A., Fujiwara, S., Matsumoto, I. and Abe, K. (2009) 'Stress repression in restrained rats by (R)-(–)-linalool inhalation and gene expression profiling of their whole blood cells.' *Journal of Agricultural and Food Chemistry 57*, 5480–5485. Cited by Trellakis, S., Fischer, C., Rydleuskaya, A., Tagay, S. *et al.* (2012) 'Subconscious olfactory influences of stimulant and relaxant odours on immune function.' *European Archives of Otorhinolaryngology 269*, 1909–1916.

Nakamura, C.V., Ishida, K., Faccin, L.C., Filho, B.P. *et al.* (2004) '*In vitro* activity of essential oil from *Ocimum gratissimum* L. against four *Candida* species.' *Research in Microbiology 155*, 7, 579–586. Cited by Abad, M.J., Ansuategui, M. and Bermejo, P. (2007) 'Active antifungal substances from natural sources.' *ARKIVOC 7*, 116–145.

Nejad, A.R. and Ismaili, A. (2013) 'Changes in growth, essential oil yield and composition of geranium (*Pelargonium graveolens* L.) as affected by growing media.' *Journal of Science of Food and Agriculture 94*, 905–910.

Ng, F., Berk, M., Dean, O. and Bush, A.I. (2008) 'Oxidative stress in psychiatric disorders: evidence base and therapeutic implications.' *International Journal of Neuropsychopharmacology 11*, 6, 851–876. Cited by Zhang, Y., Wu, Y., Chen, T., Yao, L. *et al.* (2013) 'Assessing the metabolic effects of aromatherapy in human volunteers.' *Evidence-Based Complementary and Alternative Medicine.* Available at http://dx.doi.org/10.1155/2013/356381, accessed on 7 April 2015.

Nguyen, R. and Su, J. (2011) 'Treatment of acne vulgaris.' *Paediatrics and Child Health 21*, 3, 119–125.

Niempoog, S., Siriarchavatana, P. and Kajsongkram, T. (2012) 'The efficacy of Plygersic gel for use in the treatment of osteoarthritis of the knee.' *Journal of the Medical Association of Thailand 95*, 10, 113–119.

Nikolaevskii, V., Kononova, N., Pertsovskii, A. and Shinarchuk, I. (1990) 'Effect of essential oils on the course of experimental atherosclerosis.' *Patologicheskaia Fiziologica i Eksperimental'naia Terapia 5*, 52–53. Cited by Shaaban, H.A.E., El-Ghorab, A.H. and Shibamoto, T. (2012) 'Bioactivity of essential oils and their volatile aroma components: review.' *Journal of Essential Oil Research 24*, 2, 203–212.

Nissen, L., Zatta, A., Stefanini, I., Grandi, S. *et al.* (2010) 'Characterization and antimicrobial activity of essential oils of industrial hemp varieties (*Cannabis sativa* L.).' *Fitoterapia 81*, 5, 413–419.

Oboh, G., Ademosun, A.O., Odubanjo, O.V. and Akinbola, I.A. (2013) 'Antioxidative properties and inhibition of key enzymes relevant to type-2 diabetes and hypertension by essential oils from black pepper.' *Advances in Pharmacological Sciences.* Article ID 926047. Available at http://dx.doi.org/10.1155/2013/926047, accessed on 7 April 2015.

Oboh, G., Olasehinde, T.A. and Ademosun, A.O. (2014) 'Essential oil from lemon peels inhibit key enzymes linked to neurodegenerative conditions and pro-oxidant induced lipid peroxidation.' *Journal of Oleo Science 63*, 4, 373–381.

Oh, T.H., Kim, S.S., Yoon, W.J. (2009) 'Chemical composition and biological activities of Jeju *Thymus quinquecostatus* essential oils against *Propionibacterium* species including acne.' *The Journal of General and Applied Microbiology 55*, 1, 63–68.

Okello, E.J., Dimaki, C., Howes, M.-J. R., Houghton, P.J. and Perry, E.K. (2008) '*In vitro* inhibition of human acetyl-and butyryl-cholinesterase by *Narcissus poeticus* L. (Amaryllidaceae) flower absolute.' *International Journal of Essential Oil Therapeutics 2*, 3, 105–110.

Okonogi, S. and Chaiyana, W. (2012) 'Enhancement of anti-cholinesterase activity of *Zingiber cassumunar* essential oil using a microemulsion technique.' *Drug Discoveries and Therapeutics 6*, 5, 249–255.

Oliveira, J.S., Porto, L.A., Estevam, C.S., Siqueira, R.S. *et al.* (2009) 'Phytochemical screening and anticonvulsant property of *Ocimum basilicum* leaf essential oil.' *Latin American and Caribbean Bulletin of Medicinal and Aromatic Plants 8*, 195–202. Cited by de Almeida, R.N., Agra, M.F., Maior, F.N.S. and de Sousa, D.P. (2011) 'Essential oils and their constituents: anticonvulsant activity.' *Molecules 16*, 2726–2742.

Oomah, B.D., Busson, M., Godfrey, D.V. and Drover, J.C.G. (2002) 'Characteristics of hemp (*Cannabis sativa* L.) seed oil.' *Food Chemistry 76*, 33–43.

Oprea, E., Radulescu, V., Balotescu, C., Lazar, V., Bucur, M., Mladin, P. and Farcasanu, I.C. (2008) 'Chemical and biological studies of Ribes nigrum L. buds essential oil.' *Biofactors 34*, 1, 3–12.

Ostad, S.N., Soodi, M., Shariffzadeh, M., Khorshidi, N. and Marzban, H. (2001) 'The effect of fennel essential oil on uterine contraction as a model for dysmenorrhoea, pharmacology and toxicity.' *Journal of Ethnopharmacology 76*, 3, 299–304.

Ou, M.C., Hsu, T.F., Lai, L.C., Lin, Y.T. and Lin, C.C. (2012) 'Pain relief assessment by aromatic essential oil massage on outpatients with primary dysmenorrhea: a randomised, double-blind clinical trial.' *Journal of Obstetrics and Gynaecology Research 38*, 5, 817–822.

Ou, M.C., Lee, Y.F., Li, C.C. and Wu, S.K. (2014) 'The effectiveness of essential oils for patients with neck pain: a randomised controlled study.' *Journal of Alternative and Complementary Medicine 20*, 10, 771–779.

Ozbek, H., Ugras, S., Dulger, H., Bayram, I. *et al.* (2003) 'Hepatoprotective effect of *Foeniculum vulgare* essential oil.' *Fitoterapia 74*, 3, 317–319. Cited by Edris, A.E. (2007) 'Pharmaceutical and therapeutic potentials of essential oils and their individual volatile constituents: a review.' *Phytotherapy Research 21*, 4, 308–323.

Pain, S., Altobelli, C., Boher, A., Cittadini, L. *et al.* (2011) 'Surface rejuvenating effect of *Achillea millefolium* extract.' *International Journal of Cosmetic Science 33*, 535–542.

Palouzier-Paulignan, B., Lacroix, M.-C., Aimé, P., Baly, C. *et al.* (2012) 'Olfaction under metabolic influences.' *Chemical Senses 37*, 769–797.

Papadopoulos, L., Walker, C., Aitken, D. and Bor, R. (2000) 'The relationship between body location and psychological morbidity in individuals with *acne vulgaris.' Psychology, Health and Medicine 5*, 431–438.

Patil, J.R., Jaiprakasha, G.K., Murthy, K.N.C., Tichy, S.E., Chetti, M.B. and Patil, B.S. (2009) 'Apoptosis-mediated proliferation inhibition of human colon cancer cells by volatile principles of *Citrus aurantifolia.' Food Chemistry 114*, 1351–1358.

Patnaik, G.K. *et al.* (1977) 'Spasmolytic activity of sesquiterpenes from *Cedrus deodora.' Indian Drug Manufacturing Association Bulletin* (VII) 18, 238–242. Cited by Burfield, T. (2002) 'Cedarwood oils.' *The Cropwatch Series.* Available at www.cropwatch.org, accessed on 30 November 2011.

Patra, M., Shahi, S.K., Midgley, G. and Dikshit, A. (2002) 'Utilisation of sweet fennel oil as natural antifungal against nail-infective fungi.' *Flavour and Fragrance Journal 17*, 91–94.

Pattnaik, S., Subramanyam, V.R., Bapaji, M. and Kole, C.R. (1997) 'Antibacterial and antifungal activity of aromatic constituents of essential oils.' *Microbios 89*, 39–46. Cited by Caplin, J.L., Allan, I. and Hanlon, G.W. (2009) 'Enhancing the *in vitro* activity of *Thymus* essential oils against *Staphylococcus aureus* by blending oils from specific cultivars.' *International Journal of Essential Oil Therapeutics 3*, 35–39.

Pauli, A. (2006) 'α-Bisabolol from chamomile – a specific ergosterol biosynthesis inhibitor?' *International Journal of Aromatherapy 16*, 1, 21–25.

Peana, A.T., D'Aquila, P.S., Panin, F., Serra, G., Pippia, P. and Moretti, M.D. (2002) 'Anti-inflammatory activity of linalool and linalyl acetate constituents of essential oils.' *Phytomedicine 9*, 8, 721–726. Cited by Guimarães, A.G., Quintans, J.S.S. and Quintans-Júnior, L.J. (2013) 'Monoterpenes with analgesic activity: a systematic review.' *Phytotherapy Research 27*, 1, 1–15.

Pénoël, D. (1998/1999) 'Medical aromatherapy.' *International Journal of Aromatherapy 9*, 4, 162–165.

Pénoël, D. (2005) 'Fragonia (*Agonis fragrans*). Newsletter August 15.' Cited by Turnock, S. (2006) 'Potent oil.' *Nova*, January 2006, 29–36.

Pérez-López, A., Cirio, A.T., Rivas-Galindo, V.M., Aranda, R.S. and De Torres, N.W. (2011) 'Activity against *Streptococcus pneumoniae* of the essential oil and δ-cadinene isolated from *Schinus molle* fruit.' *Journal of Essential Oil Research 23*, 5, 25–28.

Perkins, A.C., Maglione, J., Hillebrand, G.G., Miyamoto, K. and Kimball, A.B. (2012) '*Acne vulgaris* in women: prevalence across the life span.' *Journal of Women's Health 21*, 223–230.

Perry, N. and Perry, E. (2006) 'Aromatherapy in the management of psychiatric disorders: clinical and neuropharmacological perspectives.' *CNS Drugs 20*, 4, 257–280.

Perry, R., Terry, R., Watson, L.K. and Ernst, E. (2012) 'Is lavender an anxiolytic drug? A systematic review of randomised clinical trials.' *Phytomedicine 19*, 8–9, 825–835.

Perveen, T., Haider, S., Kanwal, S. and Haleem, D.J. (2009) 'Repeated administration of *Nigella sativa* decreases 5-HT turnover and produces anxiolytic effects in rats.' *Pakistani Journal of Pharmaceutical Science 22*, 139–144. Cited by Lv, X.N., Liu, Z.J., Zhang, H.J. and Tzeng, C.M. (2013) 'Aromatherapy and the central nerve system (CNS): therapeutic mechanisms and associated genes.' *Current Drug Targets 14*, 872–879.

Pinto, E., Vale-Silva, L., Cavaleiro, C. and Salguero, L. (2009) 'Antifungal activity of the clove essential oil from *Syzygium aromaticum* on *Candida, Aspergillus* and dermatophyte species.' *Journal of Medical Microbiology 58*, 11, 1454–1462

Piochon-Gauthier, M., Legault, J., Sylvestre, M. and Pichette, A. (2014) 'The essential oil of *Populus balsamifera* buds: its chemical composition and cytotoxic activity.' *Natural Products Communications* 9, 2, 257–260.

Piromrat, K., Tuchinda, M., Geadsomnuig, S. and Koysooko, R. (1986) 'Antihistaminic effect of Plai (*Zingiber cassumunar* Roxb.) on histamine skin test in asthmatic children.' *Siriraj Hospital Gazette* 38, 4, 251–256. Cited by Bhuiyan, M.N.I., Chowdhury, J.U. and Begum, J. (2008) 'Volatile constituents of essential oils isolated from leaf and rhizome of *Zingiber cassumunar* Roxb.' *Bangladesh Journal of Pharmacology 3*, 69–73.

Pithayanukul, P., Tubprasert, J. and Wuthi-Udomlert, M. (2007) '*In vitro* antimicrobial activity of *Zingiber cassumunar* (plai) oil and a 5% plai gel.' *Phytotherapy Research 21*, 2, 164–169.

Pole, S. (2006) *Ayurvedic Medicine: The Principles of Traditional Practice.* Edinburgh: Churchill Livingstone.

Politano, V.T., Diener, R.M., Christian, M.S., Hawkins, D.R., Ritacco, G. and Api, A.M. (2013). 'The pharmacokinetics of phenylethyl alcohol (PEA): safety evaluation comparisons in rats, rabbits and humans.' *International Journal of Toxicology 32*, 1, 39–47.

Porcherot, C., Delplanque, S., Raviot-Derrien, S., Le Calvé, B. *et al.* (2010) 'How do you feel when you smell this? Optimization of a verbal measurement of odor-elicited emotions.' *Food Quality and Preference 21*, 938–947.

Posadzki, P., Alotaibi, A. and Ernst, E. (2012) 'Adverse effects of aromatherapy: a systematic review of case reports and case series.' *International Journal of Risk and Safety in Medicine 24*, 147–161.

Potterton, D. (ed.) (1983) *Culpeper's Colour Herbal.* London: W. Foulsham & Company Ltd.

Prakash, P. and Gupta, N. (2005) 'Therapeutic uses of *Ocimum sanctum* Linn (Tulsi) with a note on eugenol and its pharmacological actions: a short review.' *Indian Journal of Physiology and Pharmacology 49*, 2, 125–131.

Prabhu, K.S., Lobo, R., Shirwaikar, A.A. and Shirwaikar, A. (2009) '*Ocimum gratissimum:* a review of its chemical, pharmacological and ethnomedicinal properties.' *Open Complementary Medicine Journal 1*, 1–15.

Prashar, A., Locke, I.C. and Evans, C.S. (2004) 'Cytotoxicity of lavender oil and its major components to human skin cells.' *Skin Proliferation 37*, 221–229. Cited by Baumann, L.S. (2007) 'Less-known botanical cosmeceuticals.' *Dermatologic Therapy 20*, 330–342.

Price, L. (1999) *Carrier Oils for Aromatherapy and Massage.* Stratford-upon-Avon: Riverhead.

Price, S. and Price, L. (eds) (2007) *Aromatherapy for Health Professionals.* (3rd edition.) Edinburgh: Churchill Livingstone.

Proudfoot, C.J., Garry, E.M. and Cottrell, D.F. (2006) 'Analgesia mediated by the TRPM8 cold receptor in chronic neuropathic pain.' *Current Biology 16*, 1591–1605. Cited by Guimarães, A.G., Quintans, J.S.S. and Quintans-Júnior, L.J. (2013) 'Monoterpenes with analgesic activity: a systematic review.' *Phytotherapy Research 27*, 1, 1–15.

Purvis, D., Robinson, E., Merry, S. and Watson, P. (2006) 'Acne, anxiety, depression and suicide in teenagers: a cross-sectional survey of New Zealand secondary school students.' *Journal of Paediatrics and Child Health 42*, 793–796.

Qadan, F., Thewaini, A.J., Ali, D.A., Afifi, R., Elkhawad, A. and Matalka, K.Z. (2005) 'The antimicrobial activities of *Psidium guajava* and *Juglans regia* leaf extracts to acne-developing organisms.' *American Journal of Chinese Medicine 33*, 197–204. Cited by Azimi, H., Fallah-Tafti, M., Khakshur, A.A. and Abdollahi, M. (2012) 'A review of the treatment of acne vulgaris: perspective of new pharmacological treatments.' *Fitoterapia 83*, 8, 1306–1317.

Quintans-Júnior, L.J., Souza, T.T., Leite, B.S., Lessa, N.M.N. *et al.* (2008) 'Phytochemical screening and anticonvulsant activity of *Cymbopogon winterianus* Jowitt (Poaceae) leaf essential oil in rodents.' *Phytomedicine 15*, 8, 619–624.

Quintans-Júnior, L.J., Melo, M.S., de Sousa, D.P., Araujo, A.A. *et al.* (2010) 'Anti-nociceptive activity of citronellal in formalin-, capsaicin- and glutamate-induced orofacial nociception in rodents and its action on nerve excitability.' *Journal of Orofacial Pain 24*, 305–312.

Quintans-Júnior, L.J., Rocha, L.F., Caregnato, F.F., Moreira, J.C.F. *et al.* (2011a) 'Anti-nociceptive action and redox properties of citronellal, an essential oil present in lemongrass.' *Journal of Medicinal Food 14*, 630–639.

Quintans-Júnior, L.J., Guimarães, A.G., Santana, M.T., Araujo, B.E.S. *et al.* (2011b) 'Citral reduces nociceptive and anti-inflammatory response in rodents.' *Brazilian Journal of Pharmacognosy 21*, 497–502.

Quintans-Júnior, L.J., Oliveira, M.G.B., Santana, M.F., Santgana, M.T. *et al.* (2011c) 'α-Terpineol reduces nociceptive behaviour in mice.' *Pharmaceutical Biology 49*, 583–586.

Quintans-Júnior, L., Moreira, J.C.F., Pasquali, M.A.B., Rabie, S.M.S. *et al.* (2013) 'Anti-nociceptive activity and redox potential of the monoterpenes (+)-camphene, *p*-cymene and geranyl acetate in experimental models.' *ISRN Toxicology* Article ID 459530. Available at http://dx.doi.org/10.1155/2013/459530, accessed on 20 November 2013.

Raharjo, S.J. and Fatchiyah, F. (2013) 'Virtual screening of compounds from the patchouli oil of *Pogostemon herba* for COX-1 inhibition.' *Bioinformation 9*, 6, 321–324.

Rahman, M., Rahman, A., Hashem, M.A., Ullah, M., Afroz, S. and Chaudhary, V. (2012) 'Anti-inflammatory, analgesic and GC-MS analysis of essential oil of *Alpinia calcarata* rhizome.' *International Journal of Pharma and Bio Sciences 3*, 4, 55–63.

Rahmani, A.H., Al Shabrmi, F.M. and Aly, S.M. (2014) 'Active ingredients of ginger as potential candidates in the prevention and treatment of diseases via modulation of biological activities.' *International Journal of Physiology, Pathophysiology and Pharmacology 6*, 2, 125–136.

Rahmani, A.H., Alzohairy, M.A., Khan, M.A. and Aly, S.M. (2014) 'Therapeutic implications of black seed and its constituent thymoquinone in the prevention of cancer through inactivation and activation of molecular pathways.' *Evidence-Based Complementary and Alternative Medicine.* doi: 10.1155/2014/724658.

Rakhshandah, H., Hosseini, M. and Dolati, K. (2004) 'Hypnotic effect of *Rosa damascena* in mice.' *Iranian Journal of Pharmaceutical Research 3*, 181–185.

Ramage, G., Milligan, S., Lappin, D.F., Sherry, L. *et al.* (2012) 'Antifungal, cytotoxic, and immunomodulatory properties of tea tree oil and its derivative components: potential role in management of oral candidosis in cancer patients.' *Frontiers in Microbiology 3*, 220. doi: 10.3389/fmicb.2012.00220. eCollection 2012. Cited by Saad, N.Y., Muller, C.D. and Lobstein, A. (2013) 'Major bioactivities and mechanism of action of essential oils and their components.' *Flavour and Fragrance Journal 28*, 269–279.

Rao, V.S.N., Menezes, A.M.S and Viana, G.S.B. (1990) 'Effect of myrcene on nociception in animals.' *Journal of Pharmacy and Pharmacology 42*, 877–878. Cited by Guimarães, A.G., Quintans, J.S.S. and Quintans-Júnior, L.J. (2013) 'Monoterpenes with analgesic activity: a systematic review.' *Phytotherapy Research 27*, 1, 1–15.

Rašković, A., Milanović, I., Pavlović, N., Ćebović, T., Vukmirović, S. and Mikov, M. (2014) 'Anti-oxidant activity of rosemary (*Rosmarinus officinalis* L.) essential oil and its hepatoprotective potential.' *BMC Complementary and Alternative Medicine 14*, 225. Available at www.biomedcentral.com/1472-6882/14/225, accessed on 7 April 2015.

Ravizza, R., Gariboldi, M.B., Molteni, R. and Monti, E. (2008) 'Linalool, a plant-derived monoterpene alcohol, reverses doxorubicin resistance in human breast adenocarcinoma cells.' *Oncology Reports 20*, 3, 625–30. Cited by Adorjan, B. and Buchbauer, G. (2010) 'Biological properties of essential oils: an updated review.' *Flavour and Fragrance Journal 25*, 407–426.

Rennie, D. (2001) 'CONSORT revised: improving the reporting of randomised trials.' *Journal of the American Medical Association 285*, 2006–2007.

Renzi, C., Picardi, A., Abeni, D., Agostini, E. *et al.* (2002) 'Association of dissatisfaction with care and psychiatric morbidity with poor treatment compliance.' *Archives of Dermatology 138*, 337–342.

Reuter, J., Huyke, C., Casetti, F., Theek, C. *et al.* (2008) 'Anti-inflammatory potential of a lipolotion containing coriander oil in the ultraviolet erythema test.' *Journal der Deutschen Dermatologischen Gesellschaft 6*, 847–851. Cited by Casetti, F., Bartelke, S., Biehler, K., Augustin, M., Schempp, C.M. and Frank, U. (2012) 'Antimicrobial activity against bacteria with dermatological relevance and skin tolerance of the essential oil from *Coriandrum sativum* L. fruits.' *Phytotherapy Research 26*, 3, 420–424.

Rezvanfar, M., Sadrkhanlou, R., Ahmadi, A., Shojaei-Sadee, H. *et al.* (2008) 'Protection of cyclophosphamide-induced toxicity in reproductive tract histology, sperm characteristics, and DNA damage by an herbal source: evidence for role of free-radical toxic stress.' *Human and Experimental Toxicology 27*, 12, 901–910. Cited by Adorjan, B. and Buchbauer, G. (2010) 'Biological properties of essential oils: an updated review.' *Flavour and Fragrance Journal 25*, 407–426.

Rhind, J. (2012) *Essential Oils: A Handbook for Aromatherapy Practice.* London and Philadelphia, PA: Singing Dragon.

Rhind, J. (2014) *Fragrance and Wellbeing: An Exploration of Plant Aromatics and Their Influences on the Psyche.* London: Singing Dragon.

Rivot, J.P., Montagne-Clavel, J. and Besson, J.M. (2002) 'Subcutaneous formalin and carrageenan increase nitric acid release as measured by *in vivo* voltametry in the spinal cord.' *European Journal of Pain 6*, 25–34. Cited by Guimarães, A.G., Quintans, J.S.S. and Quintans-Júnior, L.J. (2013) 'Monoterpenes with analgesic activity: a systematic review.' *Phytotherapy Research 27*, 1, 1–15.

Riyazi, A., Hensel, A., Bauer, K., Geissler, N., Schaaf, S. and Verspohl, E.J. (2007) 'The effect of the volatile oil from ginger rhizomes (*Zingiber officinale*), its fractions and isolated compounds on the 5-HT3 receptor complex and the serotoninergic system of the rat ileum.' *Planta Medica 73*, 4, 355–362.

Robbins, G. and Broughan, C. (2007) 'The effects of manipulating participant expectations of an essential oil on memory through verbal suggestion.' *International Journal of Essential Oil Therapeutics 1*, 2, 56–60.

Robert, G. (1998) 'The nose: a perfumer's tool.' *Perfumer and Flavorist 23*, 1–4.

Rojo, L.E., Villano, C.M., Joseph, G., Schmidt, B. *et al.* (2010) 'Original contribution: wound-healing properties of nut oil from *Pouteria lucuma.*' *Journal of Cosmetic Dermatology 9*, 185–195.

Romano, L., Battaglia, F., Masucci, L., Sanguinetti, M., Plotti, G., Zanetti, S. and Fadda, G. (2005) '*In vitro* activity of bergamot natural essence and furocoumarin-free and distilled extracts, and their associations with boric acid, against clinical yeast isolates.' *Journal of Antimicrobial Chemotherapy 55*, 1, 110–114.

Rosato, A., Vitali, C., Gallo, D., Balenzano, L. and Mallamaci, R. (2008) 'The inhibition of *Candida* species by selected essential oils and their synergism with amphotericin B.' *Phytomedicine 15*, 8, 635–638.

Rota, M.C., Herrera, A., Martinez, R.M., Sotomayor, J.A. and Jordán, M.J. (2008) 'Antimicrobial activity and chemical composition of *Thymus vulgaris, Thymus zygis* and *Thymus hyemalis* essential oils.' *Food Control 9*, 681–687. Cited by Caplin, J.L., Allan, I. and Hanlon, G.W. (2009) 'Enhancing the *in vitro* activity of *Thymus* essential oils against *Staphylococcus aureus* by blending oils from specific cultivars.' *International Journal of Essential Oil Therapeutics 3*, 35–39.

Russo, M., Serra, D., Suraci, F. and Postorino, S. (2012) 'Effectiveness of electronic nose systems to detect bergamot (*Citrus bergamia* Risso et Poiteau) essential oil quality and genuineness.' *Journal of Essential Oil Research 24*, 2, 137–151.

Russo, R., Ciociaro, A., Berliocchi, L., Cassiano, M.G. *et al.* (2013) 'Implication of limonene and linalyl acetate in cytotoxicity induced by bergamot essential oil in human neuroblastoma cells.' *Fitoterapia 89*, 1, 48–57.

Ryman, D. (1989) 'Preface.' In Maury, M., *Marguerite Maury's Guide to Aromatherapy – The Secret of Life and Youth: A Modern Alchemy.* Saffron Walden: C.W. Daniel Co. Ltd. (Original work published in English in 1961.)

Saab, A.M., Harb, F.Y. and Koenig, W.A. (2005) 'Essential oil components in heart wood of *Cedrus libani* and *Cedrus atlantica* from Lebanon.' *Minerva Biotecnologica 17*, 159–161.

Saab, A.M., Tundis, R., Loizzo, M.R., Lampronti, I. *et al.* (2012) 'Anti-oxidant and antiproliferative activity of *Laurus nobilis* L. (Lauraceae) leaves and seeds essential oils against K562 human chronic myelogenous cells.' *Natural Products Research 26*, 18, 1741–1745.

Saad, N.Y., Muller, C.D. and Lobstein, A. (2013) 'Major bioactivities and mechanism of action of essential oils and their components.' *Flavour and Fragrance Journal 28*, 269–279.

Sacchetti, G., Maietti, S., Muzzoli, M., Scaglianti, M. *et al.* (2005) 'Comparative evaluation of 11 essential oils of different origin as functional anti-oxidants, antiradicals and antimicrobials in foods.' *Food Chemistry 91*, 621–632.

Sachdev, M. and Friedman, A. (2010) 'Cosmeceuticals in day-to-day clinical practice.' *Journal of Drugs in Dermatology 9*, 5, 62–66.

Safayhi, H., Sabieraj, J., Sailer, E.R. and Ammon, H.P. (1994) 'Chamazulene: an anti-oxidant-type inhibitor of leukotriene B4 formation.' *Planta Medica 60*, 5, 410–413.

Saharkhiz, M.J., Motamedi, M., Zomorodian, K., Pakshir, K., Miri, R. and Hemyari, K. (2012) 'Chemical composition, antifungal and anitbiofilm activities of the essential oil of *Mentha piperita* L.' *International Scholarly Research Network*. Available at http://dx.doi.org/10.5402/2012/718645, accessed 11 June 2015.

Saiyudthong, S., Ausavarungnirun, R., Jiwajinda, S. and Turakitwanakan, W. (2009) 'Effects of aromatherapy massage with lime essential oil on stress.' *International Journal of Essential Oil Therapeutics 3*, 2, 76–80.

Sakurada, T., Kuwahata, H., Katsuyama, S., Komatsu, T. *et al.* (2009) 'Intraplantar injection of bergamot essential oil into the mouse hindpaw: effects on capsaicin-induced nociceptive behaviors.' *International Review of Neurobiology 85*, 237–248. Cited by Adorjan, B. and Buchbauer, G. (2010) 'Biological properties of essential oils: an updated review.' *Flavour and Fragrance Journal 25*, 407–426.

Samojlik, I., Lakić, N., Mimica-Dukić, N., Daković-Svajcer, K. and Bozin, B. (2010) 'Anti-oxidant and hepatoprotective potential of essential oils of coriander (*Coriandrum sativum* L.) and caraway (*Carum carvi* L.) (Apiaceae).' *Journal of Agricultural and Food Chemistry 58*, 15, 8848–8853.

Sanguinetti, M., Posteraro, B., Romano, L., Battaglia, F., Lopizzo, T., DeCarolis, E. and Fadda, G. (2007) '*In vitro* activity of *Citrus bergamia* (bergamot) oil against clinical isolates of dermatophytes.' *Journal of Antimicrobial Chemotherapy 59*, 2, 305–308.

Sanmukhani, J., Satodia, V., Trivedi, J., Patel, T. *et al.* (2014). 'Efficacy and safety of curcumin in major depressive disorder: a randomised controlled trial.' *Phytotherapy Research 28*, 4, 579–585.

Santana, M.F., Quintans-Junior, L.J., Cavalcanti, S.C.H., Oliveira, M.G.B. *et al.* (2011) '*p*-Cymene reduces orofacial nociceptive response in mice.' *Brazilian Journal of Pharmacognosy 21*, 6, 1138–1143. Cited by Guimarães, A.G., Quintans, J.S.S. and Quintans-Júnior, L.J. (2013) 'Monoterpenes with analgesic activity: a systematic review'. *Phytotherapy Research 27*, 1, 1–15.

Santos, F.A. and Rao, V.S.N. (2000) 'Anti-inflammatory and anti-nociceptive effects of 1,8-cineole, a terpenoid oxide present in many plant essential oils.' *Phytotherapy Research 14*, 4, 240–244.

Sarkar, A., Pandey, D.N. and Pant, M.C. (1990) 'A report on the effect of *Ocimum sanctum* (Tulsi) leaves and seeds on blood and urinary uric acid, urea and urine volume in normal albino rabbits.' *Indian Journal of Physiology and Pharmacology 34*, 61–62. Cited by Prakash, P. and Gupta, N. (2005) 'Therapeutic uses of *Ocimum sanctum* Linn. (Tulsi) with a note on eugenol and its pharmacological actions: a short review.' *Indian Journal of Physiology and Pharmacology 49*, 2, 125–131.

Satou, T., Kasuya, H., Takahashi, M., Murakami, S. *et al.* (2011a) 'Relationship between duration of exposure and anxiolytic-like effects of essential oil from *Alpinia zerumbet*.' *Flavour and Fragrance Journal 26*, 180–185.

Satou, T., Matsuura, M., Takahashi, M., Umezu, T. *et al.* (2011b) 'Anxiolytic-like effect of essential oil extracted from *Abies sachalinensis*.' *Flavour and Fragrance Journal 26*, 416–420.

Sayers, J. (2001) 'The world health report 2001 – mental health: new understanding, new hope.' *Bulletin of the World Health Organisation 79*, 1085.

Sayyah, M., Valizadeh, J. and Kamalinejad, M. (2002) 'Anticonvulsant activity of the leaf essential oil of *Laurus nobilis* against pentylenetetrazole- and maximal electroshock-induced seizures.' *Phytomedicine 9*, 3, 212–216.

Sayyah, M., Saroukhani, G., Peirovi, A. and Kamaladinejad, M. (2003) 'Analgesic and anti-inflammatory activity of the leaf essential oil of *Laurus nobilis* Linn.' *Phytotherapy Research 17*, 7, 733–736.

Schinde, U.A., Kulkarni, K.R., Phadke, A.S., Nair, A.M. *et al.* (1999a) 'Mast cell stabilising and lipoxygenase activity of *Cedrus deodara* (Roxb.) Loud. wood oil.' *Indian Journal of Experimental Biology 37*, 3, 258–261. Cited by Burfield, T. (2002) 'Cedarwood oils.' *The Cropwatch Series.* Available at www.cropwatch.org, accessed on 30 November 2011.

Schinde, U.A., Phadke, A.S., Nair, A.M., Mungantiwar, A.A. *et al.* (1999b) 'Studies on the anti-inflammatory and analgesic activity of *Cedrus deodara* (Roxb.) Loud. wood oil.' *Journal of Ethnopharmacology 65*, 1, 21–27. Cited by Burfield, T. (2002) 'Cedarwood oils.' *The Cropwatch Series.* Available at www.cropwatch.org, accessed on 30 November 2011

Schmidt, C., Fronza, M., Goettert, M., Geller, F., Luik, S., Flores, E.M., Bittencourt, C.F., Zanetti, G.D., Heinzmann, B.M., Laufer, S. and Merfort, I. (2009) 'Biological studies on Brazilian plants used in wound healing.' *Journal of Ethnopharmacology 122*, 3, 523–532.

Schmidt, G., Romero, A.L., Sartoretto, J.L., Caparroz-Assef, S.M., Bersani-Amado, C.A. and Cuman, R.K. (2009) 'Immunomodulatory activity of *Zingiber officinale* Roscoe, *Salvia officinalis* L. and *Syzygium aromaticum* L. essential oils: evidence for humor- and cell-mediated responses.' *Journal of Pharmacy and Pharmacology 61*, 7, 961–967.

Schnaubelt, K. (1995) *Advanced Aromatherapy.* Vermont: Healing Arts Press.

Schnaubelt, K. (1999) *Medical Aromatherapy: Healing with Essential Oils.* Berkeley, CA: Frog Ltd.

Schnaubelt, K. (2011) *The Healing Intelligence of Essential Oils: The Science of Advanced Aromatherapy.* Rochester, VT: Healing Arts Press.

Schnitzler, P., Wiesenhofer, K. and Reichling, J. (2008) 'Comparative study on the cytotoxicity of different Myrtaceae essential oils on cultured vero and RC-37 cells.' *Pharmazie 63*, 11, 830–835. Cited by Adorjan, B. and Buchbauer, G. (2010) 'Biological properties of essential oils: an updated review.' *Flavour and Fragrance Journal 25*, 407–426.

Selim, S.A., Adam, M.E., Hassan, S.M. and Albalawi, A.R. (2014) 'Chemical composition, antimicrobial and antibiofilm activity of the essential oil and methanol extract of the Mediterranean cypress (*Cupressus sempervirens* L.).' *BMC Complementary and Alternative Medicine 4*, 179. Available at www.biomedcentral.com/1472-6882/14/179, accessed on 7 April 2015.

Sen, P. (1993) 'Therapeutic potentials of Tulsi: from experience to facts.' *Drugs News and Views 1*, 2, 15–21. Cited by Prakash, P. and Gupta, N. (2005) 'Therapeutic uses of *Ocimum sanctum* Linn (Tulsi) with a note on eugenol and its pharmacological actions: a short review.' *Indian Journal of Physiology and Pharmacology 49*, 2, 125–131.

Seol, G.H., Shim, H.S., Kim, P-J., Li, K.H. *et al.* (2010) 'Antidepressant-like activity of *Salvia sclarea* is explained by modulation of dopamine activities in rats.' *Journal of Ethnopharmacology 130*, 1, 187–190.

Setzer, W.N. (2009) 'Essential oils and anxiolytic aromatherapy.' *Natural Product Communications 4*, 9, 1305–1316.

Sfeir, J., Lefrançois, C., Baudoux, D., Derbré, S. and Licznar, P. (2013) '*In vitro* antibacterial activity of essential oils against *Streptococcus pyogenes.*' *Evidence-Based Complementary and Alternative Medicine.* Available at http://dx.doi.org/10.1155/2013/269161, accessed on 11 June 2015.

Shaaban, H.A.E., El-Ghorab, A.H. and Shibamoto, T. (2012) 'Bioactivity of essential oils and their volatile aroma components: review.' *Journal of Essential Oil Research 24*, 2, 203–212.

Shafei, M.N., Rakhshande, H. and Boskabady, M.H. (2003) 'Antitussive effect of *Rosa damascena* in guinea pigs.' *Iranian Journal of Pharmaceutical Research 2*, 231–234.

Sharma, J.N., Srivastava, K.C. and Gan, E.K. (1994) 'Suppressive effects of eugenol and ginger oil on arthritic rats.' *Pharmacology 49*, 3, 314–318.

Sharma, P.R., Mondhe, D.M., Muthiah, S., Pal, H.C. *et al.* (2009) 'Anticancer activity of an essential oil from *Cymbopogon flexuosus.' Chemico-Biological Interactions 179*, 2–3, 160–168. Cited by Adorjan, B. and Buchbauer, G. (2010) 'Biological properties of essential oils: an updated review.' *Flavour and Fragrance Journal 25*, 407–426.

Shen, J., Niijima, A., Tanida, M., Horii, Y., Maeda, K. and Nagai, K. (2005a) 'Olfactory stimulation with scent of grapefruit oil affects autonomic nerves, lipolysis and appetite in rats.' *Neuroscience Letters 380*, 289–294.

Shen, J., Niijima, A., Tanida, M., Horii, Y., Maeda, K. and Nagai, K. (2005b) 'Olfactory stimulation with scent of lavender oil affects autonomic nerves, lipolysis and appetite in rats.' *Neuroscience Letters 383*, 118–193.

Shen, J., Niijima, A., Tanida, M., Horii, Y., Nakamura, T. and Nagai, K. (2007) 'Mechanism of changes induced in plasma glycerol by scent stimulation with grapefruit and lavender essential oils.' *Neuroscience Letters 416*, 241–246.

Shen, T. and Lou, H.X. (2008) 'Bioactive constituents of myrrh and frankincense, two simultaneously prescribed gum resins in Chinese traditional medicine.' *Chemistry and Biodiversity 5*, 540–553.

Shen, T., Li, G.H., Wang, X.N. and Lou, H.X. (2012) 'The genus *Commiphora*: a review of its traditional uses, phytochemistry and pharmacology.' *Journal of Ethnopharmacology 142*, 2, 319–330.

Shin, S. and Lim, S. (2004) 'Antifungal effects of herbal essential oils alone and in combination with ketoconazole against *Trichophyton* spp.' *Journal of Applied Microbiology 97*, 6, 1289–1296. Cited by Abad, M.J., Ansuategui, M. and Bermejo, P. (2007) 'Active antifungal substances from natural sources.' *ARKIVOC 7*, 116–145.

Shukla, R.R. (2013) '*Jasmine officinale* Linn. – Ayurvedic approach.' *International Journal of Ayurverdic and Herbal Medicine 3*, 1, 1114–1119.

Shukla, Y. and Singh, M. (2007) 'Cancer preventative properties of ginger: a brief review. *Food Chemistry and Toxicology 45*, 5, 683–690.

Silva, D.F., Araújo, I.G., Albuquerque, J.G., Porto, D.L. *et al.* (2011) 'Rotundifolone-induced relaxation is mediated by BK(Ca) channel activation and Ca(v) channel inactivation.' *Basic Clinical Pharmacology and Toxicology 109*, 6, 465–475.

Silva, J., Abebe, W., Sousa, S.M., Duarte, V.G., Machado, M.I.L. and Matos, F.J.A. (2003) 'Analgesic and anti-inflammatory effects of essential oils of eucalyptus.' *Journal of Ethnopharmacology 89*, 2–3, 277–283.

Silva, M.R., Oliveira, J.G., Fernández, O.F., Passos, X.S. *et al.* (2005) 'Antifungal activity of *Ocimum gratissimum* towards dermatophytes.' *Mycoses 48*, 3, 172–175. Cited by Abad, M.J., Ansuategui, M. and Bermejo, P. (2007) 'Active antifungal substances from natural sources.' *ARKIVOC 7*, 116–145.

Silva, M.R., Ximenes, R.M., da Costa, J.G.M., Leal, L.K.A.M., de Lopes, A.A. and de Barros Viana, G.S. (2010) 'Comparative anticonvulsant activities of the essential oils (EOs) from *Cymbopogon winterianus* Jowitt and *Cymbopogon citratus* (DC) Stapf. in mice.' *Naunyn-Schmiedeberg's Archives of Pharmacology 381*, 415–426.

Silva Cde, B., Guterres, S.S., Weisheimer, V. and Schapoval, E.E. (2008) 'Antifungal activity of the lemongrass oil and citral against *Candida* spp.' *Brazilian Journal of Infectious Diseases 12*, 63–66. Cited by Lang, G. and Buchbauer, G. (2012) 'A review on recent research results (2008–2010) on essential oils as antimicrobials and antifungals. A review.' *Flavour and Fragrance Journal 27*, 13–39.

Singh, P., Shukla, R., Prakash, B., Kumar, A. *et al.* (2010) 'Chemical profile, antifungal, anti-aflatoxigenic and anti-oxidant activity of *Citrus maxima* Burm. and *Citrus sinensis* L. Osbeck essential oils and their cyclic monoterpene DL-limonene.' *Journal of Chemical Toxicology 48*, 1734–1740.

Sinha, P., Srivastava, S.Mishra, N. and Yadav, N.P. (2014) 'New perspectives on antiacne plant drugs:cContribution to modern therapeutics.' *BioMed Research International.* Article ID 301304. Available at http://dx.doi.org/10.1155/2014/301304, accessed on 7 April 2015.

Soković, M.D., Brkić, D.D., Džamić, A.M., Ristić, M.S. and Marinc, P.D. (2009) 'Chemical composition and antifungal activity of *Salvia desoleana* Atzei and Picci essential oil and its major components.' *Flavour and Fragrance Journal 24*, 83–87.

Sousa, P.J.C., Linard, C.F.B.M., Azevedo-Batista, D., Oliveira, A.C., Coelho-de-Souza, A.N. and Leal-Cardoso, J.H. (2009) 'Antinociceptive effects of the essential oil of *Mentha x villosa* leaf and its major constituent piperitenone oxide in mice.' *Brazilian Journal of Medical and Biological Research 42*, 7, 655–659.

Souza, F.V., da Rocha, M.B., de Sousa, D.P. and Marçal, R.M. (2013) '(−)-Carvone: antispasmodic effect and mode of action.' *Fitoterapia 85*, 1, 20–24.

Souza, M.C., Siani, A.C., Ramos, M.F., Memezes-de-Lima, O.J. and Henriques, M.G. (2003) 'Evaluation of anti-inflammatory activity of essential oils from two Asteraceae species.' *Pharmazie 58*, 582–586. Cited by Guimarães, A.G., Quintans, J.S.S. and Quintans-Júnior, L.J. (2013) 'Monoterpenes with analgesic activity: a systematic review.' *Phytotherapy Research 27*, 1, 1–15.

Spadaro, F., Costa, R., Circosta, C. and Occhiuto, F. (2012) 'Volatile composition and biological activity of key lime *Citrus aurantifolia* essential oil.' *Natural Product Communications 7*, 11, 1523–1526.

Srisukh, V., Tribuddharat, C., Nukoolkaru, V., Bunyapraphatsara, N. *et al.* (2012) 'Antibacterial activity of essential oils from *Citrus hystrix* (makrut lime) against respiratory tract pathogens.' *Science Asia 38*, 212–217.

Stotz, S.C., Vriens, J., Martyn, D., Clardy, J. and Clapham, D.E. (2008) 'Citral sensing by TRANSient receptor potential channels in dorsal root ganglion neurons.' *PLoS One 3*, 1–14.

Su, S., Wang, T., Duan, J.A., Zhou, W. *et al.* (2011) 'Anti-inflammatory and analgesic activity of different extracts of *Commiphora myrrha*.' *Journal of Ethnopharmacology 134*, 2, 251–258.

Su, Y.W., Chao, S.H., Lee, M.H., Ou, T.Y. and Tsai, Y.C. (2010) 'Inhibitory effects of citronellol and geraniol on nitric oxide and prostaglandin E2 production in macrophages.' *Planta Medica 76*, 1666–1671.

Suanarunsawat, T., Ayutthya, W.D.N., Songsak, T., Thirawarapan, S. and Poungshompoo, S. (2010) 'Anti-oxidant activity and lipid-lowering effect of essential oils extracted from *Ocimum sanctum* L. leaves in rats fed a high cholesterol diet.' *Journal of Clinical Biochemistry and Nutrition 46*, 52–59.

Suhail, M.M., Wu, W., Mondalek, F.G., Fung, K.-M. *et al.* (2011) '*Boswellia sacra* essential oil induces tumor cell-specific apoptosis and supresses tumor aggressiveness in cultured human breast cancer cells.' *BMC Complementary and Alternative Medicine 11*, 129. doi: 10.1186/1472-6882-11-129.

Süntar, I., Akkol, E.K., Keleş, H., Oktem, A., Başer, K.H.C. and Yeşilada, E. (2011) 'A novel wound-healing ointment: a formulation of *Hypericum perforatum* oil and sage and oregano essential oils based on traditional Turkish knowledge.' *Journal of Ethnopharmacology 134*, 89–96.

Süntar, I., Tumen, I., Ustün, O., Keleş, H. and Akkol, E.K. (2012) 'Appraisal on the wound-healing and anti-inflammatory activities of the essential oils obtained from the cones and needles of *Pinus* species by *in vivo* and *in vitro* experimental models'. *Journal of Ethnopharmacology 139*, 2, 533–540.

Svoboda, K.P., Ruzickova, G., Allan, R. and Hampson, J.B. (2001) 'An investigation into drop sizes of essential oils using different dropper types.' *International Journal of Aromatherapy 10*, 3/4, 99–103.

Svoboda, R.E. (1984) *Prakruti: Your Ayurvedic Constitution.* Albuquerque, NM: Geocom.

Svoboda, R.E. (2004) *Ayurveda: Life, Health and Longevity.* Albuquerque, NM: The Ayurvedic Press.

Takahashi, Y., Inaba, N., Kuwahara, S. and Kuki, W. (2003) 'Antioxidative effect of *Citrus* essential oil components on human low-density lipoprotein *in vitro*.' *Bioscience Biotechnology and Biochemistry 67*, 195–197. Cited by Edris, A.E. (2007) 'Pharmaceutical and therapeutic potentials of essential oils and their individual volatile constituents: a review.' *Phytotherapy Research 21*, 4, 308–323.

Takahashi, M., Satou, T., Ohashi, M., Sadamoto, K. and Koike, K. (2011) 'Interspecies comparison of chemical composition and anxiolytic-like effects of lavender oils upon inhalation.' *Natural Product Communications 6*, 11, 1769–1774.

Takaki, I., Bersani-Amado, L.E., Vendruscolo, A., Sartoretto, S.M. *et al.* (2008) 'Anti-inflammatory and anti-nociceptive effects of *Rosmarinus officinalis* L. essential oil in experimental animal models.' *Journal of Medicinal Food 11*, 4, 741–746.

Takayama, K. and Nagai, T. (1994) 'Limonene and related compounds as potential skin penetration promoters.' *Drug Development and Industrial Pharmacy 20*, 4, 677–684.

Takeda, H., Tsujita, J., Kaya, M., Takemura, M. and Oku, Y. (2008) 'Differences between the physiologic and psychologic effects of aromatherapy body treatment.' *Journal of Alternative and Complementary Medicine 14*, 6, 655–661.

Takemoto, H., Ito, M., Shiraki, T., Yagura, T. and Honda, G. (2008) 'Sedative effects of vapor inhalation of agarwood oil and spikenard extract and identification of their active components.' *Journal of Natural Medicines 62*, 1, 41–46. Cited by Dobetsberger, C. and Buchbauer, G. (2011) 'Actions of essential oils on the central nervous system: an updated review.' *Flavour and Fragrance Journal 26*, 5, 300–316.

Takemoto, H., Yagura, T. and Ito, M. (2009) 'Evaluation of volatile components from spikenard: Valerena-4,7(11)-diene is a highly active sedative compound.' *Journal of Natural Medicines 63*, 4, 380–385. Cited by Dobetsberger, C. and Buchbauer, G. (2011) 'Actions of essential oils on the central nervous system: an updated review.' *Flavour and Fragrance Journal 26*, 300–316.

Talpur, N., Echard, B., Ingram, C., Bagchi, D. and Preuss, H. (2005) 'Effects of a novel formulation of essential oils on glucose-insulin metabolism in diabetic and hypertensive rats: a pilot study.' *Diabetes, Obesity and Metabolism 7*, 193–199. Cited by Edris, A.E. (2007) 'Pharmaceutical and therapeutic potentials of essential oils and their individual volatile constituents: a review.' *Phytotherapy Research 21*, 4, 308–323.

Tao, N., OuYang, O. and Jia, L. (2014) 'Citral inhibits mycelial growth of *Penicillium italicum* by a membrane damage mechanism.' *Food Control 41*, 116–121.

Thiboutot, D., Gollnick, H., Bettoli, V., Dréno, B. *et al.* (2009) 'New insights into the management of acne: an update from the Global Alliance to Improve Outcomes in Acne Group.' *Journal of the American Academy of Dermatology 60*, S1–S50.

Thornfeldt, C. (2005) 'Cosmeceuticals containing herbs: fact, fiction and future.' *Dermatologic Surgery 31*, 873–880.

Timms, R.M. (2013) 'Moderate acne as a potential barrier to social relationships: myth or reality?' *Psychology, Health and Medicine 18*, 310–320.

Tisserand, R. (1988) 'Essential oils as therapeutic agents.' In S. Van Toller and G.H. Dodd (eds) *Perfumery: The Psychology and Biology of Fragrance*. London: Chapman Hall.

Tisserand, R. (ed.) (1993) *Gattefossé's Aromatherapy*. Saffron Walden: C.W. Daniel Co. Ltd.

Tisserand, R. and Balacs, T. (1995) *Essential Oil Safety – A Guide for Health Care Professionals*. London: Churchill Livingstone.

Tisserand, R. and Young, R. (2014) *Essential Oil Safety*. (2nd edition.) Edinburgh: Churchill Livingstone.

Toda, M. and Morimoto, K. (2008) 'Effect of lavender aroma on salivary endocrinological stress markers.' *Archives of Oral Biology 53*, 10, 964–968. Cited by Dobetsberger, C. and Buchbauer, G. (2011) 'Actions of essential oils on the central nervous system: an updated review.' *Flavour & Fragrance Journal 26*, 300–316.

Tognolini, M., Barocelli, E., Ballabeni, V., Bruni, R. *et al.* (2006) 'Comparative screening of plant essential oils: phenylpropanoid moiety as basic core for antiplatelet activity.' *Life Science 78*, 13, 1419–1432.

Tognolini, M., Ballabeni, V., Bertoni, S., Bruni, R., Impicciatore, M. and Barocelli, E. (2007) 'Protective effect of *Foeniculum vulgare* essential oil and anethole in an experimental model of thrombosis.' *Pharmacology Research 56*, 3, 254–260.

Tonkal, A.M. and Morsy, T.A. (2008) 'An update review on *Commiphora molmol* and related species.' *Journal of the Egyptian Society of Parasitology 38*, 3, 763–796.

Tragoolpua, Y. and Jatisatienr, A. (2007) 'Anti-herpes simplex virus activities of *Eugenia caryophyllus* (Spreng.) Bullock and S.G. Harrison and essential oil, eugenol.' *Phytotherapy Research 21*, 12, 1153–1158. Cited by Adorjan, B. and Buchbauer, G. (2010) 'Biological properties of essential oils: an updated review.' *Flavour and Fragrance Journal 25*, 407–426.

Trellakis, S., Fischer, C., Rydleuskaya, A., Tagay, S. *et al.* (2012) 'Subconscious olfactory influences of stimulant and relaxant odors on immune function.' *European Archcives of Otorhinolaryngology 269*, 1909–1916.

Tsai, Y.-C., Hsu, H.C., Yang, W.C, Tsai, W.J., Chen, C.C. and Watanabe, T. (2007) 'α-Bulnesene, a PAF inhibitor isolated from the essential oil of *Pogostemon cablin*.' *Fitoterapia 78*, 1, 7–11. Cited by Tisserand, R. and Young, R. (2014) *Essential Oil Safety*. Edinburgh: Churchill Livingstone.

Tsang, H.W. and Ho, T.Y. (2010) 'A systematic review on the anxiolytic effects of aromatherapy on rodents under experimentally induced anxiety models.' *Reviews in the Neurosciences 21*, 2, 141–152.

Tubaro, A., Giangaspero, A., Sosa, S., Negri, R. *et al.* (2010) 'Comparative topical anti-inflammatory activity of cannabinoids and cannabivarins.' *Fitoterapia 81*, 7, 816–819.

Tucker, A., Maciarello, M.J. and Howell, J.T. (1990) 'Botanical aspects of commercial sage.' *Economic Botany 34*, 16–19. Cited by Abu-Darwish, M.S., Cabral, C., Ferreira, I.V., Gonçalves, M.J. *et al.* (2013) 'Essential oil of common sage (*Salvia officinalis* L.) from Jordan: assessment of safety in mammalian cells and its antifungal and anti-inflammatory potential.' *BioMed Research International.* doi:101155/2013/538940. Available at www.ncbi.nlm.nih.gov/pmc/articles/PMC3809930, accessed on 7 April 2015.

Tumen, I., Hafizoglu, H., Dönmez, I.E., Sivrikaya, H. and Reunanen, M. (2010) 'Yields and constituents of essential oil from cones of *Pinacea* spp. natively grown in Turkey.' *Molecules 15*, 5797–5806. Cited by Süntar, I., Tumen, I., Ustün, O., Keleş, H. and Akkol, E.K. (2012) 'Appraisal on the wound-healing and anti-inflammatory activities of the essential oils obtained from the cones and needles of *Pinus* species by *in vivo* and *in vitro* experimental models.' *Journal of Ethnopharmacology 139*, 533–540.

Tumen, I., Akkol, E.K., Süntar, I. and Keleş, H. (2011) 'Wound repair and anti-inflammatory potential of essential oils from cones of Pinacea: preclinical experimental research in animal models.' *Journal of Ethnopharmacology 137*, 3, 1215–1220.

Tumen, I., Süntar, I., Keleş, H. and Akkol, E.K. (2012) 'A therapeutic approach for wound healing by using essential oils of *Cupressus* and *Juniperus* species growing in Turkey.' *Evidence-Based Complementary and Alternative Medicine.* Available at www.ncbi.nlm.nih.gov/pmc/articles/PMC3175711, accessed on 7 April 2015.

Tumen, I., Süntar, I., Eller, F.J., Keleş, H. and Akkol, E.K. (2013) 'Topical wound-healing effects and phytochemical composition of heartwood essential oils of *Juniperus virginiana* L., *Juniperus occidentalis* Hook., and *Juniperus ashei* J. Buchholz.' *Journal of Medicinal Food 16*, 1, 48–55.

Turnock, S. (2006) 'Potent oil.' *Nova*, January 2006, 29–36.

Twetrakul, S. and Subhadhirasakul, S. (2007) 'Anti-allergic activity of some selected plants in the Zingiberaceae family.' *Journal of Ethnopharmacology 109*, 3, 535–538.

Ulmer, W.T. and Schott, D. (1991) 'Chronic obstructive bronchitis: effect of Gelomyrtol in a placebo-controlled double-blind study.' *Fortschritte der Medizin 109*, 27, 547–550. Cited by Bowles, E.J. (2003) *The Chemistry of Aromatherapeutic Oils.* (3rd edition.) Crows Nest: Allen and Unwin.

Ulusoy, S., Boşgelmez-Tinaz, G. and Secilmis-Canbay, H. (2009) 'Tocopherol, carotene, phenolic contents and antibacterial properties of rose essential oil, hydrosol and absolute.' *Current Microbiology 59*, 554–558.

Uysal, B., Sozmen, F., Aktas, O., Oksal, B.S. and Kose, E.O. (2011) 'Essential oil composition and antibacterial activity of the grapefruit *(Citrus paradisi* L) peel essential oils obtained by solvent-free microwave extraction: comparison with hydrodistillation.' *International Journal of Food Science and Technology 46*, 1455–1461.

Uzun, Ö., Başoğlu, C., Akar, A., Cansever, A. *et al.* (2003) 'Body dysmorphic disorder in patients with acne.' *Comprehensive Psychiatry 44*, 415–419.

Valente, J., Zuzarte, M., Gonçalves, M.J., Lopez, M.C. *et al.* (2013) 'Antifungal, anti-oxidant and anti-inflammatory activities of *Oenathe crocata* L. essential oil.' *Food Chemistry and Toxicology 62*, 349–354.

Vallianou, I., Peroulis, N., Pantaziz, P. and Hadzopoulou-Cladaras, M. (2011) 'Camphene, a plant-derived monoterpene, reduces plasma cholesterol and triglycerides in hyperlipidemic rats independently of HMG-CoA reductase activity.' *PLoS ONE 6*, 11, e20516.

Vats, A. and Sharma, P. (2012) 'Formulation and evaluation of topical anti acne formulation of coriander extract.' *International Journal of Pharmaceutical Sciences Review and Research 16*, 97–103.

Verma, M., Singh, S.K., Bhushan, S., Pal, H.C. *et al.* (2008) 'Induction of mitochondrial-dependent apoptosis by an essential oil from *Tanacetum gracile.*' *Planta Medica 74*, 5, 515–520.

Villa, C., Trucchi, B., Bertoli, A., Pistelli, L., Parodi, A., Bassi, A.M. and Ruffoni, B. (2009) '*Salvia somalensis* essential oil as a potential cosmetic ingredient: solvent-free microwave extraction, hydrodistillation, GC-MS analysis, odour evaluation and in vitro cytotoxicity assays.' *International Journal of Cosmetic Science 31*, 1, 55–61.

Vimala, S., Norhanom, A.W. and Yadav, M. (1999) 'Anti-tumour promoter activity in Malaysian ginger rhizobia used in traditional medicine.' *British Journal of Cancer 80*, 1/2, 110–116.

Voinchet, V. and Giraud-Robert, A.-M. (2007) 'Utilisation de l'huile essentielle d'hélichryse italienne et de l'huile végétale de rose musquée après intervention de chirurgie plastique réparatrice et esthétique.' *Phytothérapie 2*, 67–72.

Wahab, A., Ul Haq, R., Ahmed, A., Khan, R.A. and Raza, M. (2009) 'Anticonvulsant activities of nutmeg oil of *Myristica fragrans.*' *Phytotherapy Research 23*, 2, 153–158.

Wajs, A., Bonikowski, R. and Kalemba, D. (2008) 'Composition of essential oil from seeds of *Nigella sativa* L. cultivated in Poland.' *Flavour and Fragrance Journal 23*, 126–132.

Warren, C. and Warrenburg, S. (1993) 'Mood benefits of fragrance.' *International Journal of Aromatherapy 5*, 2, 12–16.

Wei, A. and Shibamoto, T. (2010a) 'Anti-oxidant/lipoxygenase inhibitory activities and chemical compositions of selected essential oils.' *Journal of Agricultural and Food Chemistry 57*, 1655–7225. Cited by Shaaban, H.A.E., El-Ghorab, A.H. and Shibamoto, T. (2012) 'Bioactivity of essential oils and their volatile aroma components: review.' *Journal of Essential Oil Research 24*, 2, 203–212.

Wei, A. and Shibamoto, T. (2010b) 'Anti-oxidant/lipoxygenase inhibitory activities and chemical compositions of selected essential oils.' *Journal of Agricultural and Food Chemistry 57*, 1655–7225.

Weiss, E.A. (1997) *Essential Oil Crops.* Wallingford: CAB International.

Wildwood, C. (1996) *The Encyclopedia of Aromatherapy.* Rochester, VT: Healing Arts Press. Cited by Wu, Y., Zhang, Y., Zhao, A., Pan, X. *et al.* (2012) 'The metabolic responses to aerial diffusion of essential oils.' *PLoS ONE 7*, 9, e44830.

Williams, H.C., Dellavalle, R.P. and Garner, S. (2012) 'Acne vulgaris.' *Lancet 379*, 361–372.

Williamson, E.M. (2001) 'Synergy and other interactions in phytomedicines.' *Phytomedicine 8*, 5, 401–409.

Woelk, H. and Schläfke, S. (2010) 'A multi-center, double-blind, randomised study of the Lavender oil preparation Silexan in comparison to Lorazepam for generalized anxiety disorder.' *Phytomedicine 17*, 2, 94–99. Cited by Dobetsberger, C. and Buchbauer, G. (2011) 'Actions of essential oils on the central nervous system: an updated review.' *Flavour and Fragrance Journal 26*, 5, 300–316.

Woolley, C.L., Suhail, M.M., Smith, B.L., Boren, K.E. *et al.* (2012) 'Chemical differentiation of *Boswellia sacra* and *Boswellia carterii* essential oils by gas chromatography and chiral gas chromatography–mass spectrometry.' *Journal of Chromatography A 1261*, 158–163.

World Health Organization (2001) 'The World Health Report. Mental Health: New Understanding New Hope.' Geneva: WHO.

Wu, X., Li, X., Xiao, F., Zhang, Z., Xu, Z. and Wang, H. (2004) 'Studies on the analgesic and anti-inflammatory effect of bornyl acetate in volatile oil from *Amomum villosum.*' *Zong Yao Cai 27*, 6, 438–439. (Article in Chinese.) Abstract available from www.ncbi.nlm.nih.gov/pubmed/15524301, accessed on 7 April 2015.

Wu, Y., Zhang, Y., Zhao, A., Pan, X. *et al.* (2012) 'The metabolic responses to aerial diffusion of essential oils.' *PLoS ONE 7*, 9, e44830.

Xu, H., Delling, M., Jun, J.C. and Clapham, D.E. (2008) 'Oregano, thyme and clove-derived flavors and skin sensitizers activate specific TRP channels.' *Nature Neuroscience 9*, 628–635. Cited by Guimarães, A.G., Quintans, J.S.S. and Quintans-Júnior, L.J. (2013) 'Monoterpenes with analgesic activity: a systematic review.' *Phytotherapy Research 27*, 1–15.

Yamada, K., Mimaki, Y. and Sashida, Y. (1994) 'Anticonvulsive effects of inhaling lavender oil vapour.' *Biological and Pharmaceutical Bulletin 17*, 359–360. Cited by de Almeida, R.N., Agra, M.F., Maior, F.N.S. and de Sousa, D.P. (2011) 'Essential oils and their constituents: anticonvulsant activity.' *Molecules 16*, 2726–2742.

Yang, S.-A., Jeon, S.-K., Lee, E.-J., Im, N.-K. *et al.* (2009) 'Radical scavenging activity of the essential oil of silver fir (*Abies alba*).' *Journal of Clinical Biochemistry and Nutrition 44*, 3, 253–259.

Yang, S.-A., Jeon, S.-K., Lee, E.-J., Shim, E.-H. and Lee, I.-S. (2010) 'Comparative study of the chemical composition and anti-oxidant activity of six essential oils and their components.' *Natural Products Research 24*, 140–151.

Yang, X., Zhang, X., Yang, S.-P. and Liu, W-Q. (2013) 'Evaluation of the antibacterial activity of patchouli oil.' *Iranian Journal of Pharmaeutical Research 12*, 3, 307–316.

Yap, P.S.X., Yiap, B.C., Ping, H.C. and Lim, S.H.E. (2014) 'Essential oils, a new horizon in combatting bacterial antibiotic resistance.' *Open Microbiology Journal 8*, 6–14.

Yi, L.T., Li, J., Geng, D., Liu, B.B., Fu, Y., Tu, J.Q., Liu, Y. and Weng, L.J. (2013) 'Essential oil of *Perilla frutescens*-induced changes in hippocampal expression of brain-derived neurotrophic factor in chronic unpredictable stress in mice.' *Journal of Ethnopharmacology 147*, 1, 245–253.

Yim, V.W.C., Ng, A.K.Y., Tsang, H.W.H. and Leung, A.Y. (2009) 'A review on the effects of aromatherapy for patients with depressive symptoms.' *Journal of Alternative and Complementarity Medicine 15*, 2, 187–195.

Yoon, W.-J., Kim, S.-S., Oh, T.-H., Lee, N.H. and Hyun, C.-G. (2009a) '*Abies koreana* essential oil inhibits drug-resistant skin pathogen growth and LPS-induced inflammatory effects of murine macrophage.' *Lipids 44*, 471–476.

Yoon, W.-J., Kim, S.-S., Oh, T.-H., Lee, N.H. and Hyun, C.-G. (2009b) '*Cryptomeria japonica* essential oil inhibits the growth of drug-resistant skin pathogens and LPS-induced nitric oxide and pro-inflammatory cytokine production.' *Polish Journal of Microbiology 58*, 1, 61–68.

Yu, L.L., Zhou, K.K. and Parry, J. (2005) 'Anti-oxidant properties of cold-pressed black caraway, carrot, cranberry and hemp seed oils.' *Food Chemistry 91*, 723–729.

Yvon, Y., Raoelison, E.G., Razafindrazaka, R., Randriantsoa, A. *et al.* (2012) 'Relation between chemical composition or anti-oxidant activity and anti-hypertensive activity for six essential oils.' *Journal of Food Science 77*, 8, 184–191.

Zaveri, M., Khandhar, A., Patel, S. and Patel, A. (2010) 'Chemistry and pharmacology of *Piper longum* L.' *International Journal of Pharmaceutical Sciences Review and Research 5*, 1, 67–76.

Zhang, Y., Wu, Y., Chen, T., Yao, L. *et al.* (2013) 'Assessing the metabolic effects of aromatherapy in human volunteers.' *Evidence-Based Complementary and Alternative Medicine.* Available at http://dx.doi.org/10.1155/2013/356381, accessed on 10 June 2015.

Zhou, J., Qu, F., Sang, X., Burrows, E. and Nan, R. (2008) 'Auricular acupressure may improve absorption of flavanones in the extracts from *Citrus aurantium* L. in the human body.' *Journal of Alternative and Complementary Medicine 14*, 4, 423–425.

Zu, Y., Yu, H. and Liang, L. (2010) 'Activities of ten essential oils towards *Propionibacterium acnes* and PC-3, A-549 and MCF-7 cancer cells.' *Molecules 15*, 3200–3210.

RESOURCES

UK: Essential oils and aromatic plant materials

Aqua Oleum www.aqua-oleum.co.uk
Ellwoods of Dumfries www.ellwoodsofdumfries.co.uk
Oshadhi UK www.oshadhi.co.uk
Quinessence www.quinessence.co.uk

USA: Essential oils and aromatic plant materials

Eden Botanicals www.edenbotanicals.com
Oshadhi USA www.oshadhiusa.com
Snow Lotus Inc. www.snowlotus.org
White Lotus Aromatics www.whitelotusaromatics.com

Australia: Essential oils and aromatic plant materials

Sydney Essential Oil Co. www.seoc.com.au

Animal welfare (UK and International)

People for the Ethical Treatment of Animals (PETA) www.peta.org.uk
Humane Society International www.hsi.org
Dr Hadwen Trust www.drhadwentrust.org

ESSENTIAL OILS INDEX

SUBJECT INDEX

AUTHOR INDEX